A Tale of Two Surrogates

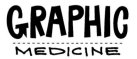

Susan Merrill Squier, Juliet McMullin, and Brian Callender, *General Editors*

CO-FOUNDING EDITORS
Ian Williams
Susan Merrill Squier

Books in the Graphic Medicine series reflect the value of comics as a resource for communicating about medicine and health. For healthcare practitioners, patients, family members, and caregivers dealing with illness and disability, graphic narratives enlighten complicated or difficult experiences. They can also communicate the scaled meanings of health, from the molecular to the human and to the planetary, including works addressing climate change, environmental pollution, zoonotic diseases, and other complex problems not commonly conceptualized as "medical." For scholars in literary, cultural, and comics studies, the medium articulates a complex and powerful rethinking of the boundaries of medicine and the expansive meanings of health. The series includes monographs and edited collections from scholars, practitioners, and medical educators as well as collections of comics used in medical training and education.

OTHER TITLES IN THE SERIES:

MK Czerwiec, Ian Williams, Susan Merrill Squier, Michael J. Green, Kimberly R. Myers, and Scott T. Smith, *Graphic Medicine Manifesto*

Ian Williams, *The Bad Doctor: The Troubled Life and Times of Dr. Iwan James*

Peter Dunlap-Shohl, *My Degeneration: A Journey Through Parkinson's*

Aneurin Wright, *Things to Do in a Retirement Home Trailer Park: . . . When You're 29 and Unemployed*

Dana Walrath, *Aliceheimers: Alzheimer's Through the Looking Glass*

Lorenzo Servitje and Sherryl Vint, eds., *The Walking Med: Zombies and the Medical Image*

Henny Beaumont, *Hole in the Heart: Bringing Up Beth*

MK Czerwiec, *Taking Turns: Stories from HIV/AIDS Care Unit 371*

Paula Knight, *The Facts of Life*

Gareth Brookes, *A Thousand Coloured Castles*

Jenell Johnson, ed., *Graphic Reproduction: A Comics Anthology*

Olivier Kugler, *Escaping Wars and Waves: Encounters with Syrian Refugees*

Judith Margolis, *Life Support: Invitation to Prayer*

Ian Williams, *The Lady Doctor*

Sarah Lightman, *The Book of Sarah*

Benjamin Dix and Lindsay Pollock, *Vanni: A Family's Struggle through the Sri Lankan Conflict*

Ephameron, *Us Two Together*

Scott T. Smith and José Alaniz, eds., *Uncanny Bodies: Superhero Comics and Disability*

MK Czerwiec, ed., *Menopause: A Comic Treatment*

Susan Merrill Squier and Irmela Marei Krüger-Fürhoff, eds., *PathoGraphics: Narrative, Aesthetics, Contention, Community*

Swann Meralli and Deloupy, *Algériennes: The Forgotten Women of the Algerian Revolution*

Aurélien Ducoudray and Jeff Pourquié, *The Third Population*

Abby Hershler, Lesley Hughes, Patricia Nguyen, and Shelley Wall, eds., *Looking at Trauma: A Tool Kit for Clinicians*

Kimberly R. Myers, Molly L. Osborne, and Charlotte A. Wu, Illustrations by Zoe Schein, *Clinical Ethics: A Graphic Medicine Casebook*

Meredith Li-Vollmer, *Graphic Public Health: A Comics Anthology and Road Map*

Monica Chiu, *Show Me Where It Hurts: Manifesting Illness and Impairment in Graphic Pathography*

A Tale of Two Surrogates

A Graphic Narrative on Assisted Reproduction

Elly Teman and Zsuzsa Berend
Art by Andrea Scebba

The Pennsylvania State University Press
University Park, Pennsylvania

Library of Congress Cataloging-in-Publication
data is on file.

Copyright © 2025 Elly Teman, Zsuza Berend, and
Andrea Scebba
All rights reserved
Printed in the United States of America
Published by The Pennsylvania
State University Press,
University Park, PA 16802–1003

The Pennsylvania State University Press is a
member of the Association of University Presses.

It is the policy of The Pennsylvania State
University Press to use acid-free paper.
Publications on uncoated stock satisfy the
minimum requirements of American National
Standard for Information Sciences—Permanence
of Paper for Printed Library Material,
ANSI Z39.48–1992.

Elly—In memory of my dad, Nissan Teman, whom I miss every single day

Zsuzsa—To my sons, Benjamin and Daniel, with tremendous love and appreciation

Contents

Acknowledgments (viii)
Introduction (xi)

Prologue (2)

1. **Thinking It Through (Dana)** (8)

2. **Getting the Hubby on Board (Jenn)** (14)

   Interlude: Moscow, Russia (21)

3. **Baby Steps (Dana)** (22)

4. **First Date (Jenn)** (32)

   Interlude: Mumbai, India (41)

5. **Weighing the Risks (Dana)** (42)

6. **Contract (Jenn)** (48)

   Interlude: St. Petersburg, Russia (59)

7. **The State (Dana)** (60)

8. **Transfer (Jenn)** (64)

   Interlude: Bangkok, Thailand (75)

9. **Roller Coaster (Dana)** (76)

10. **The Ferris Wheel (Jenn)** (86)

    Interlude: Gujarat, India (93)

11. **Heartbeat (Dana)** (94)

12. **Telling the Kids (Jenn)** (100)

    Interlude: Bangalore, India (105)

13. **Testing Boundaries (Dana)** (106)

14. **Babysitting (Jenn)** (116)

    Interlude: Bangkok, Thailand (125)

15. **Birth Plan (Dana)** (126)

16. **The Gift (Jenn)** (132)

    Interlude: Delhi, India (137)

17. **The Choice (Dana)** (138)

18. **Delivery (Jenn)** (146)

    Interlude: Tabasco, Mexico (155)

19. **Acknowledgment (Dana)** (156)

20. **Postpartum (Jenn)** (162)

    Interlude: Southern California (169)

21. **The Story (Dana)** (170)

Afterword (176)
Discussion Guide (185)
Notes (186)
Bibliography (188)
Contributor Bios (190)

Acknowledgments

This work could not have been completed without the support of an HBI Research Award from the Hadassah-Brandeis Institute honoring the memory of Frances Leder Kornmehl, as well as the support of the Ruppin Academic Center and the Katz Center for Jewish Studies at the University of Pennsylvania. The preparation and publication of this work was also supported by the Memorial Foundation for Jewish Culture.

We would like to thank comic artist Andrea Scebba for working with us on this project, which took over three years. We wrote a full script and storyboarded the entire book before we began our search through hundreds of online portfolios of comic artists to find someone with the style that we imagined. Andrea's work was what we had been looking for, and we were lucky that he agreed to work with us on all stages of creation of every page of this book: sketching, inking, shading, lettering. Each illustrated page began with Andrea's initial sketched interpretation of our storyboard, followed by many messages and emails back and forth among the three of us about multiple things that needed to be clarified, shortened, and reinterpreted. Our collaboration spanned three locations—Andrea in Sicily, Elly in Israel, and Zsuzsa in Los Angeles—as well as different time zones, languages, and perspectives. Grazie, Andrea, for your patience, creative interpretations and ideas, and artistic skills.

We gratefully acknowledge the surrogates for their openness and willingness to tell their stories during our fieldwork upon which this work is based. The manuscript benefited from the comments and suggestions of Susan Squier, the anonymous reviewers, Kendra Boileau, and the members of the editorial board at Penn State University Press. We were very lucky to have the technical advice and last-minute help of graphic artist Shunit Ben-Chaim.

We are thankful for the close reading of our manuscript by Eitan Schechtman-Drayman, Orit Chorowicz Bar-Am, Meira Weiss, Dominique and Fiorella Mennesson, Natalie B. Dohrmann, Sarah Zager, Noemie Duhaut, Tsofia Gabay, Nielufar Varjavand, Rogers Brubaker, Adrea Veszits, and Nina Eliasoph.

Our families have been generous with their support and encouragement, as well as being sounding boards for our ideas. Zsuzsa's sister, Dora Gyarmati, has been an early supporter of a more popular work on surrogacy. Elly's husband, Avi Solomon, gave us tech support and invaluable advice throughout, especially making sure that we made and perfected our storyboard before taking this project further. Zsuzsa's sons, Benjamin and Daniel Brubaker, and Elly's mother, Rhisa Teman, read different drafts of our manuscript and made important comments. Elly's godfathers, David B. Sherman and Roberto Benitez, commented, encouraged, and contributed to the completion of this project. Elly's children, Uriel, Rachela, and Gabriella, made helpful suggestions.

We are grateful for advice along this journey from Ann Brackenbury, Stacey Leigh Pigg, Hadas Shveky-Teman, Merav Levi, Matthew Noe, Aomar Baum, Yael Hashiloni-Dolev, Jacqueline Adams, Simon J. Bronner, Susan Kahn, Efrat Ben-Zeev, Caren Weinberg, Daphna Birenbaum-Carmeli, Robbie Davis-Floyd, and Ron Poole-Dayan. Other friends have encouraged us along the way: Svetta Roberman, Rinat Zohar-Menachem, Tafat Hacohen, Helene Goldberg, Sophie Fellman Rafalovitz, Lisa Carlsson, Danny Kaplan, Katya Rice, Noosh Green, and Joan Waugh.

Finally, Zsuzsa is grateful to Elly for her zany idea to write a graphic novel, and Elly thanks Zsuzsa for rolling with that idea. This effort carried us both through the pandemic years and gave us a shared project to keep us on our toes. We have loved working together on several academic articles and on this book, bouncing ideas off each other, arguing over interpretations, and each listening to and incorporating the other's perspective to create this story. If this book isn't dramatic enough, it's Zsuzsa's fault, and if it's too dramatic, it's Elly's fault!

TERMINOLOGY YOU SHOULD KNOW **BEFORE** CONTINUING TO READ

SURROGACY: A CONTRACTUAL AGREEMENT IN WHICH A WOMAN AGREES TO CARRY AND BIRTH A BABY (OR BABIES) FOR A COUPLE OR SINGLE PERSON WHO WILL RAISE THE BABY. SURROGATES ARE USUALLY FINANCIALLY COMPENSATED.

TRADITIONAL SURROGACY

THE SURROGATE BECOMES PREGNANT BY ARTIFICIAL INSEMINATION (IT IS HER EGG).

INTENDED PARENT/S (IPs)
OR DONOR/S
SURROGATE
PROCESS

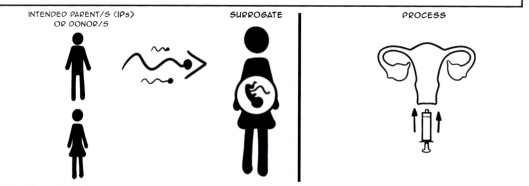

GESTATIONAL SURROGACY

THE SURROGATE BECOMES PREGNANT FOLLOWING EMBRYO TRANSFER OF A FERTILIZED EGG CREATED THROUGH IN VITRO FERTILIZATION (**IVF**)

INTENDED PARENT/S (IPs)
OR DONOR/S
SURROGATE
PROCESS

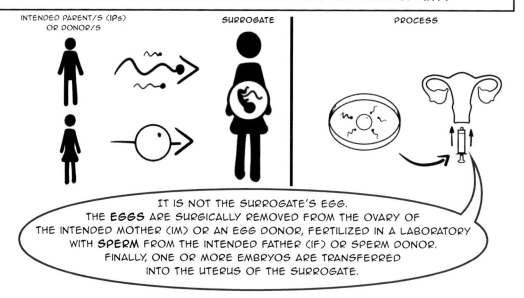

IT IS NOT THE SURROGATE'S EGG.
THE **EGGS** ARE SURGICALLY REMOVED FROM THE OVARY OF THE INTENDED MOTHER (IM) OR AN EGG DONOR, FERTILIZED IN A LABORATORY WITH **SPERM** FROM THE INTENDED FATHER (IF) OR SPERM DONOR. FINALLY, ONE OR MORE EMBRYOS ARE TRANSFERRED INTO THE UTERUS OF THE SURROGATE.

IPs: INTENDED PARENTS; *IM*: INTENDED MOTHER; *IF*: INTENDED FATHER

Introduction

A Tale of Two Surrogates is the first graphic novel about the controversial topic of surrogacy. The book is a collaboration between sociologist Zsuzsa Berend and anthropologist Elly Teman, who have each devoted two decades of their careers to ethnographic research on surrogacy. Illustrated by comic artist Andrea Scebba, the storyline follows two surrogates in alternating chapters—Jenn in the United States and Dana in Israel. Their stories show the striking similarities and differences in the way surrogacy plays out in these two countries in particular, and, at the same time, they situate the storyline in an international context.

Publicly available stories about surrogacy most often focus on extreme legal cases, celebrity intended parents (IPs), or babies in transnational surrogacy arrangements stranded because of bureaucratic hurdles, natural disasters, the pandemic, or war. Our graphic novel focuses on the much less sensational everyday stories of surrogates and the important practical and ethical questions those stories raise. Jenn and Dana are composite fictional characters, but their words, actions, and interactions come from qualitative data from our respective ethnographic studies. Ethnographers study people in social context, often for long periods of time, and observe their interactions and behaviors. They also usually talk to people in these social settings to hear their individual and collective interpretations of their reality.

DANA
JENN
ARTIST
ANDREA SCEBBA

Jenn's story is based on Zsuzsa's online ethnographic research on Surrogate Mothers Online (SMO), a virtual meeting place where surrogates constructed a distinct culture of surrogacy. Dana's story is based on Elly's ethnographic research among Israeli surrogates and IPs. More about these studies and their methods can be found in our separate and joint publications.[1] This graphic novel condenses the most important themes and ideas that emerged from our studies and from our joint comparative publications on US and Israeli surrogates' responses to legal regulations, articulations of kinship and

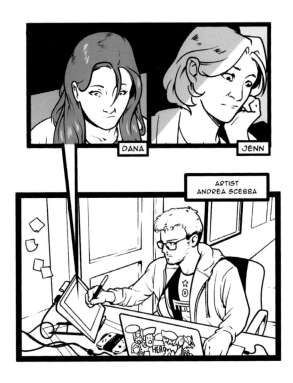

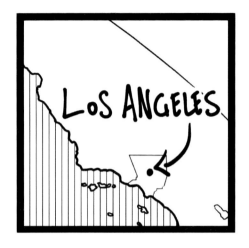

motherhood, and negotiations of surrogacy with their husbands and children as a "family project."

Jenn's and Dana's stories are situated in the United States and Israel, which are outliers in relation to the rest of the world in terms of surrogacy. These are the only two highly developed countries where compensated surrogacy has remained legal for over two decades, throughout a period in which the international surrogacy industry became something of a "Wild West." Some countries allowed surrogacy "under the radar" for short-lived, unregulated periods that resulted in complications, scandals, and eventual criminalization.[2] Each ban, in succession, pushed the industry to the next country (India, Thailand, Nepal, Mexico, Cambodia). Current unregulated markets include Russia, Ukraine, and Georgia. A few countries continue to permit uncompensated surrogacy arrangements (Canada, Australia, UK), and many have banned surrogacy altogether (most of Europe).

The United States and Israel legislate compensated surrogacy in very different ways. Our comparative approach invites readers to think about the repercussions of these regulatory differences. The United States does not have a federal law; surrogacy is regulated state by state and is open to noncitizens. Private agencies and clinics function with little or no state oversight.[3] California, where Jenn lives, has long been the center of this booming industry and is known as a surrogacy-friendly state.

Conversely, Israel's surrogacy law closely regulates the process via a government-appointed committee that must approve all applicants and contracts. Surrogacy is formulated as a last resort for Israeli citizens or permanent residents who satisfy a long list of criteria for approval. Medical and psychological screening and other contractual protections are mandated. Further complicating the Israeli surrogacy law are provisions for making surrogacy compatible with Jewish law.

For instance, surrogacy parties cannot be related, because some rabbis view intrafamilial surrogacy as a form of incest. Moreover, parties must share the same religion, unless none of them is Jewish. This is because cross-religious surrogacy can have religious repercussions for the recognition of the baby as a Jew.[4]

Surrogacy is prohibited in Islam, so Israeli surrogacy occurs primarily between Jews. Accordingly, the characters of Dana and her IPs are Jewish. They are not religiously observant, but like many Jewish-Israeli families, they honor Jewish life cycle rituals and holidays. Jenn and her family are Christian, reflecting a prominent demographic among surrogates in the United States.

The majority of surrogates in the United States and Israel are heterosexual and married.[5] A growing number of US surrogates carry for same-sex couples and single persons, yet the majority of IPs they work with are straight, married couples. In Israel, the surrogacy law prevented single women from contracting with a surrogate until 2018 and prevented single men and same-sex couples from entering these arrangements until 2022, a social inequality addressed in the story.

In keeping with our and others' scholarly findings on the demographics of surrogacy in these two countries, we chose to depict both surrogates and their IPs as married, heterosexual couples. The two surrogates are middle-class, working mothers. They represent the majority of surrogates in the United States and Israel, who are lower-middle to middle class and are most often not financially needy. Most have complex reasons for becoming a surrogate, in which financial reasons, although relevant, are not necessarily dominant. These reasons include doing something important and meaningful, creating life and families, becoming one of a select group of women, and earning money that helps their families achieve their goals. Surrogates in both countries tend to conceptualize surrogacy as a family project undertaken openly in their communities, and they usually form a relationship with their IPs.

In order to highlight the often-neglected reality of family members' involvement in surrogacy, we depict Jenn and Dana each interacting with a husband, three children, a sister, and other family members.

US surrogates and IPs are predominantly white. Jenn and her IPs are white, reflecting the majority of empirical evidence. There are some Latina but still very few African American and almost no Asian surrogates in the United States. Surrogates do carry babies for couples of various racial, ethnic, and national backgrounds, including many Europeans, an increasing number of Chinese, and other foreign nationals who cannot pursue surrogacy in their countries because of legal barriers.[6]

Throughout the story, Jenn and Dana participate in online social networks, giving us a vehicle to portray how surrogates share information, advice, and support in online communities. Through these networks we introduce the different voices and range of approaches, outcomes, and opinions they represent. The surrogates Jenn meets online carry babies for a diverse group of people involved in surrogacy, including single persons, same-sex couples, and international IPs.

Jenn's online world of US surrogates is represented as a modern version of a classical Greek chorus commenting on and underscoring themes of her story. The chorus, like the online surrogacy network (SMO) that it represents, vocalizes a particular image of surrogacy that aligns with the collective meanings and norms of

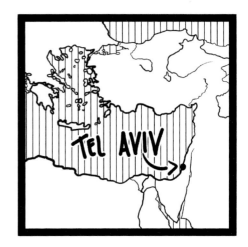

CAST OF CHARACTERS

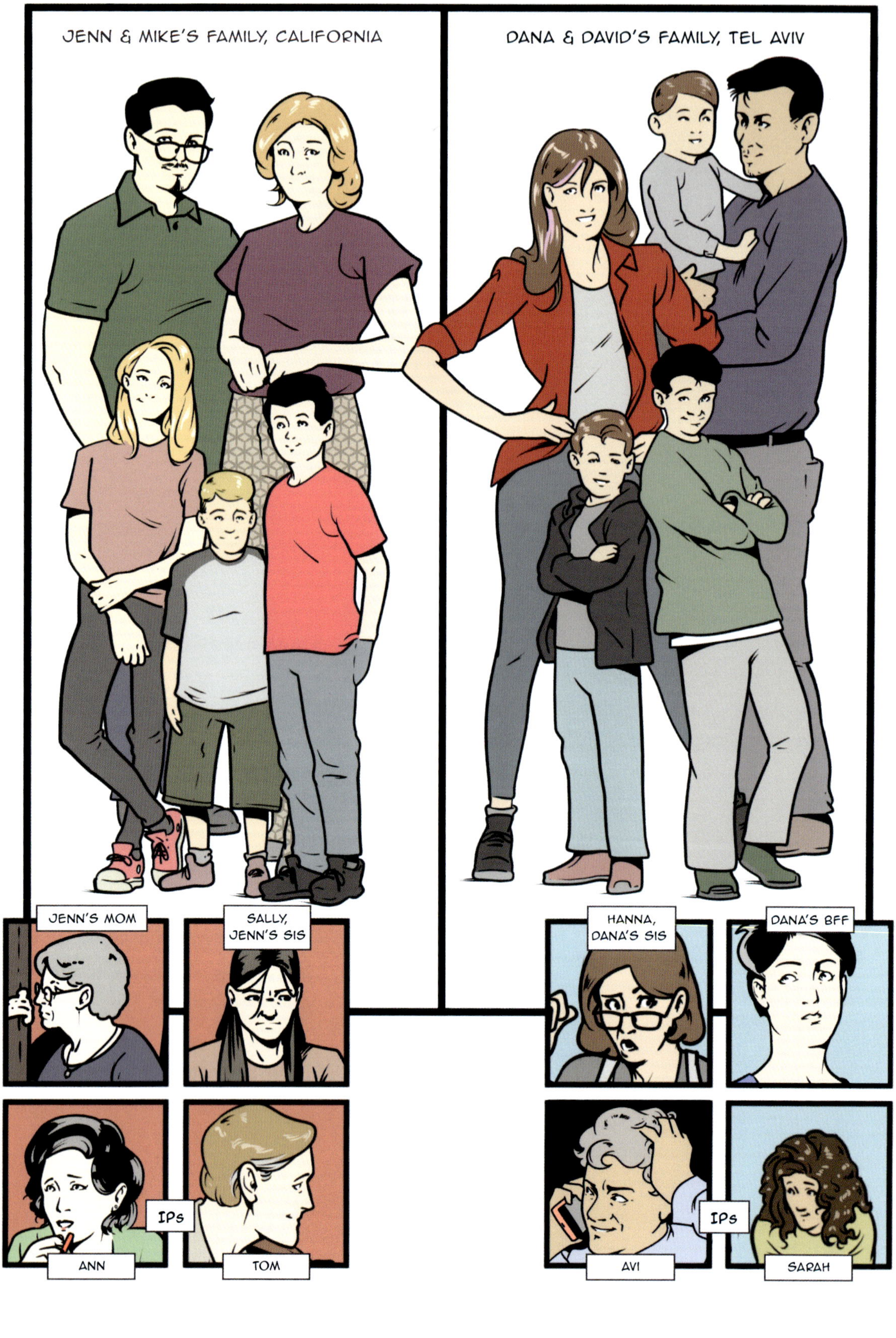
JENN & MIKE'S FAMILY, CALIFORNIA
DANA & DAVID'S FAMILY, TEL AVIV
JENN'S MOM
SALLY, JENN'S SIS
HANNA, DANA'S SIS
DANA'S BFF
ANN
IPs
TOM
AVI
IPs
SARAH

the group, which are shaped by online discussions and debates. We portray the chorus in shades of gray, representing their symbolic nature in the story.

HONOR THE JOURNEY

In turn, Dana's online network of Israeli surrogates is represented as competitors surmounting the challenges of an obstacle course. This depiction highlights Dana's athletic lifestyle as well as the selective nature of Israeli surrogacy screening; only women who satisfy the physical and mental criteria outlined in the law can become surrogates. It also connotes the hero's journey, a narrative trope that Israeli surrogates often draw upon to tell their stories as tough, determined adventurers who bravely choose to face risks and surmount obstacles to complete their mission. All of the advice and opinions shared with Jenn and Dana through their social networks represent the diverse voices of surrogates in our research. All names used in this book are fictional.

WE CAN DO IT!

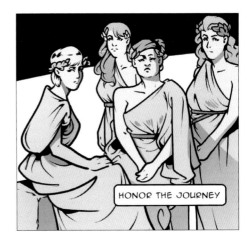

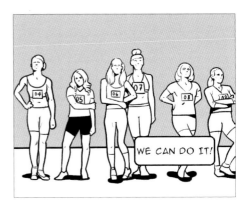

We have included interludes throughout the book, representing some of the research findings on transnational surrogacy in other scholars' work.[7] Each interlude depicts a place where fertility clinics once catered to international surrogacy clients, such as different locations in India. The one-page vignettes include a snapshot of a monument or setting in that specific part of the world, as well as quotes from participants in the surrogacy process from relevant publications. The interludes are not meant to present a comprehensive picture but to spark comparative conversation. They provide a brief glimpse into the medical, interpersonal, and legal situations of surrogates in the few countries where surrogacy has been documented by other researchers.

Juxtaposed with themes from Jenn's and Dana's stories, they illuminate major differences in surrogates' situations in different social and cultural contexts. For example, the scholarship on women who became surrogates in Russia, India, Mexico, and Thailand suggests they did so primarily because surrogacy paid significantly more than the jobs available to them. These surrogates hoped to accomplish goals such as repaying debt, buying a house, and paying for their children's education.

Surrogates documented in these places often lived separately from their partners, children, and community for the duration of the pregnancy and kept their involvement in surrogacy a secret, sometimes out of shame, because the practice was stigmatized. They rarely met or directly communicated with the IPs, and many did not even know who they were carrying the baby for.

Yet scholars described not only these surrogates' vulnerability but also their subjectivity and agency. Surrogates in these studies expressed awareness that their lives in the reproductive market were "discounted," their "womb work" objectified and invisible. Nevertheless, they did not view themselves as victims but as making use of opportunities to better their lives.

We urge readers to pause during the interludes, to think about the institutional arrangements that constrain Jenn's and Dana's actions as well and how their impact unfolds in the two stories.

This graphic novel has found its home in a series on graphic medicine, a term coined by Ian Williams to denote the intersection between comics and the discourse of healthcare. Several books in this series are based on personal memoirs of the authors' encounters with reproductive health issues, such as infertility, miscarriage, and menopause.[8] Our ethnographic contribution to graphic medicine brings it into dialogue with the anthropology of reproduction and is inspired by recent works in anthropology that communicate scholarly research findings through comics in order to make the findings more broadly accessible.[9] Our story uses fictional characters based on many women's stories as a means to introduce readers to the practice of surrogacy and its social implications, including different medical and legal practices and the diverse interests and perspectives of the participants involved.

We do not advocate for or against any of the practices we present in these stories. These are all real practices we encountered during our years of research. We believe these stories can help readers understand surrogacy from the surrogate's perspective, better grasp the potential difficulties, and form a realistic assessment of the complexities. In line with the vision of graphic medicine, we hope this book will be useful and informative for medical providers, healthcare workers, people interested in pursuing surrogacy, public health and legal decision-makers, students, and anyone curious about what many US and Israeli surrogates grapple with during their "journeys." While reading, we encourage readers to think about some of the questions below.

What draws Jenn and Dana to surrogacy? How do they imagine surrogacy and what do they discover?

What is the impact of each woman's family on her decisions and experience? What are the implications of surrogacy for her family?

How do Jenn and Dana exercise agency and negotiate bodily autonomy throughout the surrogacy process?

Which issues do they view as their own responsibility and what are their expectations, if any, of the state?

What kind of relationship do the surrogates develop with their IPs? What expectations do the surrogates have about this relationship?

What recurrent metaphors shape the surrogates' experience?

What role do gifts and reciprocity play in surrogacy?

What role do their online communities have in shaping their expectations and interpretations?

A Tale of Two Surrogates

-PROLOGUE-
JENN, CALIFORNIA

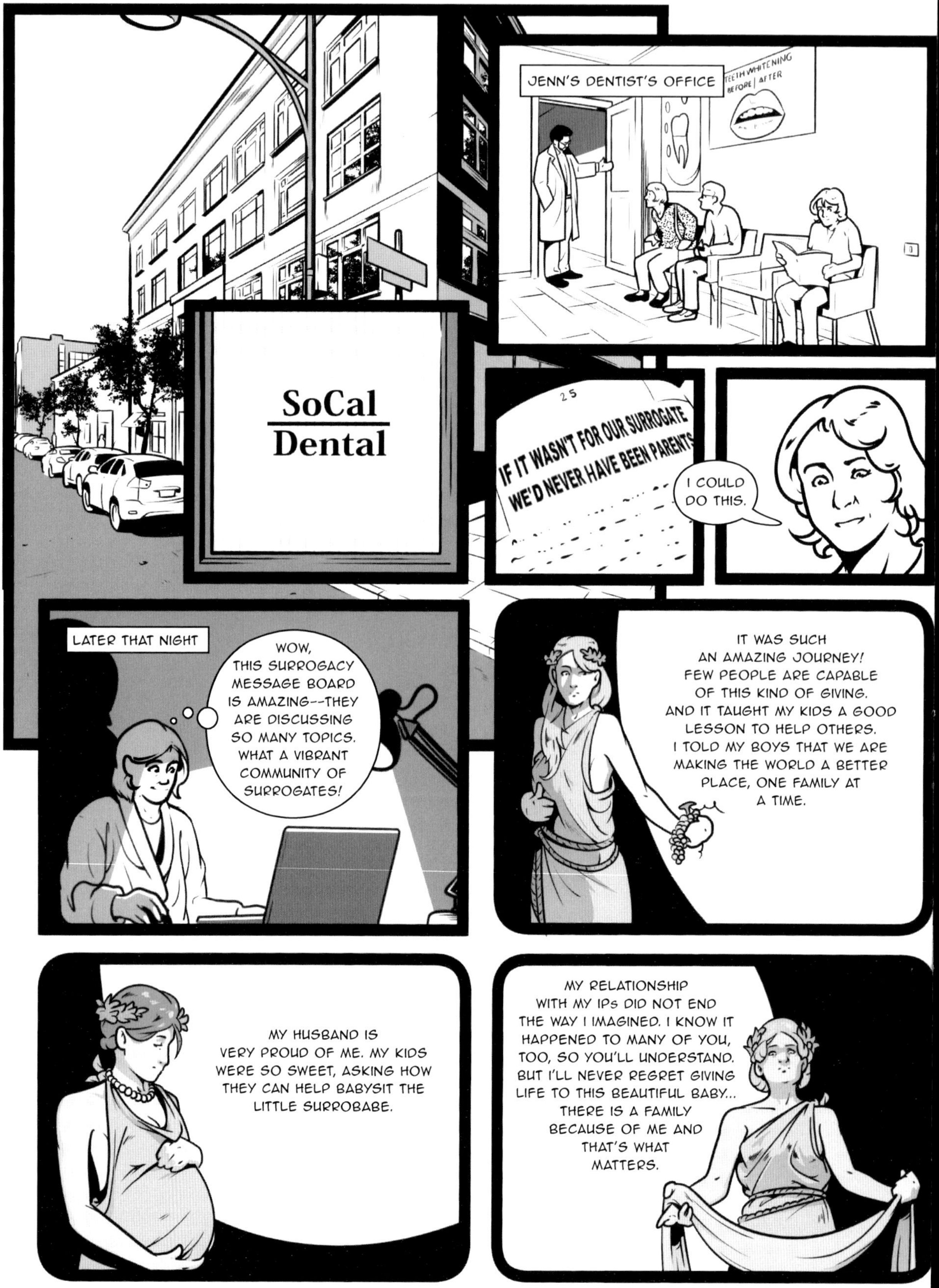
JENN'S DENTIST'S OFFICE
TEETH WHITENING
BEFORE | AFTER
SoCal
Dental
25
IF IT WASN'T FOR OUR SURROGATE
WE'D NEVER HAVE BEEN PARENTS
I COULD DO THIS.
LATER THAT NIGHT
WOW, THIS SURROGACY MESSAGE BOARD IS AMAZING--THEY ARE DISCUSSING SO MANY TOPICS. WHAT A VIBRANT COMMUNITY OF SURROGATES!
IT WAS SUCH AN AMAZING JOURNEY! FEW PEOPLE ARE CAPABLE OF THIS KIND OF GIVING. AND IT TAUGHT MY KIDS A GOOD LESSON TO HELP OTHERS. I TOLD MY BOYS THAT WE ARE MAKING THE WORLD A BETTER PLACE, ONE FAMILY AT A TIME.
MY HUSBAND IS VERY PROUD OF ME. MY KIDS WERE SO SWEET, ASKING HOW THEY CAN HELP BABYSIT THE LITTLE SURROBABE.
MY RELATIONSHIP WITH MY IPs DID NOT END THE WAY I IMAGINED. I KNOW IT HAPPENED TO MANY OF YOU, TOO, SO YOU'LL UNDERSTAND. BUT I'LL NEVER REGRET GIVING LIFE TO THIS BEAUTIFUL BABY... THERE IS A FAMILY BECAUSE OF ME AND THAT'S WHAT MATTERS.

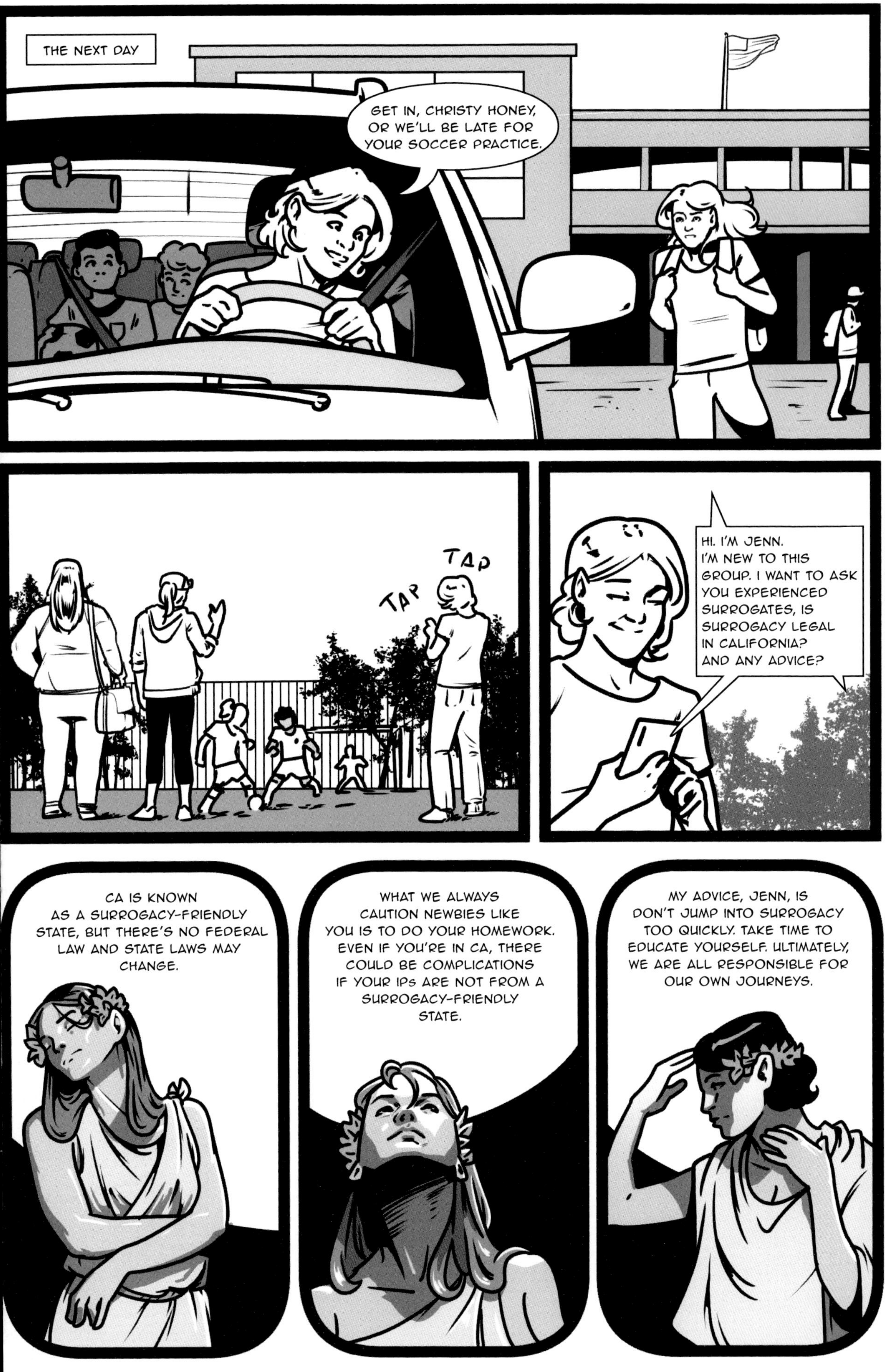
THE NEXT DAY
GET IN, CHRISTY HONEY, OR WE'LL BE LATE FOR YOUR SOCCER PRACTICE.
TAP
TAP
HI. I'M JENN. I'M NEW TO THIS GROUP. I WANT TO ASK YOU EXPERIENCED SURROGATES, IS SURROGACY LEGAL IN CALIFORNIA? AND ANY ADVICE?
CA IS KNOWN AS A SURROGACY-FRIENDLY STATE, BUT THERE'S NO FEDERAL LAW AND STATE LAWS MAY CHANGE.
WHAT WE ALWAYS CAUTION NEWBIES LIKE YOU IS TO DO YOUR HOMEWORK. EVEN IF YOU'RE IN CA, THERE COULD BE COMPLICATIONS IF YOUR IPs ARE NOT FROM A SURROGACY-FRIENDLY STATE.
MY ADVICE, JENN, IS DON'T JUMP INTO SURROGACY TOO QUICKLY. TAKE TIME TO EDUCATE YOURSELF. ULTIMATELY, WE ARE ALL RESPONSIBLE FOR OUR OWN JOURNEYS.

MEANWHILE...
DANA, TEL AVIV

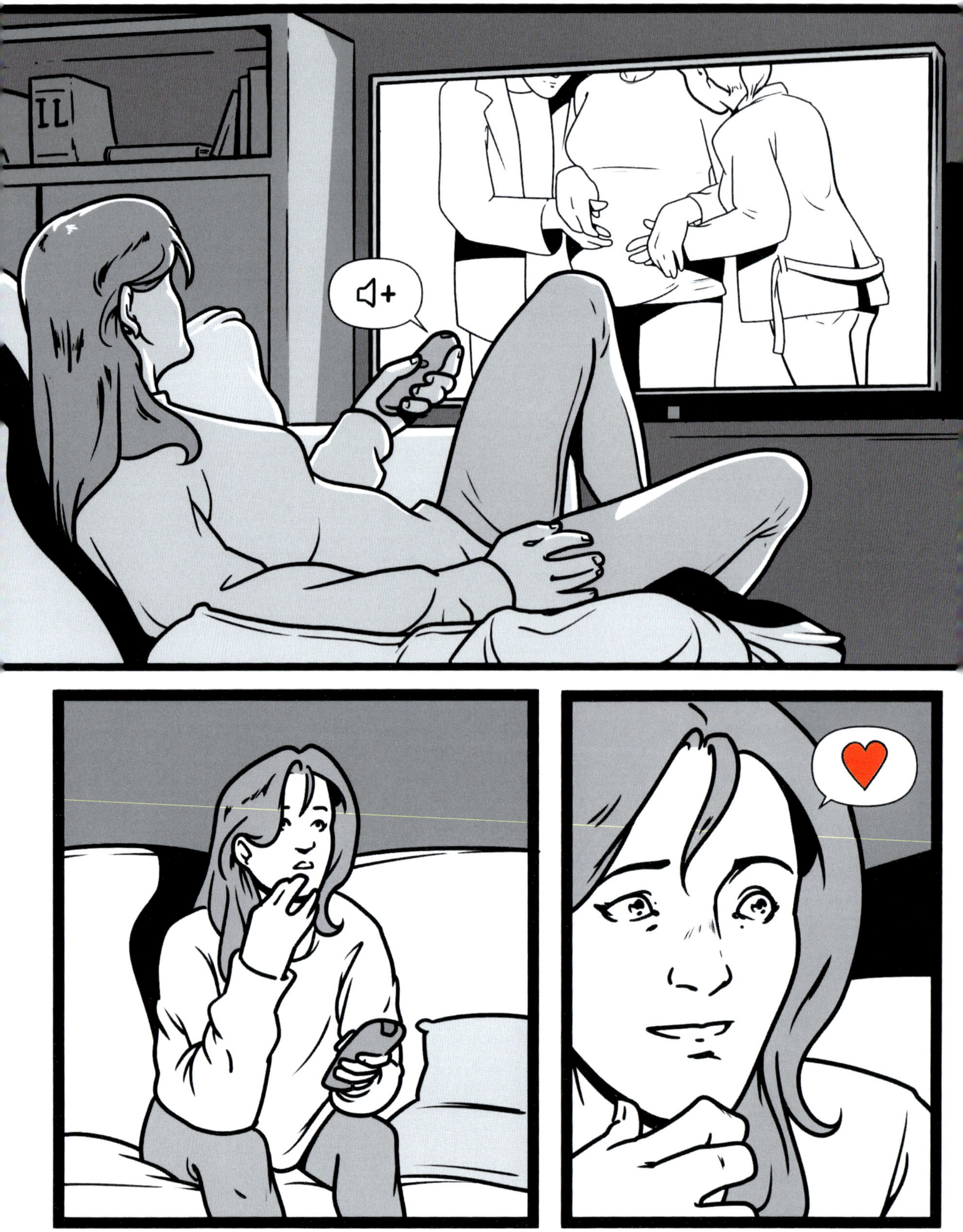

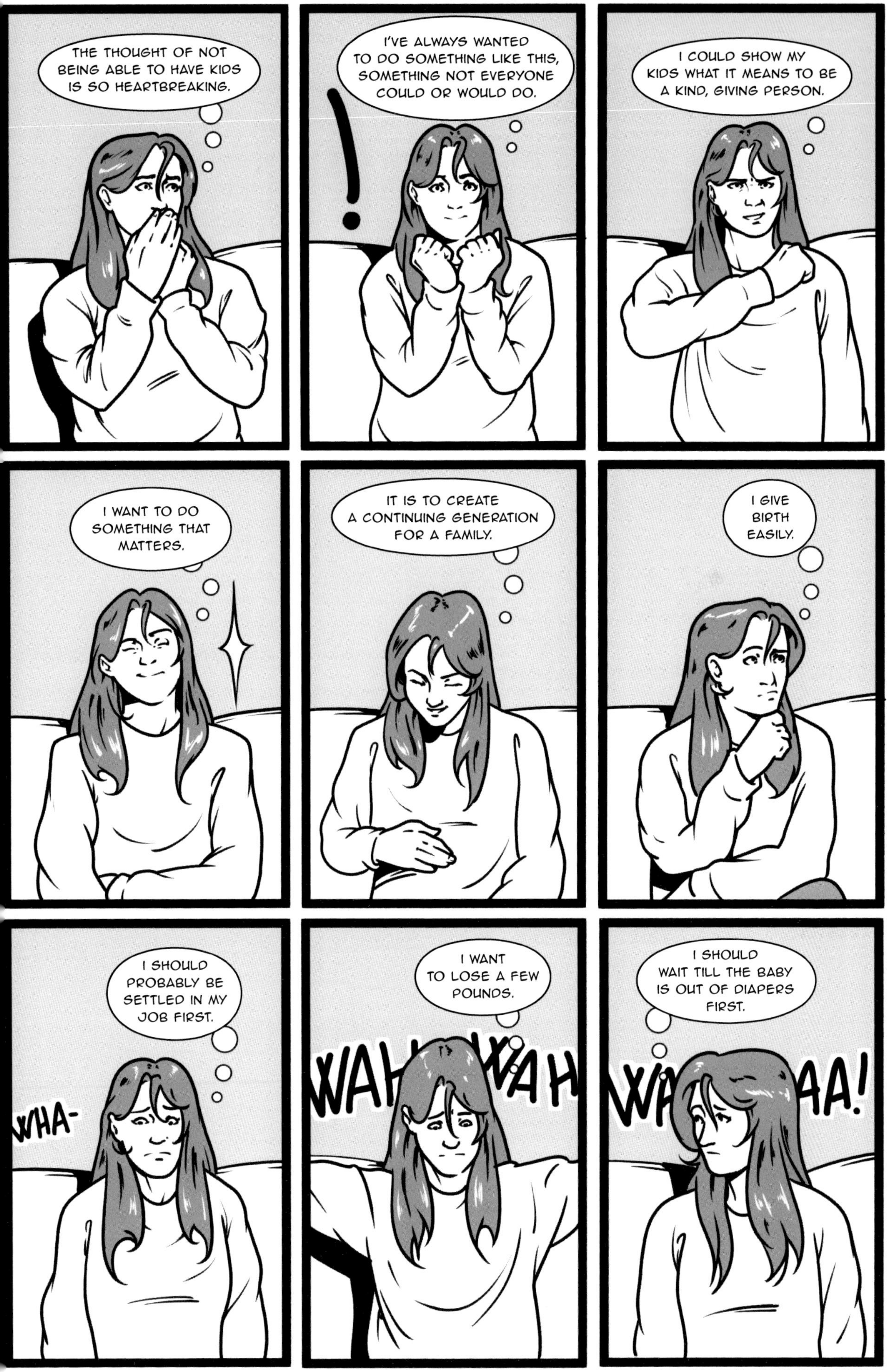
THE THOUGHT OF NOT BEING ABLE TO HAVE KIDS IS SO HEARTBREAKING.
I'VE ALWAYS WANTED TO DO SOMETHING LIKE THIS, SOMETHING NOT EVERYONE COULD OR WOULD DO.
!
I COULD SHOW MY KIDS WHAT IT MEANS TO BE A KIND, GIVING PERSON.
I WANT TO DO SOMETHING THAT MATTERS.
IT IS TO CREATE A CONTINUING GENERATION FOR A FAMILY.
I GIVE BIRTH EASILY.
I SHOULD PROBABLY BE SETTLED IN MY JOB FIRST.
WHA-
I WANT TO LOSE A FEW POUNDS.
WAH
WAH
I SHOULD WAIT TILL THE BABY IS OUT OF DIAPERS FIRST.
WA
AA!

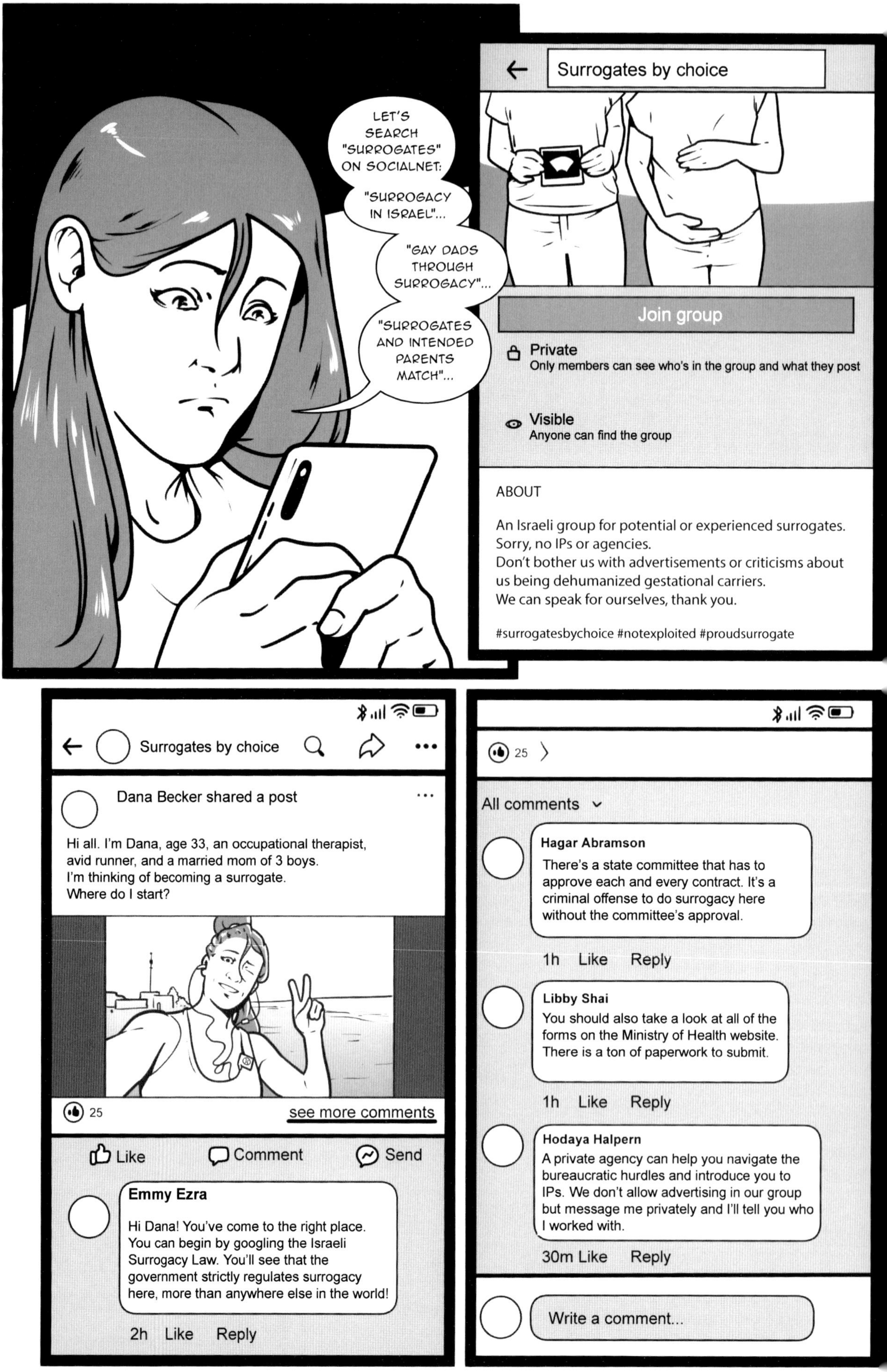
LET'S SEARCH "SURROGATES" ON SOCIALNET:
"SURROGACY IN ISRAEL"...
"GAY DADS THROUGH SURROGACY"...
"SURROGATES AND INTENDED PARENTS MATCH"...
Surrogates by choice
Join group
Private
Only members can see who's in the group and what they post
Visible
Anyone can find the group
ABOUT
An Israeli group for potential or experienced surrogates.
Sorry, no IPs or agencies.
Don't bother us with advertisements or criticisms about us being dehumanized gestational carriers.
We can speak for ourselves, thank you.
#surrogatesbychoice #notexploited #proudsurrogate
Surrogates by choice
Dana Becker shared a post
Hi all. I'm Dana, age 33, an occupational therapist, avid runner, and a married mom of 3 boys.
I'm thinking of becoming a surrogate.
Where do I start?
25
see more comments
Like
Comment
Send
Emmy Ezra
Hi Dana! You've come to the right place. You can begin by googling the Israeli Surrogacy Law. You'll see that the government strictly regulates surrogacy here, more than anywhere else in the world!
2h Like Reply
25
All comments
Hagar Abramson
There's a state committee that has to approve each and every contract. It's a criminal offense to do surrogacy here without the committee's approval.
1h Like Reply
Libby Shai
You should also take a look at all of the forms on the Ministry of Health website. There is a ton of paperwork to submit.
1h Like Reply
Hodaya Halpern
A private agency can help you navigate the bureaucratic hurdles and introduce you to IPs. We don't allow advertising in our group but message me privately and I'll tell you who I worked with.
30m Like Reply
Write a comment...

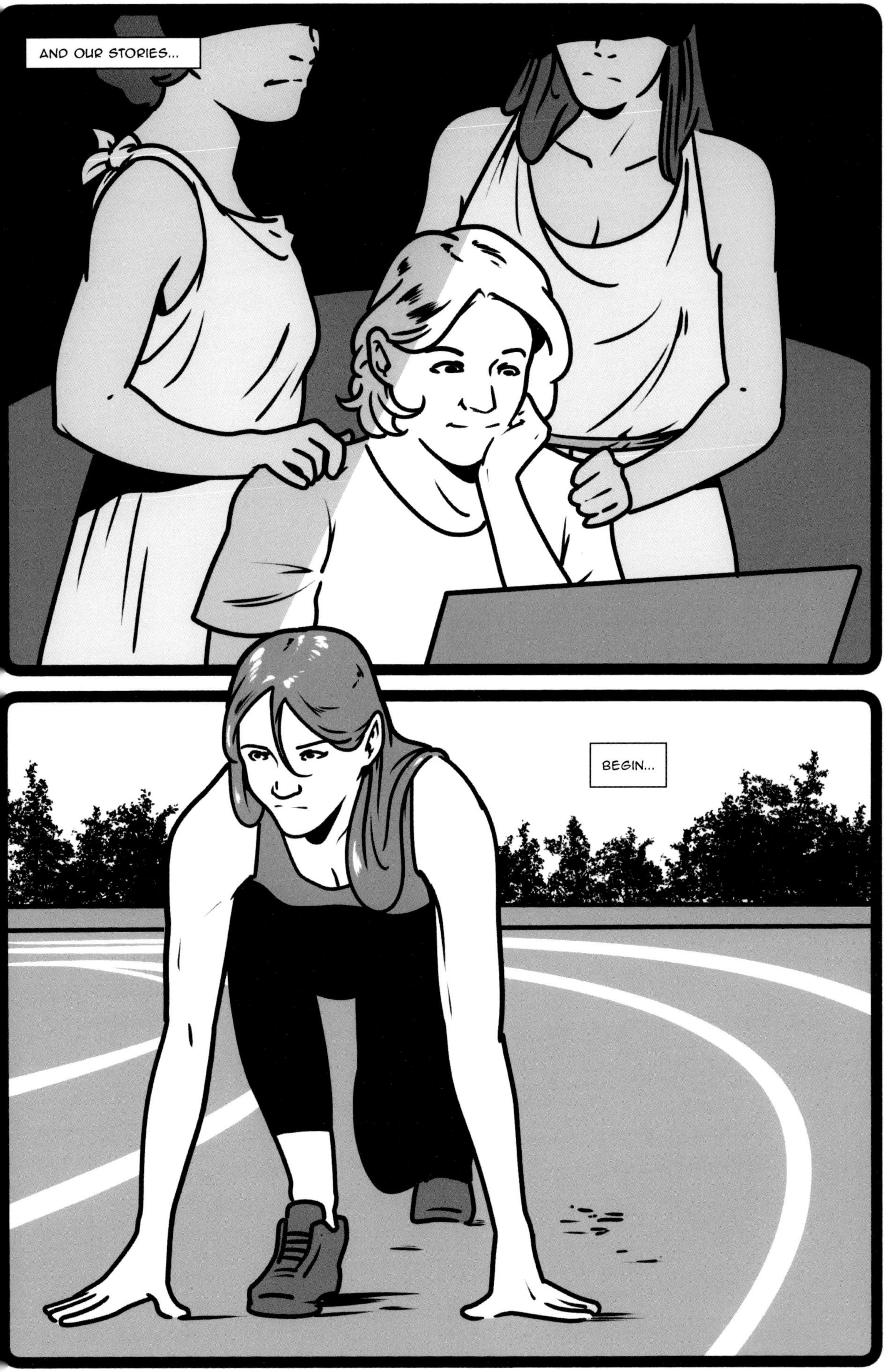
AND OUR STORIES...
BEGIN...

-CHAPTER 1-
THINKING IT THROUGH

-DANA-

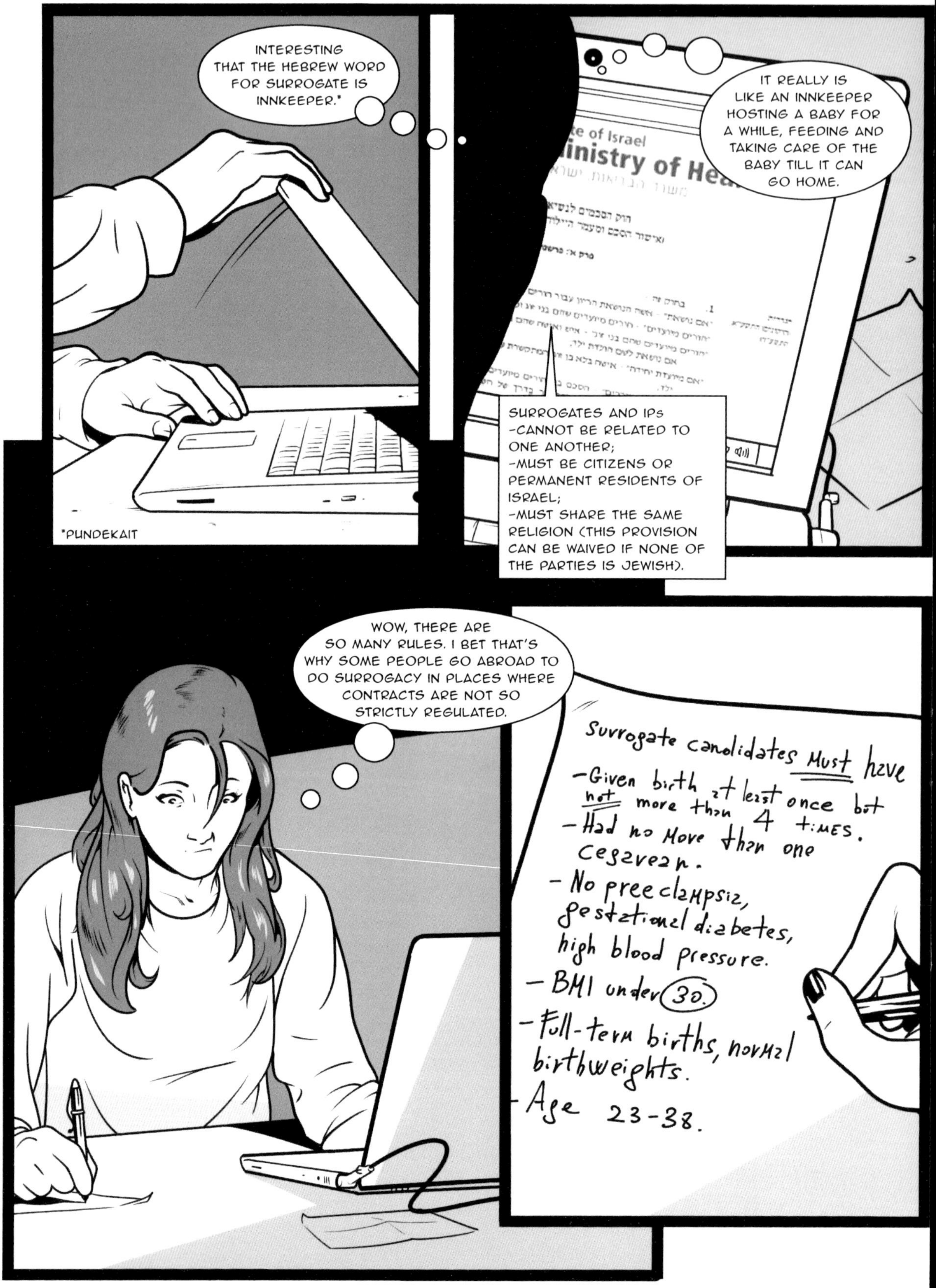
INTERESTING THAT THE HEBREW WORD FOR SURROGATE IS INNKEEPER.*
*PUNDEKAIT
IT REALLY IS LIKE AN INNKEEPER HOSTING A BABY FOR A WHILE, FEEDING AND TAKING CARE OF THE BABY TILL IT CAN GO HOME.
SURROGATES AND IPs
-CANNOT BE RELATED TO ONE ANOTHER;
-MUST BE CITIZENS OR PERMANENT RESIDENTS OF ISRAEL;
-MUST SHARE THE SAME RELIGION (THIS PROVISION CAN BE WAIVED IF NONE OF THE PARTIES IS JEWISH).
WOW, THERE ARE SO MANY RULES. I BET THAT'S WHY SOME PEOPLE GO ABROAD TO DO SURROGACY IN PLACES WHERE CONTRACTS ARE NOT SO STRICTLY REGULATED.
Surrogate candidates Must have
-Given birth at least once but not more than 4 times.
-Had no More than one cesarean.
- No preeclampsia, gestational diabetes, high blood pressure.
- BMI under 30.
-Full-term births, normal birthweights.
-Age 23-38.

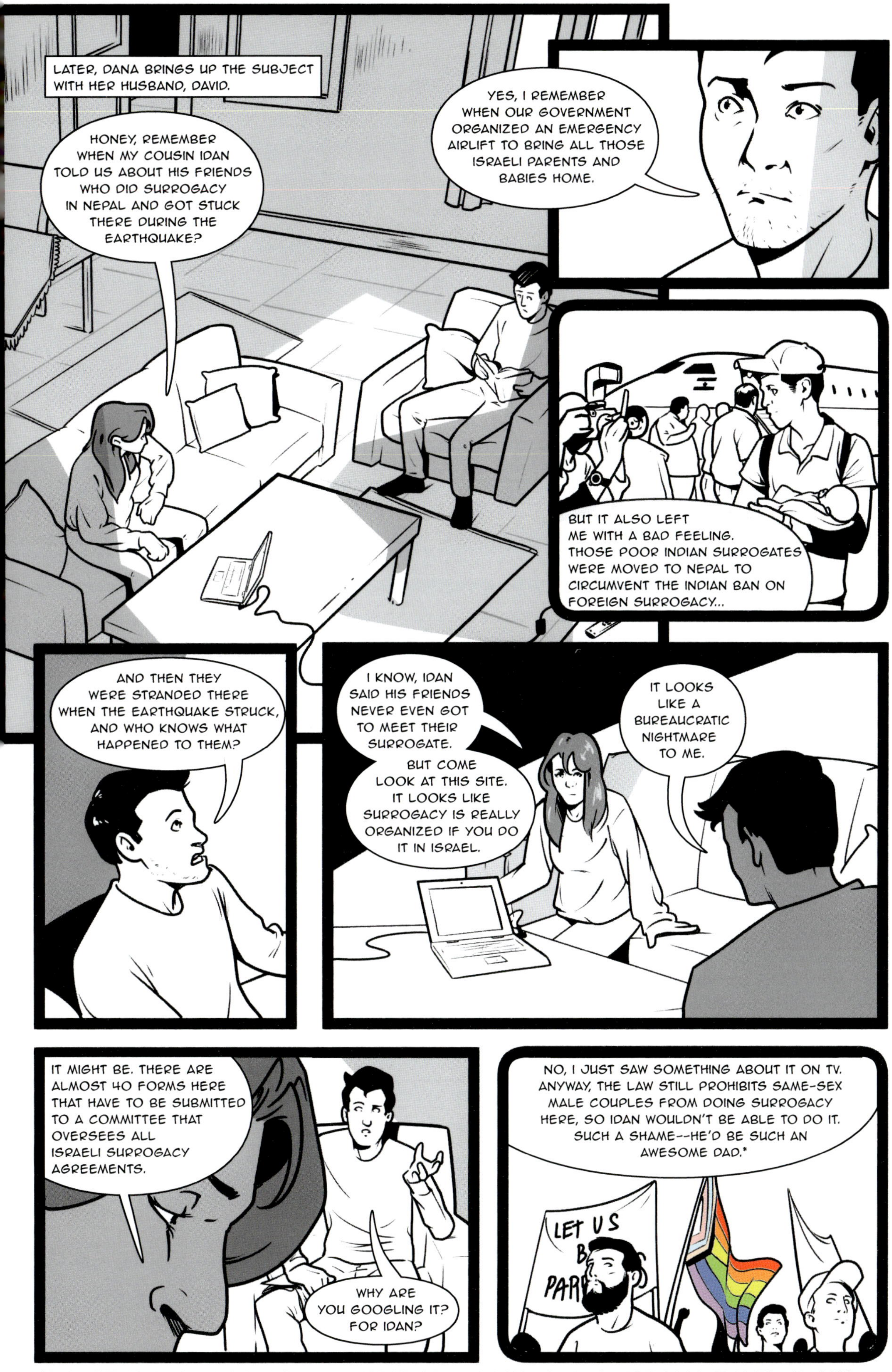
LATER, DANA BRINGS UP THE SUBJECT WITH HER HUSBAND, DAVID.
HONEY, REMEMBER WHEN MY COUSIN IDAN TOLD US ABOUT HIS FRIENDS WHO DID SURROGACY IN NEPAL AND GOT STUCK THERE DURING THE EARTHQUAKE?
YES, I REMEMBER WHEN OUR GOVERNMENT ORGANIZED AN EMERGENCY AIRLIFT TO BRING ALL THOSE ISRAELI PARENTS AND BABIES HOME.
BUT IT ALSO LEFT ME WITH A BAD FEELING. THOSE POOR INDIAN SURROGATES WERE MOVED TO NEPAL TO CIRCUMVENT THE INDIAN BAN ON FOREIGN SURROGACY...
AND THEN THEY WERE STRANDED THERE WHEN THE EARTHQUAKE STRUCK, AND WHO KNOWS WHAT HAPPENED TO THEM?
I KNOW, IDAN SAID HIS FRIENDS NEVER EVEN GOT TO MEET THEIR SURROGATE.
BUT COME LOOK AT THIS SITE. IT LOOKS LIKE SURROGACY IS REALLY ORGANIZED IF YOU DO IT IN ISRAEL.
IT LOOKS LIKE A BUREAUCRATIC NIGHTMARE TO ME.
IT MIGHT BE. THERE ARE ALMOST 40 FORMS HERE THAT HAVE TO BE SUBMITTED TO A COMMITTEE THAT OVERSEES ALL ISRAELI SURROGACY AGREEMENTS.
WHY ARE YOU GOOGLING IT? FOR IDAN?
NO, I JUST SAW SOMETHING ABOUT IT ON TV. ANYWAY, THE LAW STILL PROHIBITS SAME-SEX MALE COUPLES FROM DOING SURROGACY HERE, SO IDAN WOULDN'T BE ABLE TO DO IT. SUCH A SHAME--HE'D BE SUCH AN AWESOME DAD.*
LET US

*SAME-SEX COUPLES AND SINGLE MEN WERE NOT PERMITTED TO ENTER ISRAELI SURROGACY AGREEMENTS UNTIL 2022.

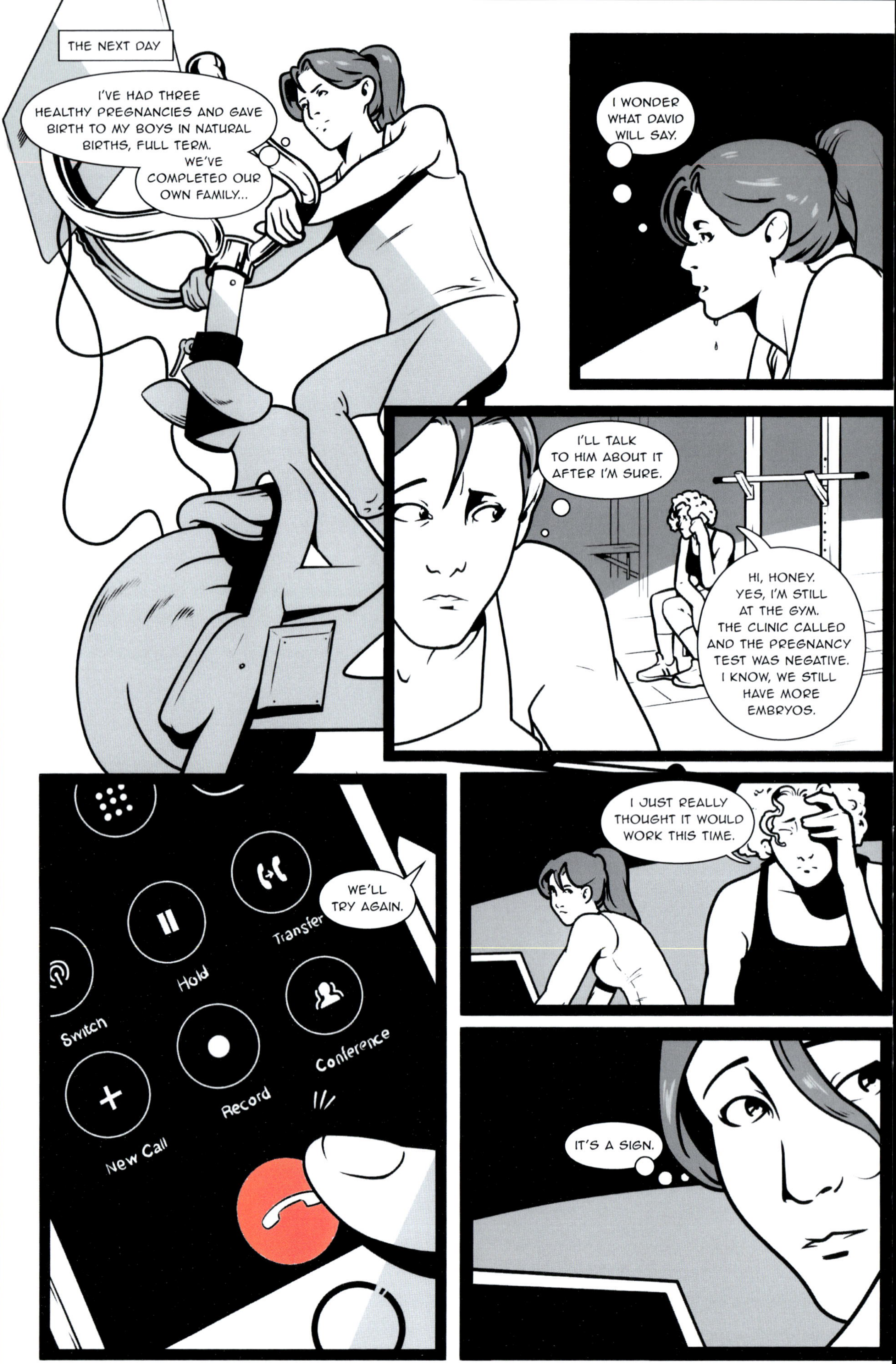
THE NEXT DAY
I'VE HAD THREE HEALTHY PREGNANCIES AND GAVE BIRTH TO MY BOYS IN NATURAL BIRTHS, FULL TERM.
WE'VE COMPLETED OUR OWN FAMILY...
I WONDER WHAT DAVID WILL SAY.
I'LL TALK TO HIM ABOUT IT AFTER I'M SURE.
HI, HONEY. YES, I'M STILL AT THE GYM. THE CLINIC CALLED AND THE PREGNANCY TEST WAS NEGATIVE. I KNOW, WE STILL HAVE MORE EMBRYOS.
Transfer
Hold
Switch
Record
Conference
New Call
WE'LL TRY AGAIN.
I JUST REALLY THOUGHT IT WOULD WORK THIS TIME.
IT'S A SIGN.

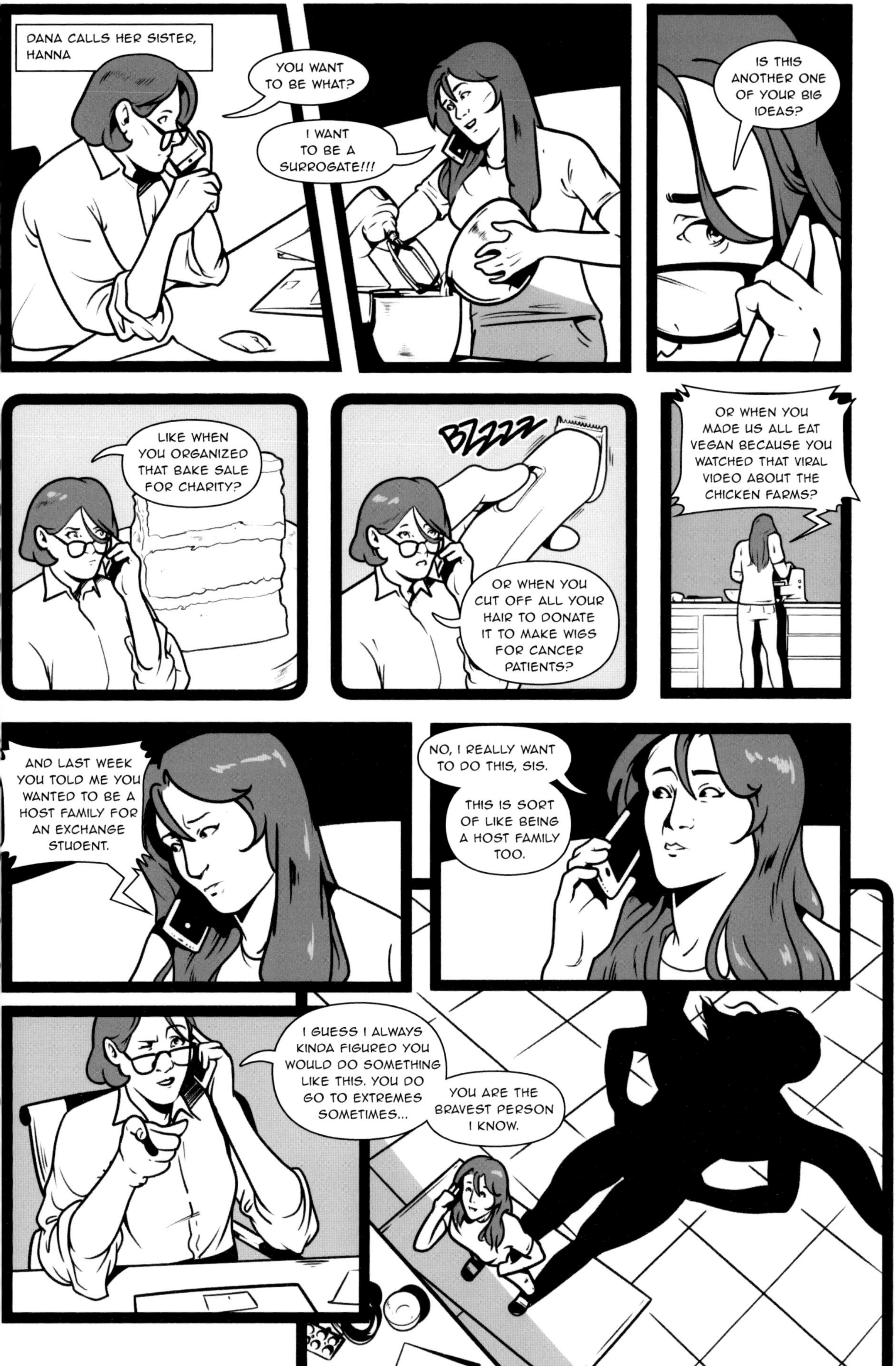
DANA CALLS HER SISTER, HANNA
YOU WANT TO BE WHAT?
I WANT TO BE A SURROGATE!!!
IS THIS ANOTHER ONE OF YOUR BIG IDEAS?
LIKE WHEN YOU ORGANIZED THAT BAKE SALE FOR CHARITY?
BZZZZ
OR WHEN YOU CUT OFF ALL YOUR HAIR TO DONATE IT TO MAKE WIGS FOR CANCER PATIENTS?
OR WHEN YOU MADE US ALL EAT VEGAN BECAUSE YOU WATCHED THAT VIRAL VIDEO ABOUT THE CHICKEN FARMS?
AND LAST WEEK YOU TOLD ME YOU WANTED TO BE A HOST FAMILY FOR AN EXCHANGE STUDENT.
NO, I REALLY WANT TO DO THIS, SIS.
THIS IS SORT OF LIKE BEING A HOST FAMILY TOO.
I GUESS I ALWAYS KINDA FIGURED YOU WOULD DO SOMETHING LIKE THIS. YOU DO GO TO EXTREMES SOMETIMES...
YOU ARE THE BRAVEST PERSON I KNOW.

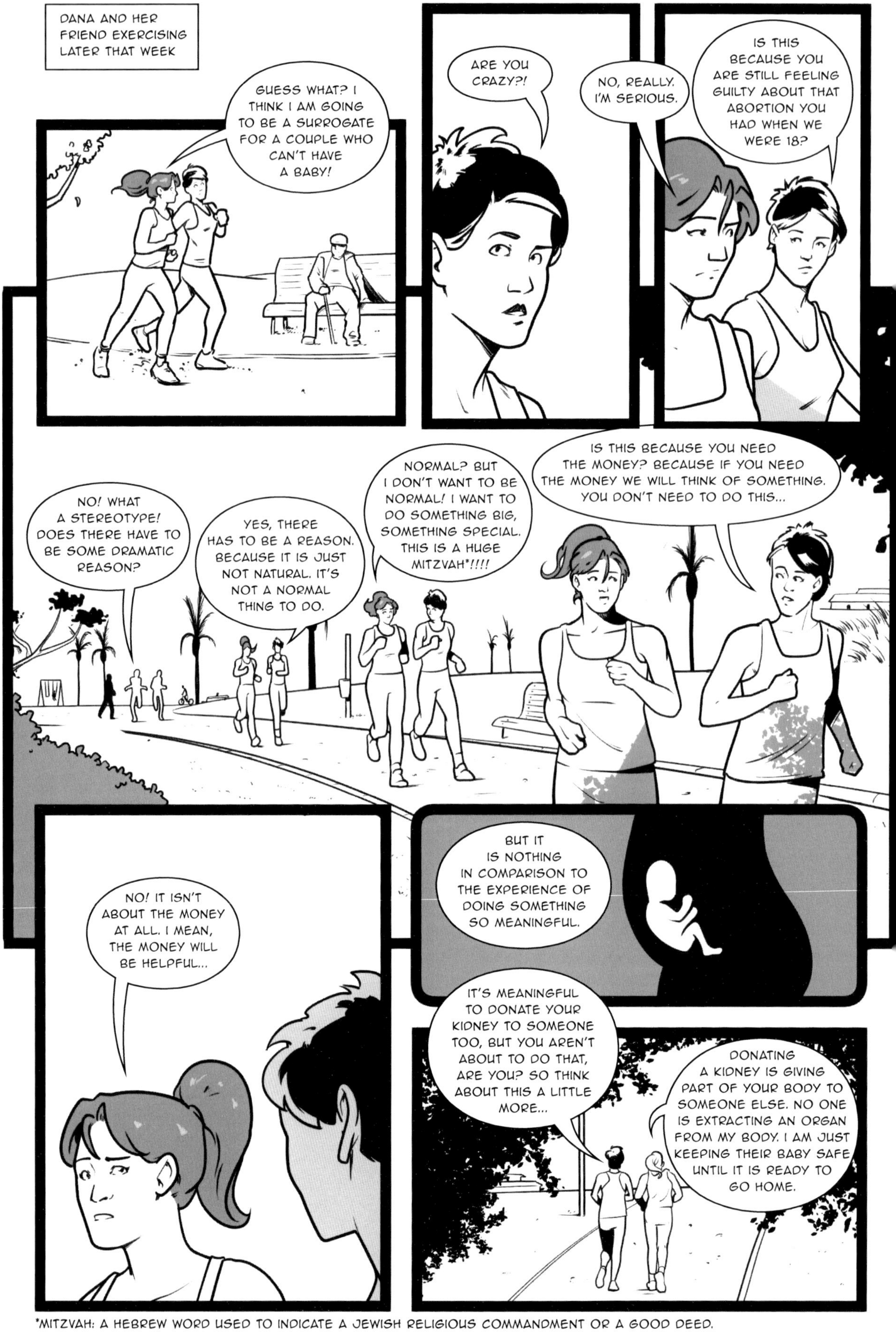
DANA AND HER FRIEND EXERCISING LATER THAT WEEK
GUESS WHAT? I THINK I AM GOING TO BE A SURROGATE FOR A COUPLE WHO CAN'T HAVE A BABY!
ARE YOU CRAZY?!
NO, REALLY. I'M SERIOUS.
IS THIS BECAUSE YOU ARE STILL FEELING GUILTY ABOUT THAT ABORTION YOU HAD WHEN WE WERE 18?
NO! WHAT A STEREOTYPE! DOES THERE HAVE TO BE SOME DRAMATIC REASON?
YES, THERE HAS TO BE A REASON. BECAUSE IT IS JUST NOT NATURAL. IT'S NOT A NORMAL THING TO DO.
NORMAL? BUT I DON'T WANT TO BE NORMAL! I WANT TO DO SOMETHING BIG, SOMETHING SPECIAL. THIS IS A HUGE MITZVAH*!!!!
IS THIS BECAUSE YOU NEED THE MONEY? BECAUSE IF YOU NEED THE MONEY WE WILL THINK OF SOMETHING. YOU DON'T NEED TO DO THIS...
NO! IT ISN'T ABOUT THE MONEY AT ALL. I MEAN, THE MONEY WILL BE HELPFUL...
BUT IT IS NOTHING IN COMPARISON TO THE EXPERIENCE OF DOING SOMETHING SO MEANINGFUL.
IT'S MEANINGFUL TO DONATE YOUR KIDNEY TO SOMEONE TOO, BUT YOU AREN'T ABOUT TO DO THAT, ARE YOU? SO THINK ABOUT THIS A LITTLE MORE...
DONATING A KIDNEY IS GIVING PART OF YOUR BODY TO SOMEONE ELSE. NO ONE IS EXTRACTING AN ORGAN FROM MY BODY. I AM JUST KEEPING THEIR BABY SAFE UNTIL IT IS READY TO GO HOME.

*MITZVAH: A HEBREW WORD USED TO INDICATE A JEWISH RELIGIOUS COMMANDMENT OR A GOOD DEED.

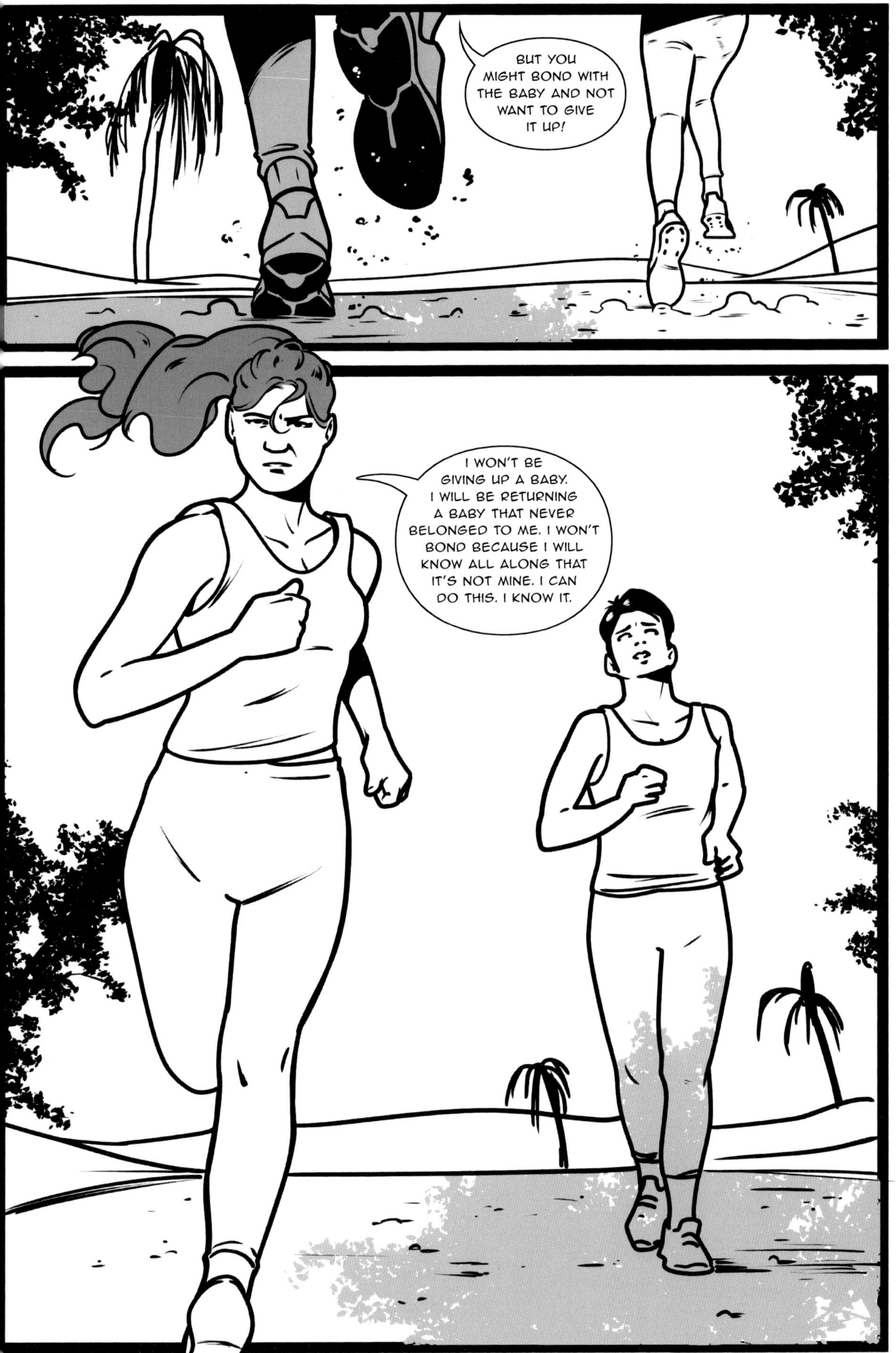
BUT YOU MIGHT BOND WITH THE BABY AND NOT WANT TO GIVE IT UP!
I WON'T BE GIVING UP A BABY. I WILL BE RETURNING A BABY THAT NEVER BELONGED TO ME. I WON'T BOND BECAUSE I WILL KNOW ALL ALONG THAT IT'S NOT MINE. I CAN DO THIS. I KNOW IT.

-CHAPTER 2-
GETTING THE HUBBY ON BOARD

-JENN-

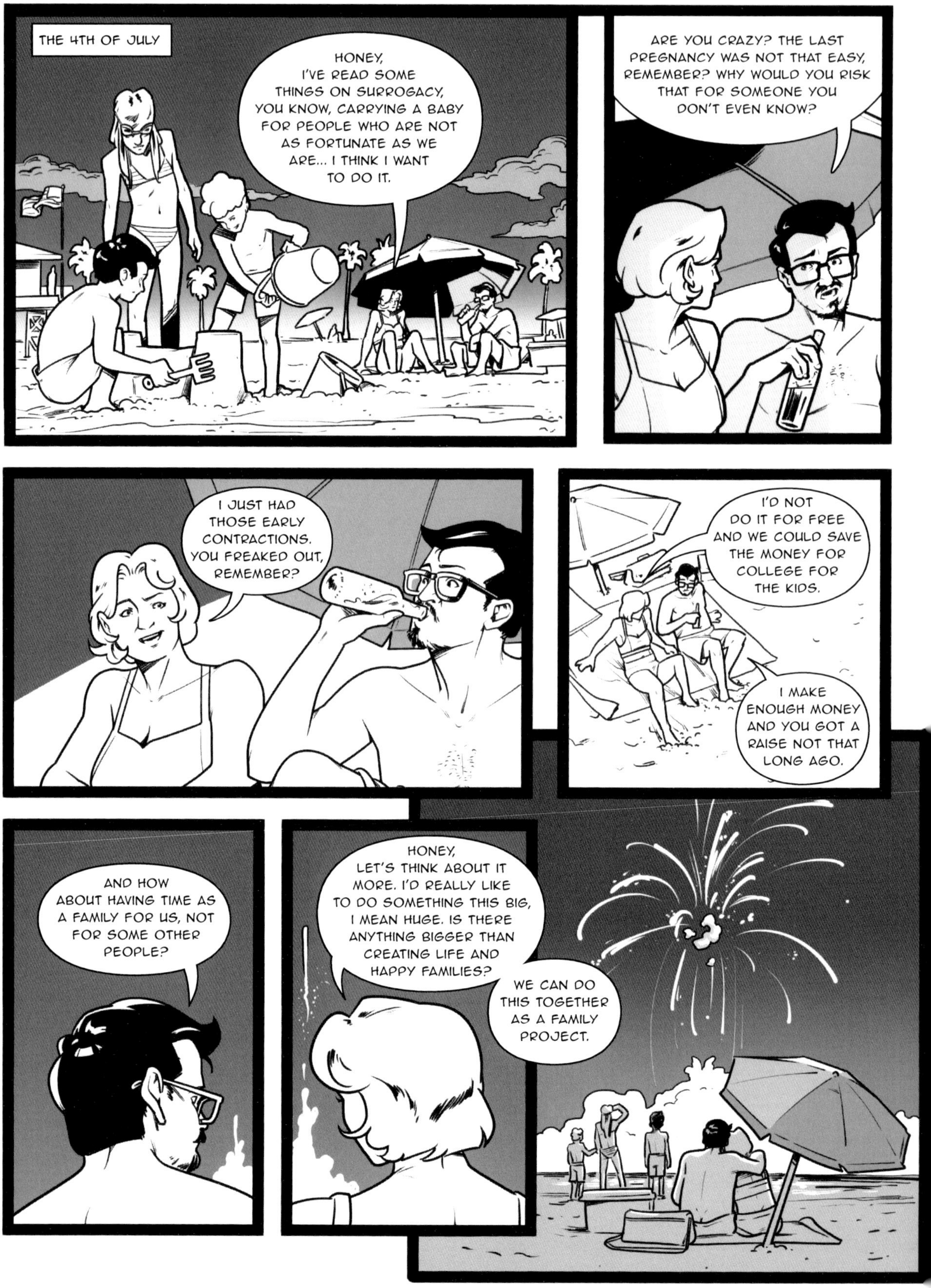

THE 4TH OF JULY
HONEY, I'VE READ SOME THINGS ON SURROGACY, YOU KNOW, CARRYING A BABY FOR PEOPLE WHO ARE NOT AS FORTUNATE AS WE ARE... I THINK I WANT TO DO IT.
ARE YOU CRAZY? THE LAST PREGNANCY WAS NOT THAT EASY, REMEMBER? WHY WOULD YOU RISK THAT FOR SOMEONE YOU DON'T EVEN KNOW?
I JUST HAD THOSE EARLY CONTRACTIONS. YOU FREAKED OUT, REMEMBER?
I'D NOT DO IT FOR FREE AND WE COULD SAVE THE MONEY FOR COLLEGE FOR THE KIDS.
I MAKE ENOUGH MONEY AND YOU GOT A RAISE NOT THAT LONG AGO.
AND HOW ABOUT HAVING TIME AS A FAMILY FOR US, NOT FOR SOME OTHER PEOPLE?
HONEY, LET'S THINK ABOUT IT MORE. I'D REALLY LIKE TO DO SOMETHING THIS BIG, I MEAN HUGE. IS THERE ANYTHING BIGGER THAN CREATING LIFE AND HAPPY FAMILIES?
WE CAN DO THIS TOGETHER AS A FAMILY PROJECT.

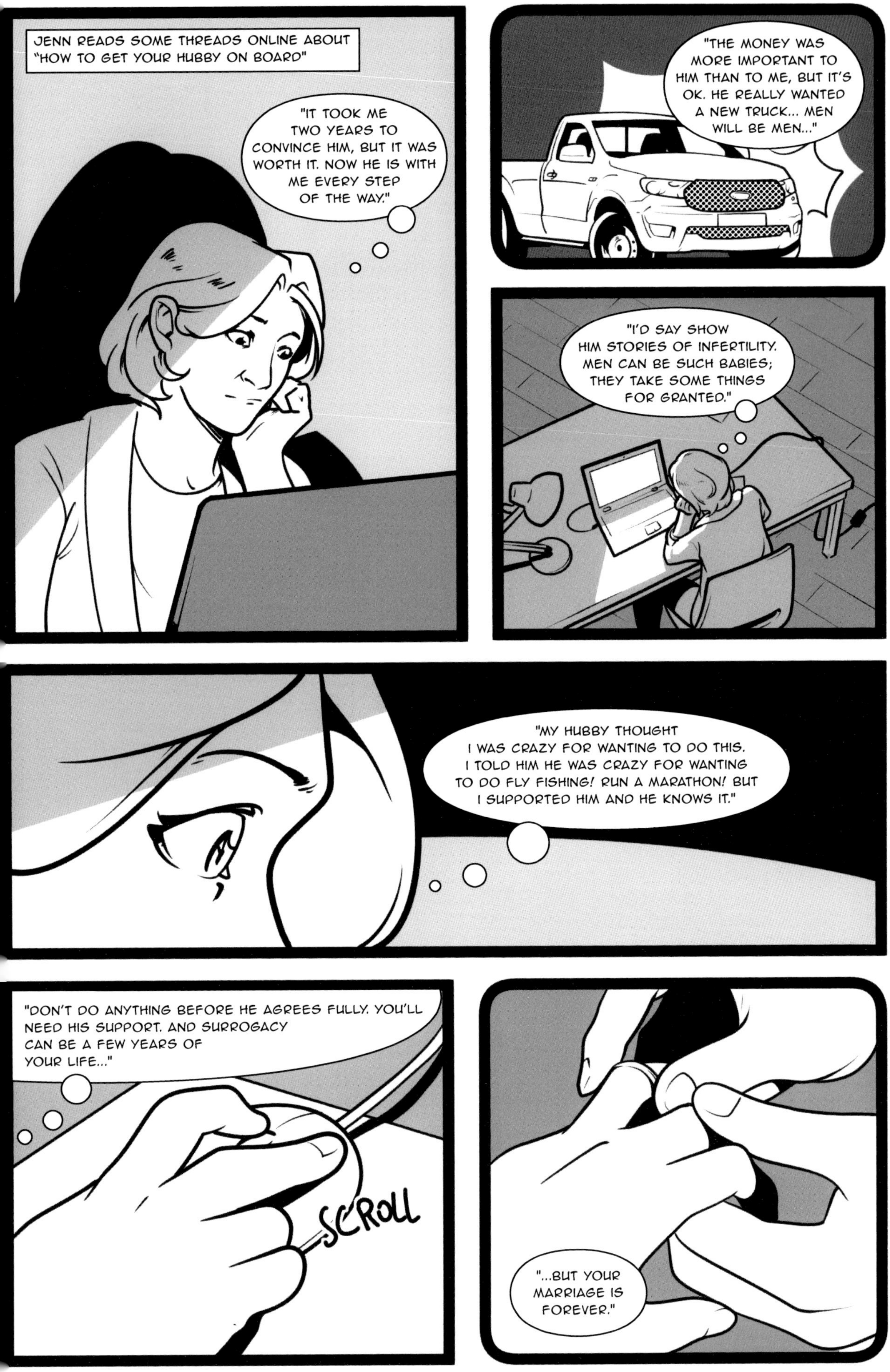
JENN READS SOME THREADS ONLINE ABOUT "HOW TO GET YOUR HUBBY ON BOARD"
"IT TOOK ME TWO YEARS TO CONVINCE HIM, BUT IT WAS WORTH IT. NOW HE IS WITH ME EVERY STEP OF THE WAY."
"THE MONEY WAS MORE IMPORTANT TO HIM THAN TO ME, BUT IT'S OK. HE REALLY WANTED A NEW TRUCK... MEN WILL BE MEN..."
"I'D SAY SHOW HIM STORIES OF INFERTILITY. MEN CAN BE SUCH BABIES; THEY TAKE SOME THINGS FOR GRANTED."
"MY HUBBY THOUGHT I WAS CRAZY FOR WANTING TO DO THIS. I TOLD HIM HE WAS CRAZY FOR WANTING TO DO FLY FISHING! RUN A MARATHON! BUT I SUPPORTED HIM AND HE KNOWS IT."
"DON'T DO ANYTHING BEFORE HE AGREES FULLY. YOU'LL NEED HIS SUPPORT. AND SURROGACY CAN BE A FEW YEARS OF YOUR LIFE..."
SCROLL
"...BUT YOUR MARRIAGE IS FOREVER."

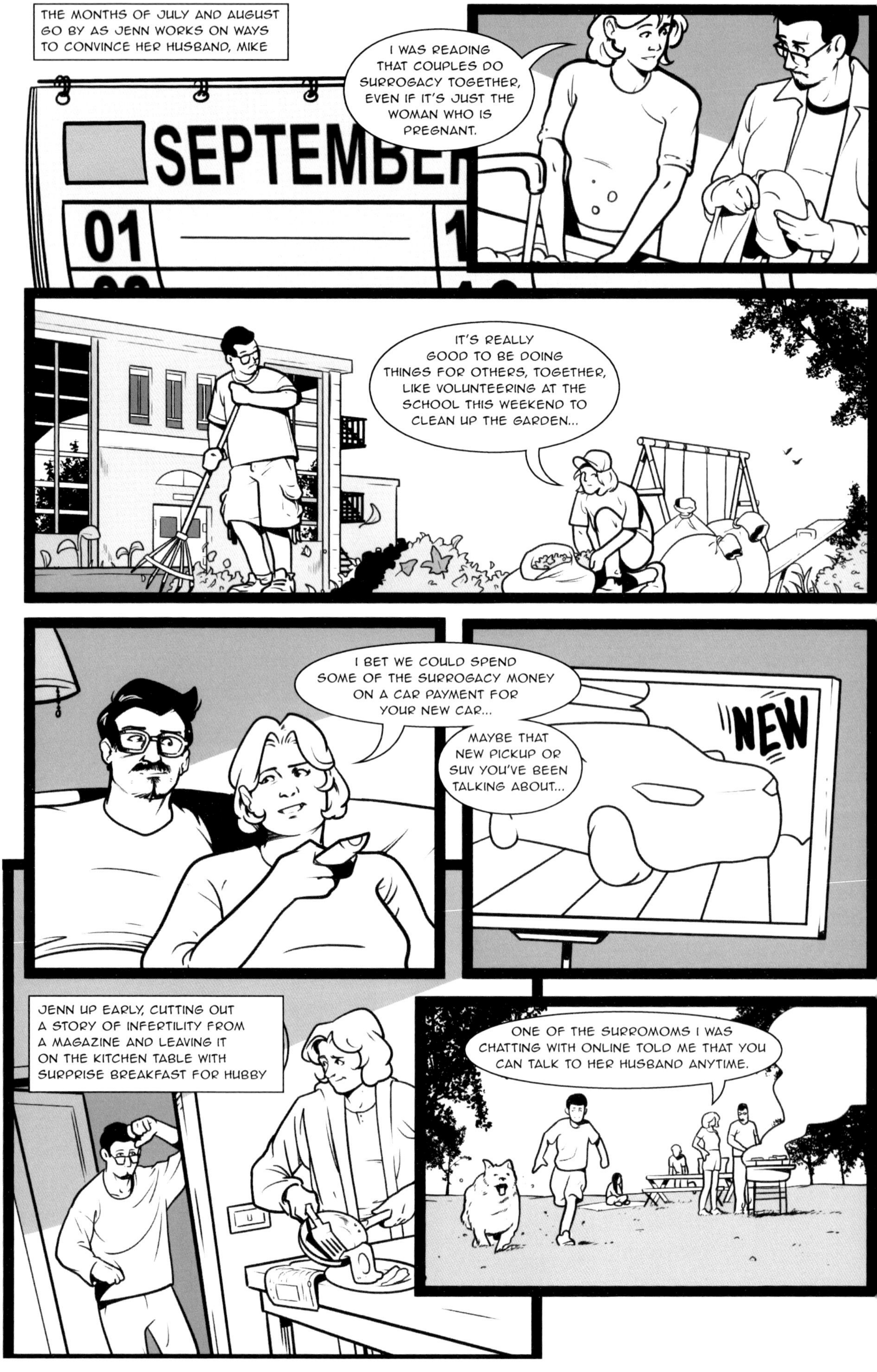
THE MONTHS OF JULY AND AUGUST GO BY AS JENN WORKS ON WAYS TO CONVINCE HER HUSBAND, MIKE
SEPTEMBER
01
I WAS READING THAT COUPLES DO SURROGACY TOGETHER, EVEN IF IT'S JUST THE WOMAN WHO IS PREGNANT.
IT'S REALLY GOOD TO BE DOING THINGS FOR OTHERS, TOGETHER, LIKE VOLUNTEERING AT THE SCHOOL THIS WEEKEND TO CLEAN UP THE GARDEN...
I BET WE COULD SPEND SOME OF THE SURROGACY MONEY ON A CAR PAYMENT FOR YOUR NEW CAR...
MAYBE THAT NEW PICKUP OR SUV YOU'VE BEEN TALKING ABOUT...
NEW
JENN UP EARLY, CUTTING OUT A STORY OF INFERTILITY FROM A MAGAZINE AND LEAVING IT ON THE KITCHEN TABLE WITH SURPRISE BREAKFAST FOR HUBBY
ONE OF THE SURROMOMS I WAS CHATTING WITH ONLINE TOLD ME THAT YOU CAN TALK TO HER HUSBAND ANYTIME.

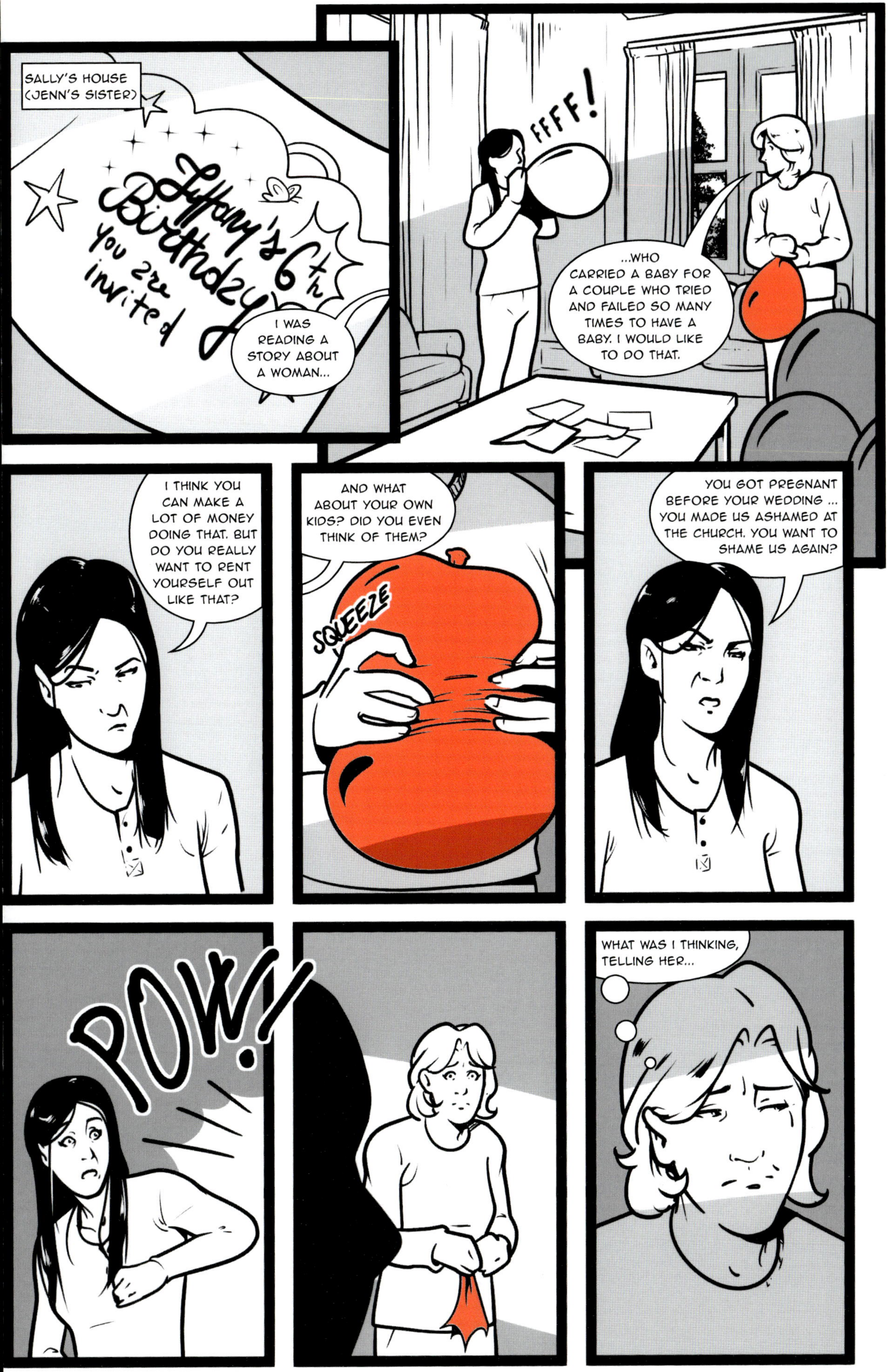
SALLY'S HOUSE (JENN'S SISTER)
Tiffany's 6th Birthday you are invited
I WAS READING A STORY ABOUT A WOMAN...
FFFF!
...WHO CARRIED A BABY FOR A COUPLE WHO TRIED AND FAILED SO MANY TIMES TO HAVE A BABY. I WOULD LIKE TO DO THAT.
I THINK YOU CAN MAKE A LOT OF MONEY DOING THAT. BUT DO YOU REALLY WANT TO RENT YOURSELF OUT LIKE THAT?
AND WHAT ABOUT YOUR OWN KIDS? DID YOU EVEN THINK OF THEM?
SQUEEZE
YOU GOT PREGNANT BEFORE YOUR WEDDING ... YOU MADE US ASHAMED AT THE CHURCH. YOU WANT TO SHAME US AGAIN?
POW!
WHAT WAS I THINKING, TELLING HER...

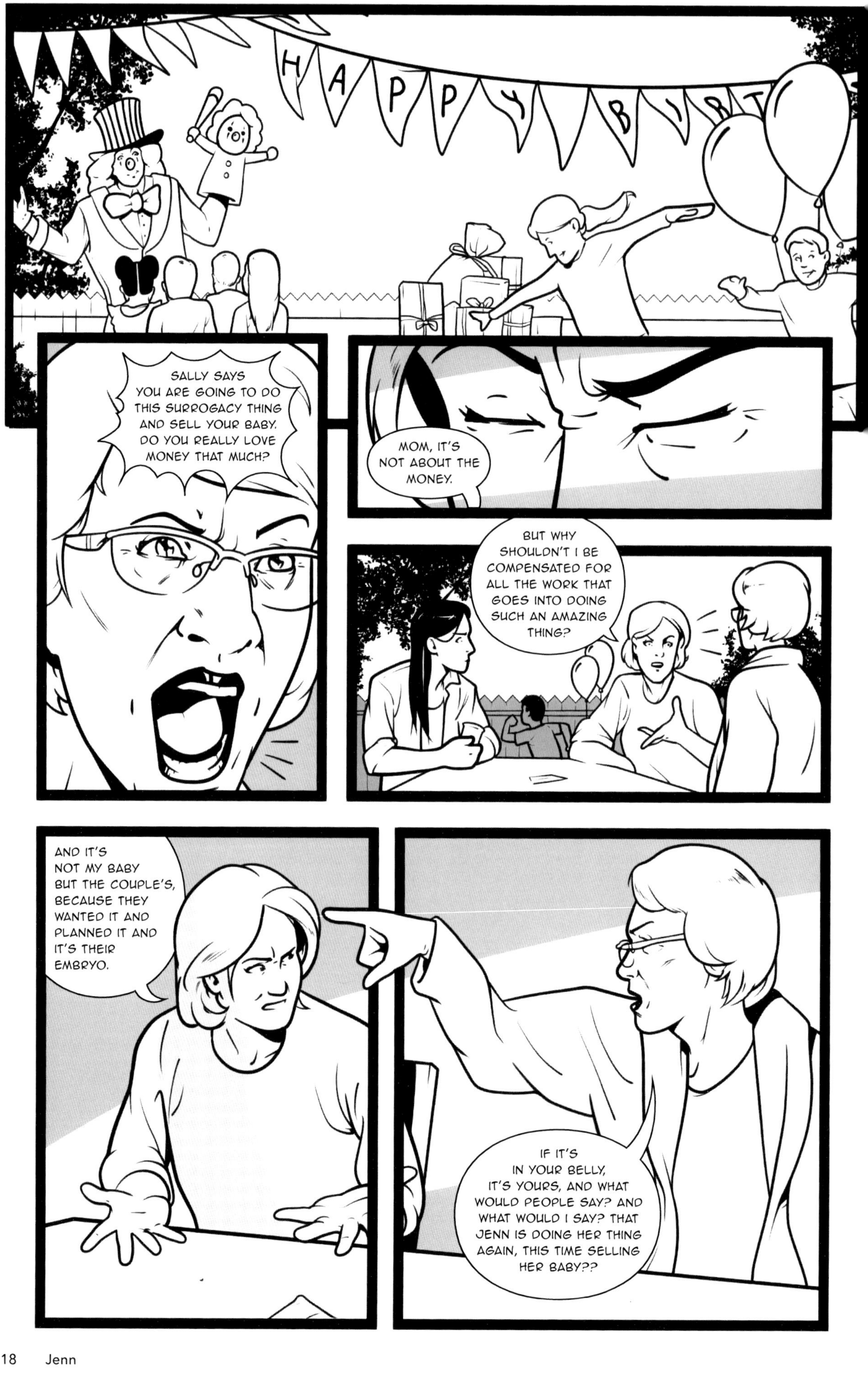
HAPPY BIRT
SALLY SAYS YOU ARE GOING TO DO THIS SURROGACY THING AND SELL YOUR BABY. DO YOU REALLY LOVE MONEY THAT MUCH?
MOM, IT'S NOT ABOUT THE MONEY.
BUT WHY SHOULDN'T I BE COMPENSATED FOR ALL THE WORK THAT GOES INTO DOING SUCH AN AMAZING THING?
AND IT'S NOT MY BABY BUT THE COUPLE'S, BECAUSE THEY WANTED IT AND PLANNED IT AND IT'S THEIR EMBRYO.
IF IT'S IN YOUR BELLY, IT'S YOURS, AND WHAT WOULD PEOPLE SAY? AND WHAT WOULD I SAY? THAT JENN IS DOING HER THING AGAIN, THIS TIME SELLING HER BABY??

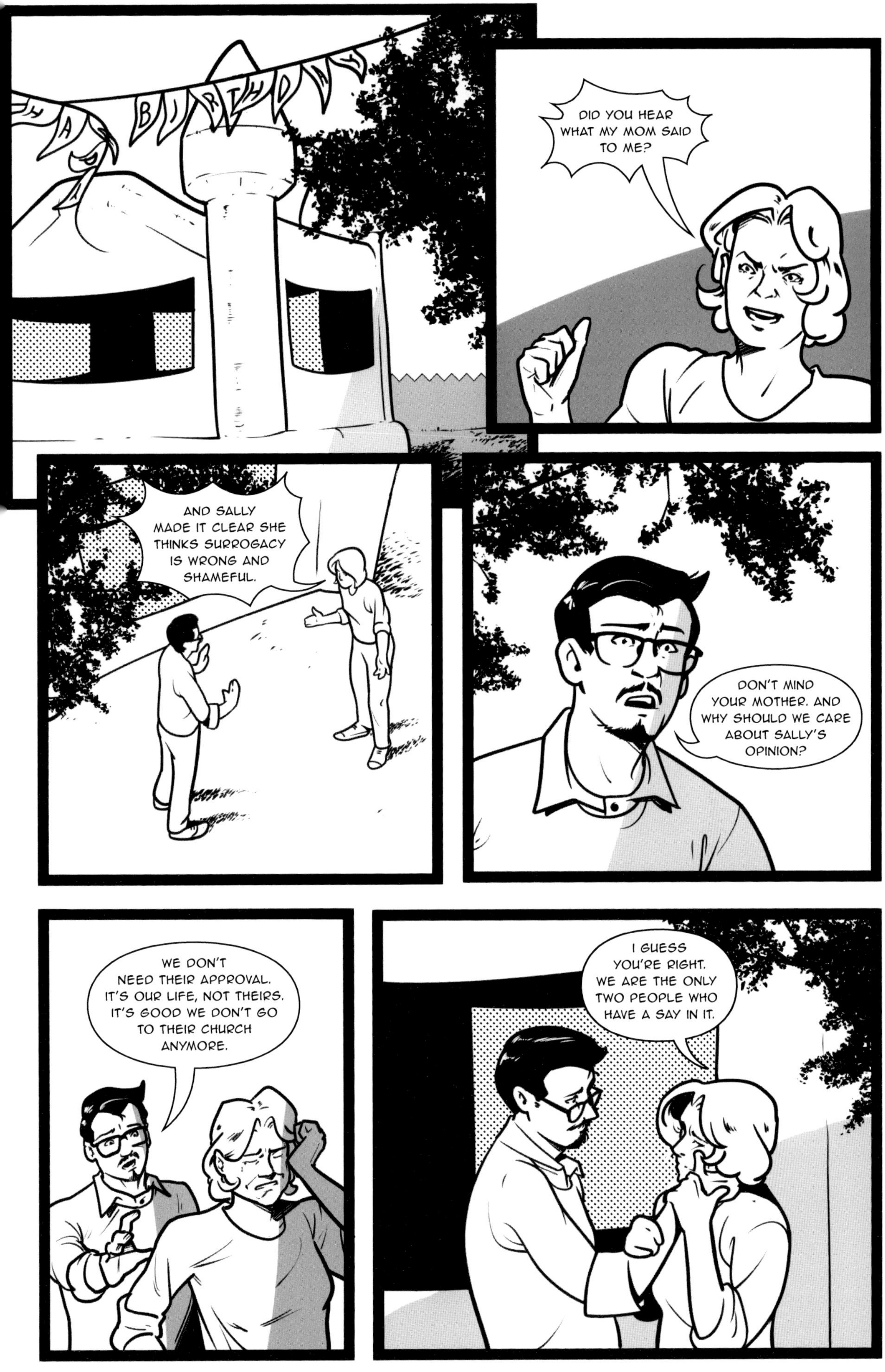
HAPPY BIRTHDAY
DID YOU HEAR WHAT MY MOM SAID TO ME?
AND SALLY MADE IT CLEAR SHE THINKS SURROGACY IS WRONG AND SHAMEFUL.
DON'T MIND YOUR MOTHER. AND WHY SHOULD WE CARE ABOUT SALLY'S OPINION?
WE DON'T NEED THEIR APPROVAL. IT'S OUR LIFE, NOT THEIRS. IT'S GOOD WE DON'T GO TO THEIR CHURCH ANYMORE.
I GUESS YOU'RE RIGHT. WE ARE THE ONLY TWO PEOPLE WHO HAVE A SAY IN IT.

INTERLUDE: ANONYMOUS MEMBERS OF A RUSSIAN-LANGUAGE SURROGACY SUPPORT GROUP

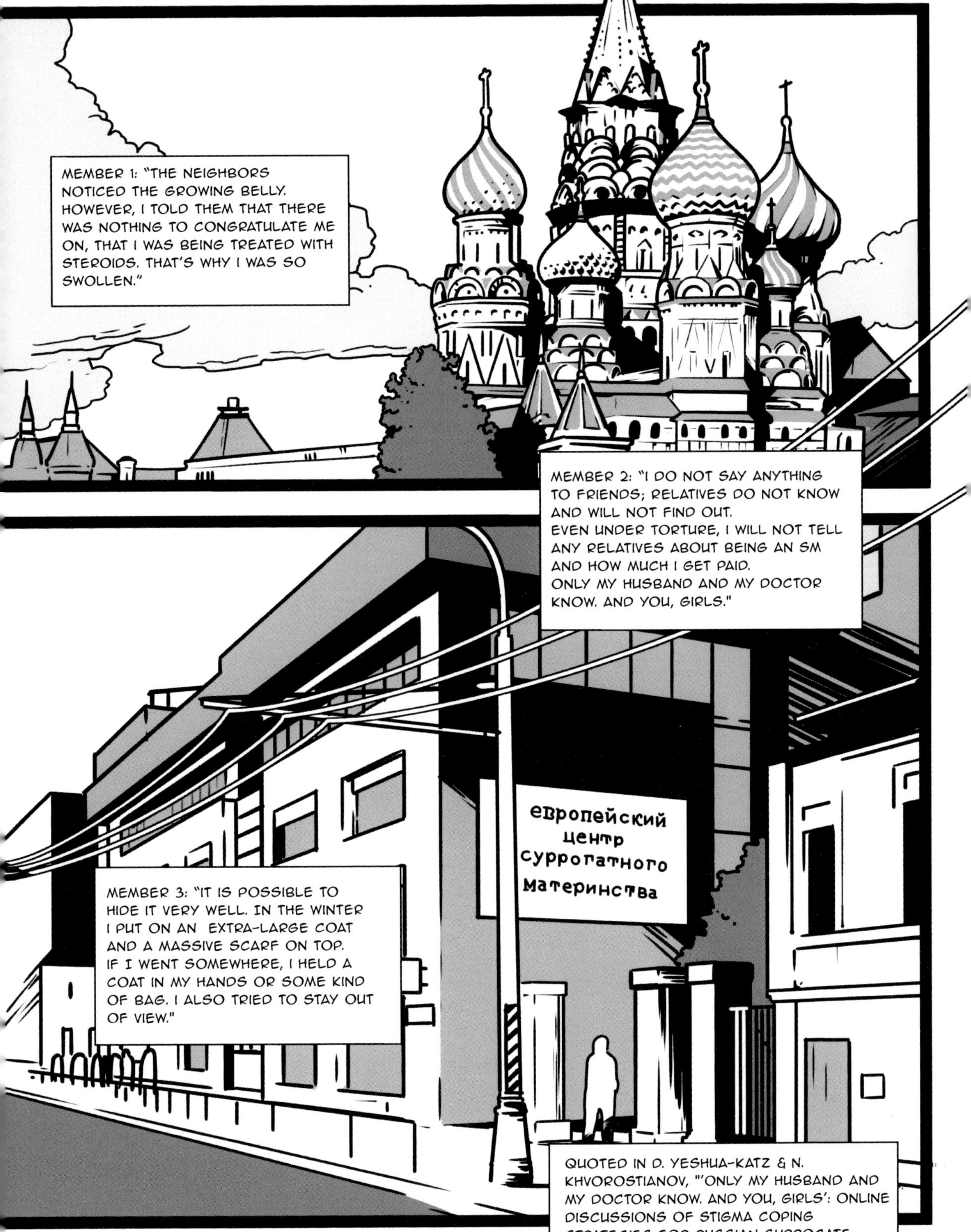
MEMBER 1: "THE NEIGHBORS NOTICED THE GROWING BELLY. HOWEVER, I TOLD THEM THAT THERE WAS NOTHING TO CONGRATULATE ME ON, THAT I WAS BEING TREATED WITH STEROIDS. THAT'S WHY I WAS SO SWOLLEN."
MEMBER 2: "I DO NOT SAY ANYTHING TO FRIENDS; RELATIVES DO NOT KNOW AND WILL NOT FIND OUT. EVEN UNDER TORTURE, I WILL NOT TELL ANY RELATIVES ABOUT BEING AN SM AND HOW MUCH I GET PAID. ONLY MY HUSBAND AND MY DOCTOR KNOW. AND YOU, GIRLS."
европейский центр суррогатного материнства
MEMBER 3: "IT IS POSSIBLE TO HIDE IT VERY WELL. IN THE WINTER I PUT ON AN EXTRA-LARGE COAT AND A MASSIVE SCARF ON TOP. IF I WENT SOMEWHERE, I HELD A COAT IN MY HANDS OR SOME KIND OF BAG. I ALSO TRIED TO STAY OUT OF VIEW."

QUOTED IN D. YESHUA-KATZ & N. KHVOROSTIANOV, "'ONLY MY HUSBAND AND MY DOCTOR KNOW. AND YOU, GIRLS': ONLINE DISCUSSIONS OF STIGMA COPING STRATEGIES FOR RUSSIAN SURROGATE MOTHERS," INTERNATIONAL JOURNAL OF ENVIRONMENTAL RESEARCH AND PUBLIC HEALTH 18, NO. 21 (2021): 11325.

-CHAPTER 3-
BABY STEPS

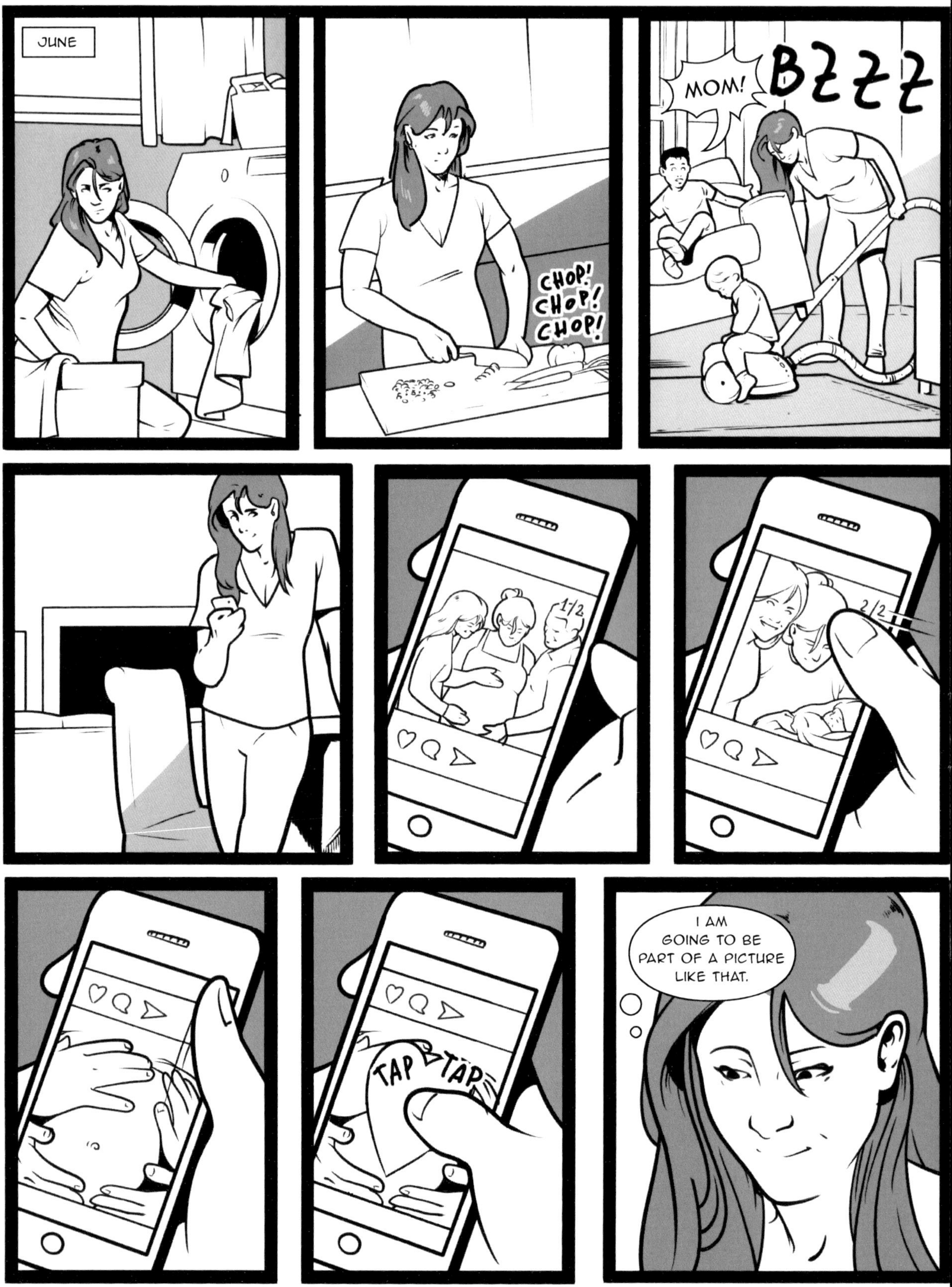

JUNE
CHOP! CHOP! CHOP!
MOM!
BZZZ
1/2
2/2
TAP TAP
I AM GOING TO BE PART OF A PICTURE LIKE THAT.

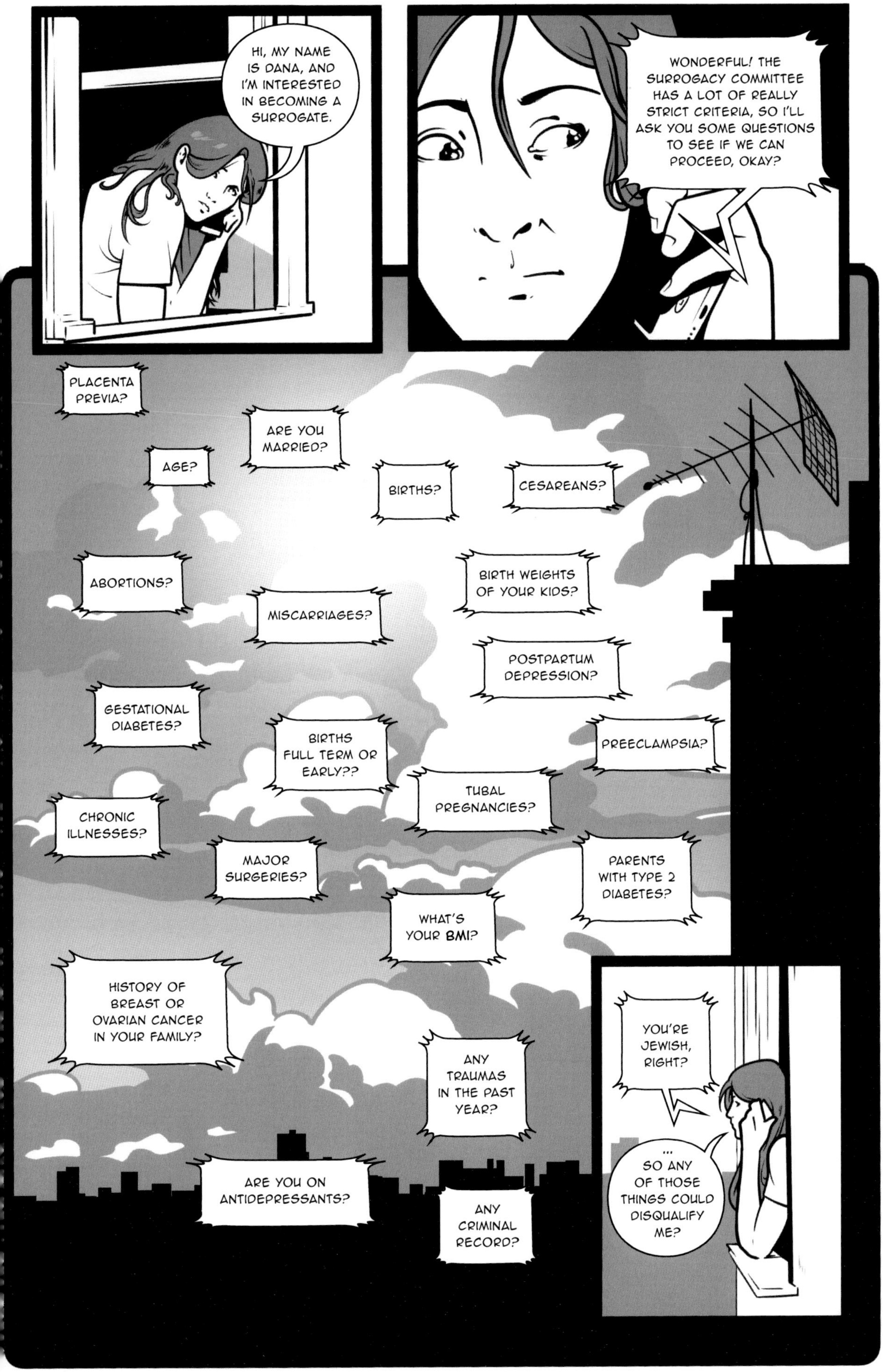
HI, MY NAME IS DANA, AND I'M INTERESTED IN BECOMING A SURROGATE.
WONDERFUL! THE SURROGACY COMMITTEE HAS A LOT OF REALLY STRICT CRITERIA, SO I'LL ASK YOU SOME QUESTIONS TO SEE IF WE CAN PROCEED, OKAY?
PLACENTA PREVIA?
ARE YOU MARRIED?
AGE?
BIRTHS?
CESAREANS?
ABORTIONS?
BIRTH WEIGHTS OF YOUR KIDS?
MISCARRIAGES?
POSTPARTUM DEPRESSION?
GESTATIONAL DIABETES?
BIRTHS FULL TERM OR EARLY??
PREECLAMPSIA?
TUBAL PREGNANCIES?
CHRONIC ILLNESSES?
MAJOR SURGERIES?
PARENTS WITH TYPE 2 DIABETES?
WHAT'S YOUR BMI?
HISTORY OF BREAST OR OVARIAN CANCER IN YOUR FAMILY?
ANY TRAUMAS IN THE PAST YEAR?
YOU'RE JEWISH, RIGHT?
ARE YOU ON ANTIDEPRESSANTS?
ANY CRIMINAL RECORD?
... SO ANY OF THOSE THINGS COULD DISQUALIFY ME?

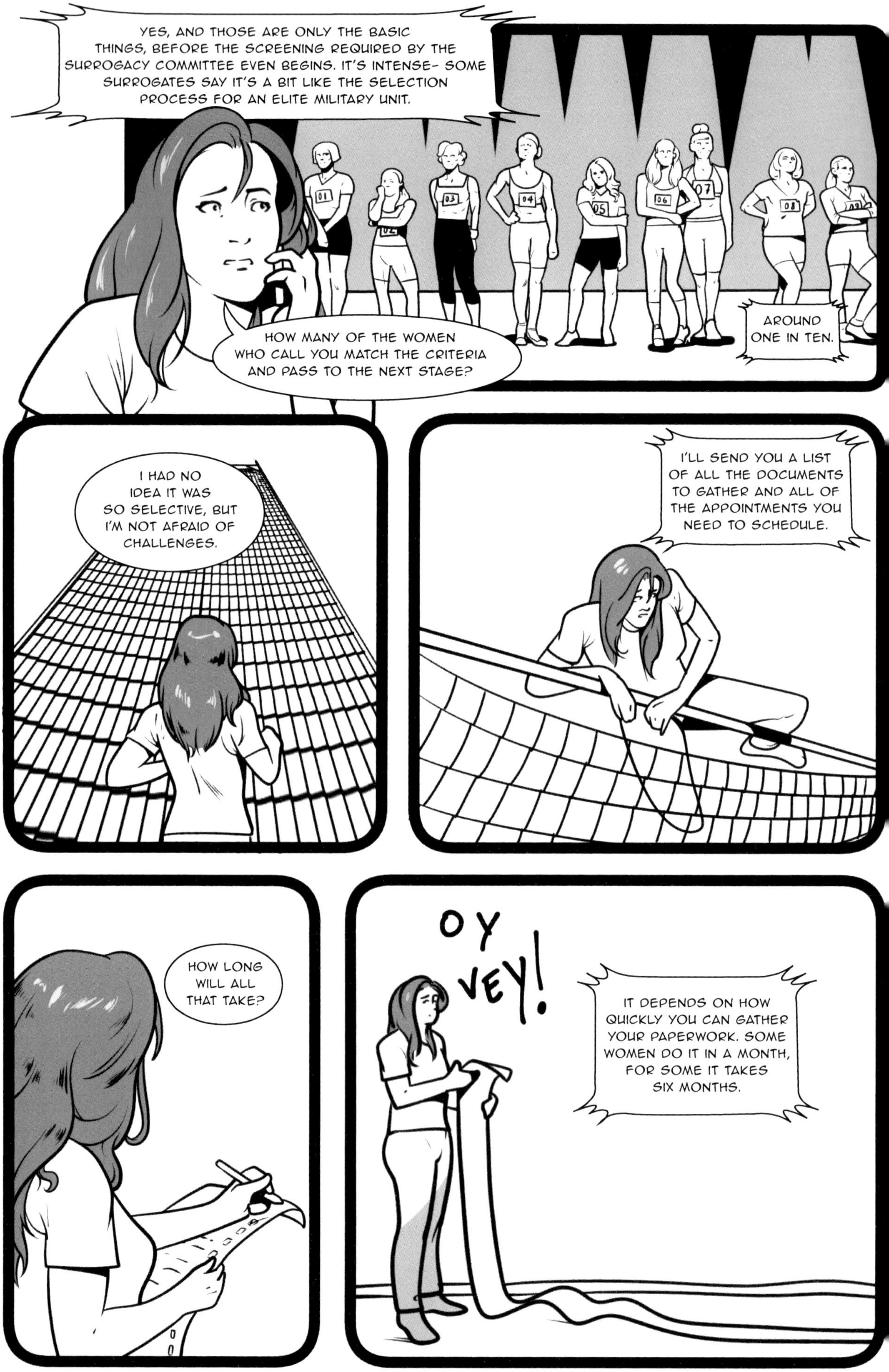

YES, AND THOSE ARE ONLY THE BASIC THINGS, BEFORE THE SCREENING REQUIRED BY THE SURROGACY COMMITTEE EVEN BEGINS. IT'S INTENSE- SOME SURROGATES SAY IT'S A BIT LIKE THE SELECTION PROCESS FOR AN ELITE MILITARY UNIT.
01
02
03
04
05
06
07
08
HOW MANY OF THE WOMEN WHO CALL YOU MATCH THE CRITERIA AND PASS TO THE NEXT STAGE?
AROUND ONE IN TEN.
I HAD NO IDEA IT WAS SO SELECTIVE, BUT I'M NOT AFRAID OF CHALLENGES.
I'LL SEND YOU A LIST OF ALL THE DOCUMENTS TO GATHER AND ALL OF THE APPOINTMENTS YOU NEED TO SCHEDULE.
HOW LONG WILL ALL THAT TAKE?
OY VEY!
IT DEPENDS ON HOW QUICKLY YOU CAN GATHER YOUR PAPERWORK. SOME WOMEN DO IT IN A MONTH, FOR SOME IT TAKES SIX MONTHS.

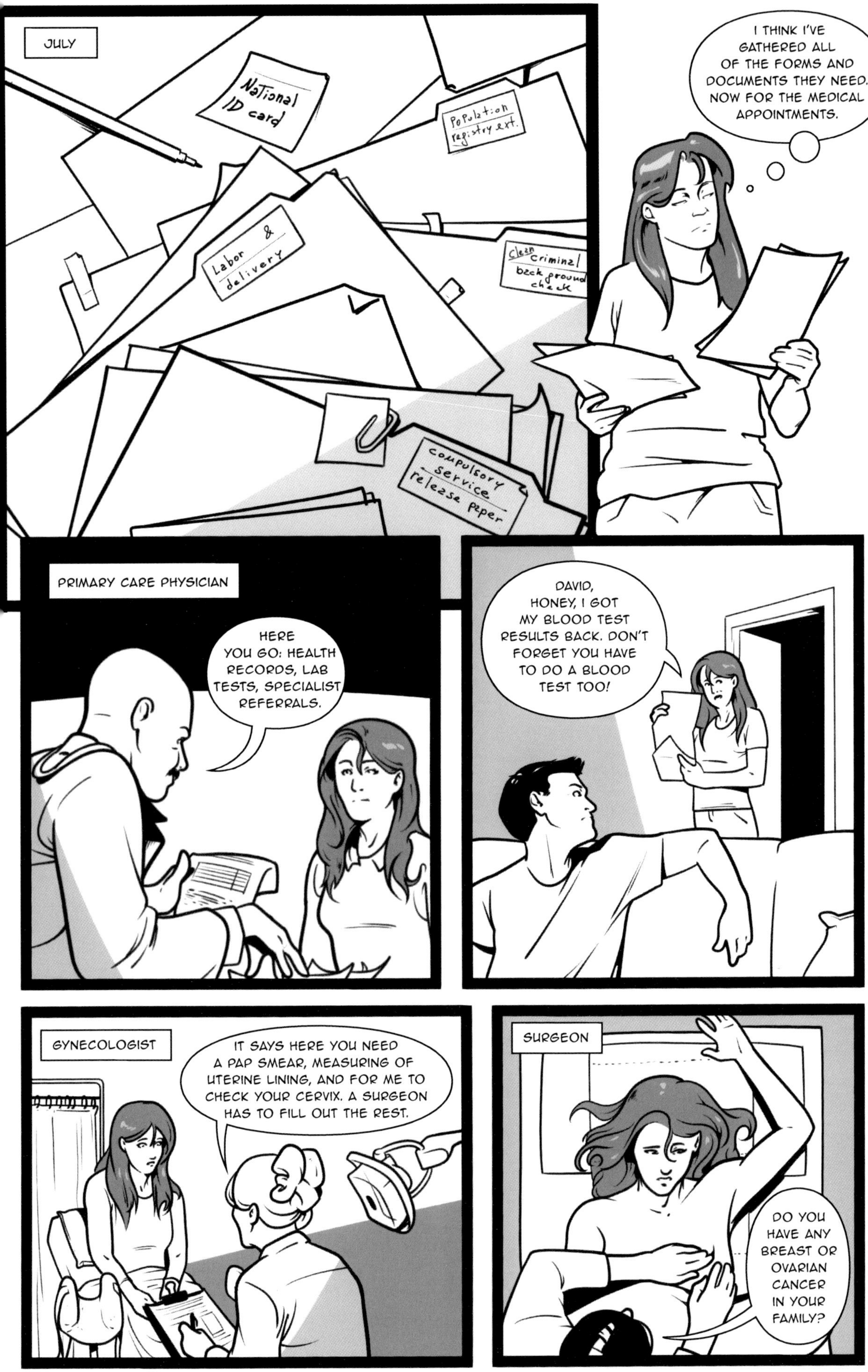
JULY
National ID card
Population registry ext.
Labor & delivery
Clean criminal background check
compulsory service release paper
I THINK I'VE GATHERED ALL OF THE FORMS AND DOCUMENTS THEY NEED. NOW FOR THE MEDICAL APPOINTMENTS.
PRIMARY CARE PHYSICIAN
HERE YOU GO: HEALTH RECORDS, LAB TESTS, SPECIALIST REFERRALS.
DAVID, HONEY, I GOT MY BLOOD TEST RESULTS BACK. DON'T FORGET YOU HAVE TO DO A BLOOD TEST TOO!
GYNECOLOGIST
IT SAYS HERE YOU NEED A PAP SMEAR, MEASURING OF UTERINE LINING, AND FOR ME TO CHECK YOUR CERVIX. A SURGEON HAS TO FILL OUT THE REST.
SURGEON
DO YOU HAVE ANY BREAST OR OVARIAN CANCER IN YOUR FAMILY?

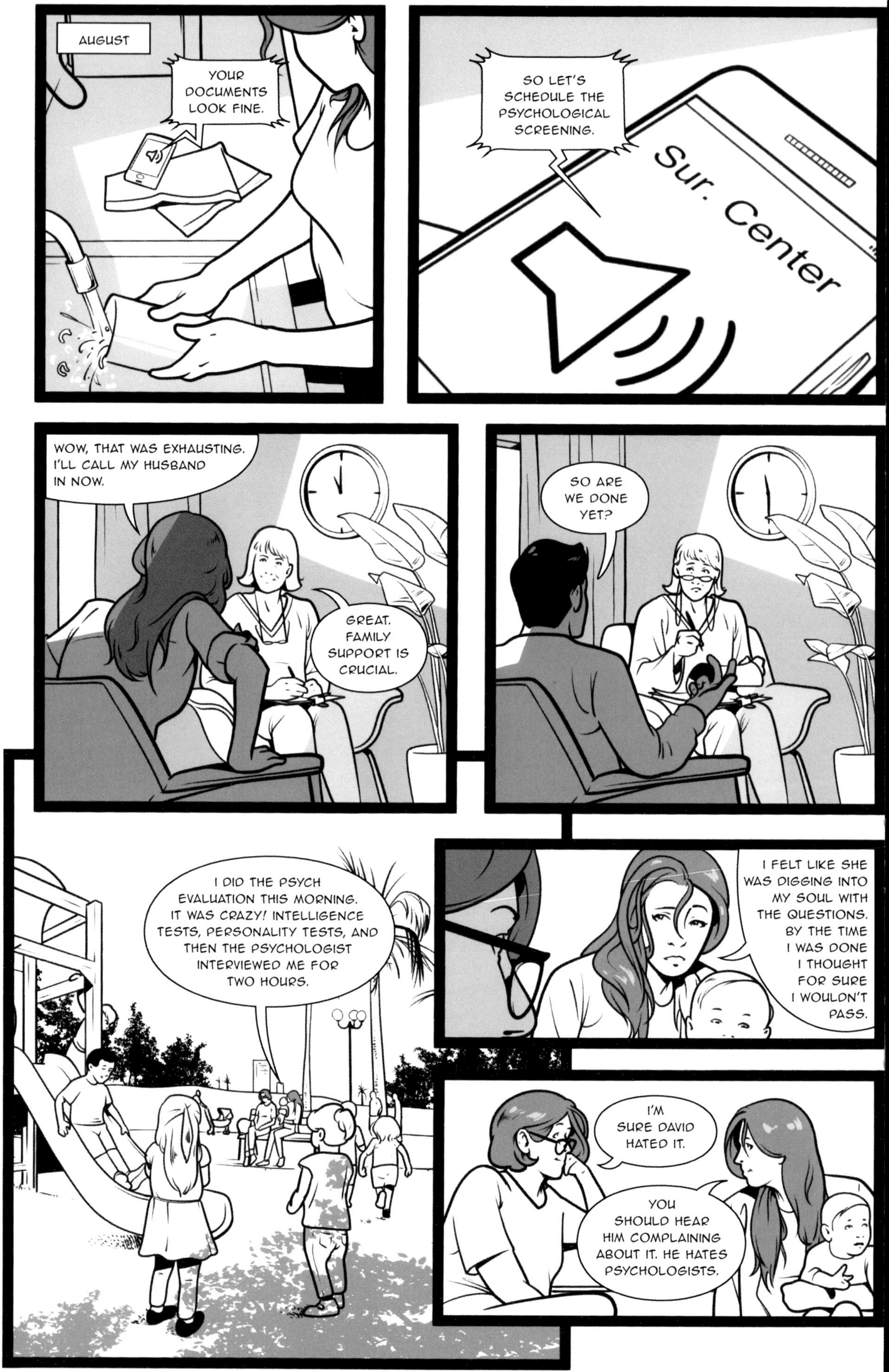
AUGUST
YOUR DOCUMENTS LOOK FINE.
SO LET'S SCHEDULE THE PSYCHOLOGICAL SCREENING.
Sur. Center
WOW, THAT WAS EXHAUSTING. I'LL CALL MY HUSBAND IN NOW.
GREAT. FAMILY SUPPORT IS CRUCIAL.
SO ARE WE DONE YET?
I DID THE PSYCH EVALUATION THIS MORNING. IT WAS CRAZY! INTELLIGENCE TESTS, PERSONALITY TESTS, AND THEN THE PSYCHOLOGIST INTERVIEWED ME FOR TWO HOURS.
I FELT LIKE SHE WAS DIGGING INTO MY SOUL WITH THE QUESTIONS. BY THE TIME I WAS DONE I THOUGHT FOR SURE I WOULDN'T PASS.
I'M SURE DAVID HATED IT.
YOU SHOULD HEAR HIM COMPLAINING ABOUT IT. HE HATES PSYCHOLOGISTS.

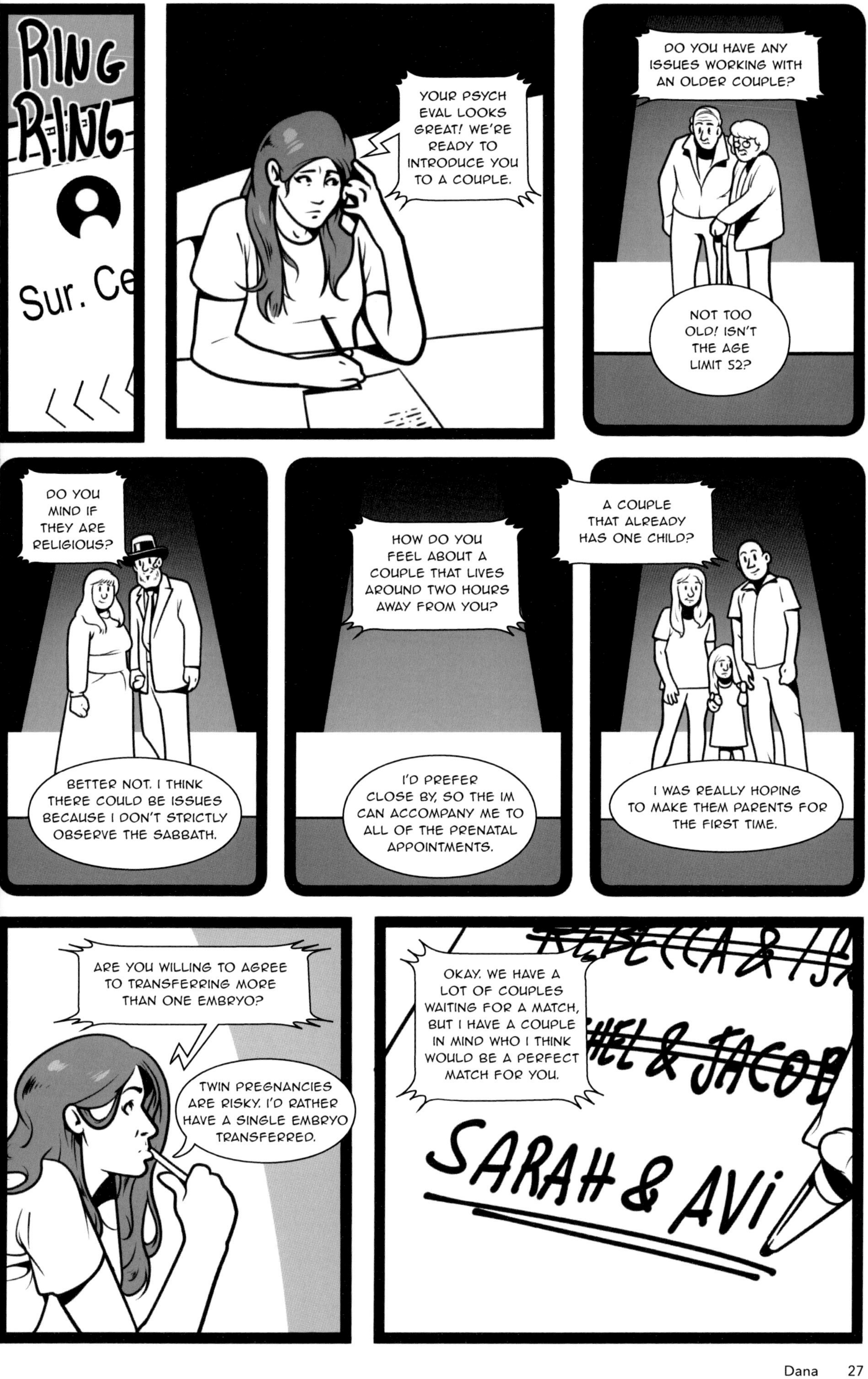
RING RING
Sur. Ce
YOUR PSYCH EVAL LOOKS GREAT! WE'RE READY TO INTRODUCE YOU TO A COUPLE.
DO YOU HAVE ANY ISSUES WORKING WITH AN OLDER COUPLE?
NOT TOO OLD! ISN'T THE AGE LIMIT 52?
DO YOU MIND IF THEY ARE RELIGIOUS?
BETTER NOT. I THINK THERE COULD BE ISSUES BECAUSE I DON'T STRICTLY OBSERVE THE SABBATH.
HOW DO YOU FEEL ABOUT A COUPLE THAT LIVES AROUND TWO HOURS AWAY FROM YOU?
I'D PREFER CLOSE BY, SO THE IM CAN ACCOMPANY ME TO ALL OF THE PRENATAL APPOINTMENTS.
A COUPLE THAT ALREADY HAS ONE CHILD?
I WAS REALLY HOPING TO MAKE THEM PARENTS FOR THE FIRST TIME.
ARE YOU WILLING TO AGREE TO TRANSFERRING MORE THAN ONE EMBRYO?
TWIN PREGNANCIES ARE RISKY. I'D RATHER HAVE A SINGLE EMBRYO TRANSFERRED.
OKAY. WE HAVE A LOT OF COUPLES WAITING FOR A MATCH, BUT I HAVE A COUPLE IN MIND WHO I THINK WOULD BE A PERFECT MATCH FOR YOU.
HEL & JACOB
SARAH & AVI

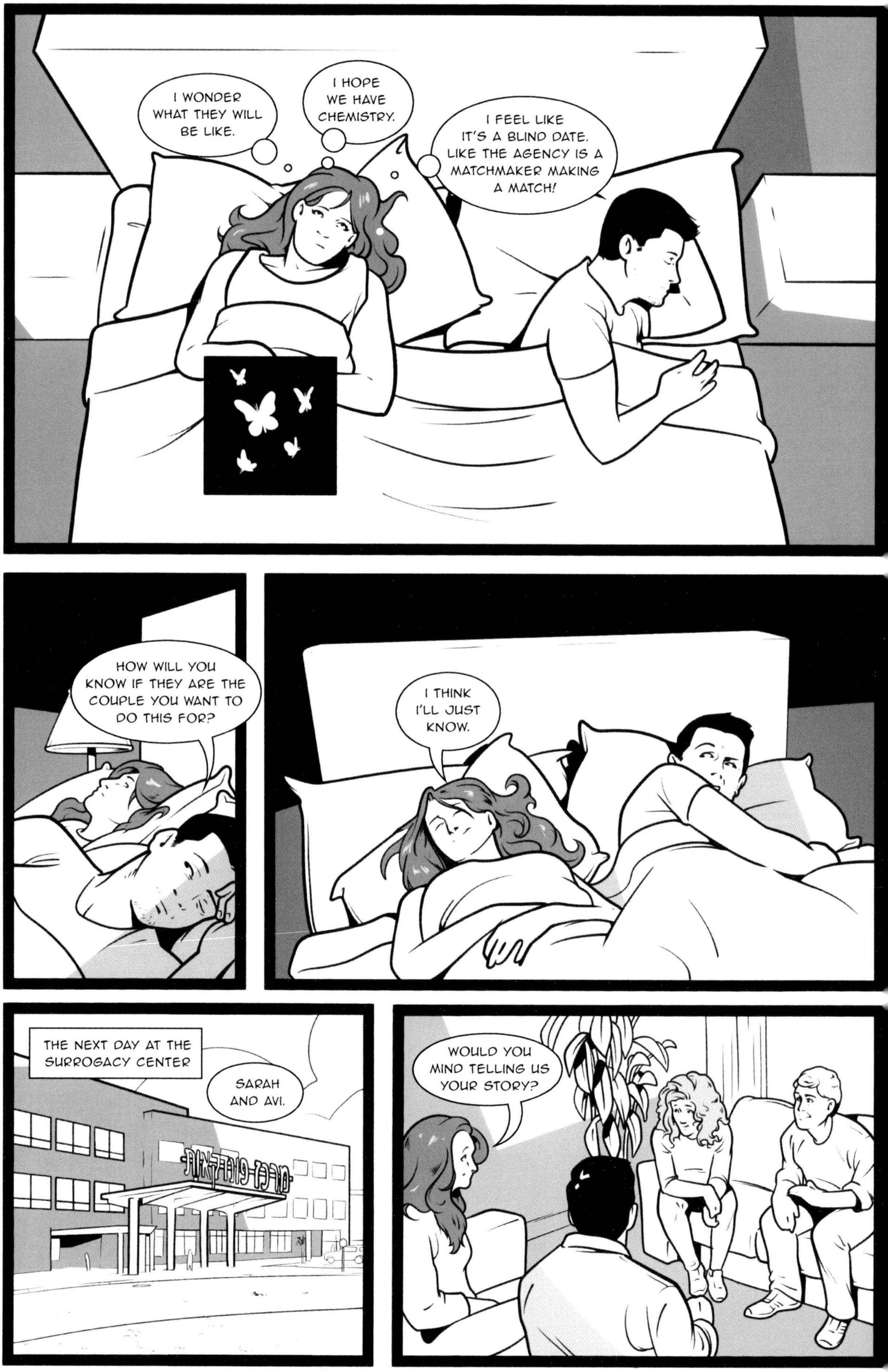
I WONDER WHAT THEY WILL BE LIKE.
I HOPE WE HAVE CHEMISTRY.
I FEEL LIKE IT'S A BLIND DATE. LIKE THE AGENCY IS A MATCHMAKER MAKING A MATCH!
HOW WILL YOU KNOW IF THEY ARE THE COUPLE YOU WANT TO DO THIS FOR?
I THINK I'LL JUST KNOW.
THE NEXT DAY AT THE SURROGACY CENTER
SARAH AND AVI.
WOULD YOU MIND TELLING US YOUR STORY?

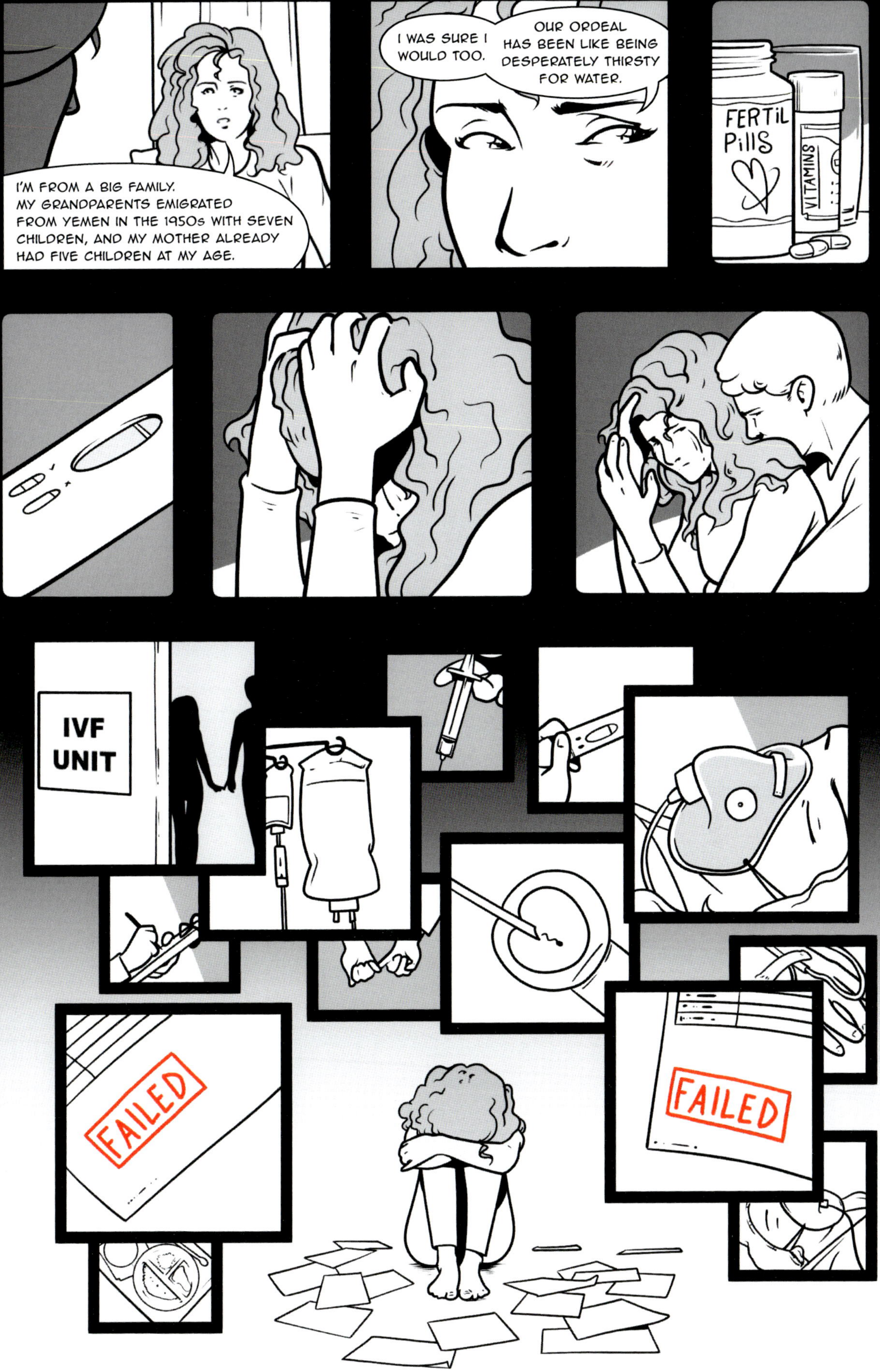
I'M FROM A BIG FAMILY. MY GRANDPARENTS EMIGRATED FROM YEMEN IN THE 1950s WITH SEVEN CHILDREN, AND MY MOTHER ALREADY HAD FIVE CHILDREN AT MY AGE.
I WAS SURE I WOULD TOO.
OUR ORDEAL HAS BEEN LIKE BEING DESPERATELY THIRSTY FOR WATER.
FERTIL PILLS
VITAMINS
IVF UNIT
FAILED
FAILED

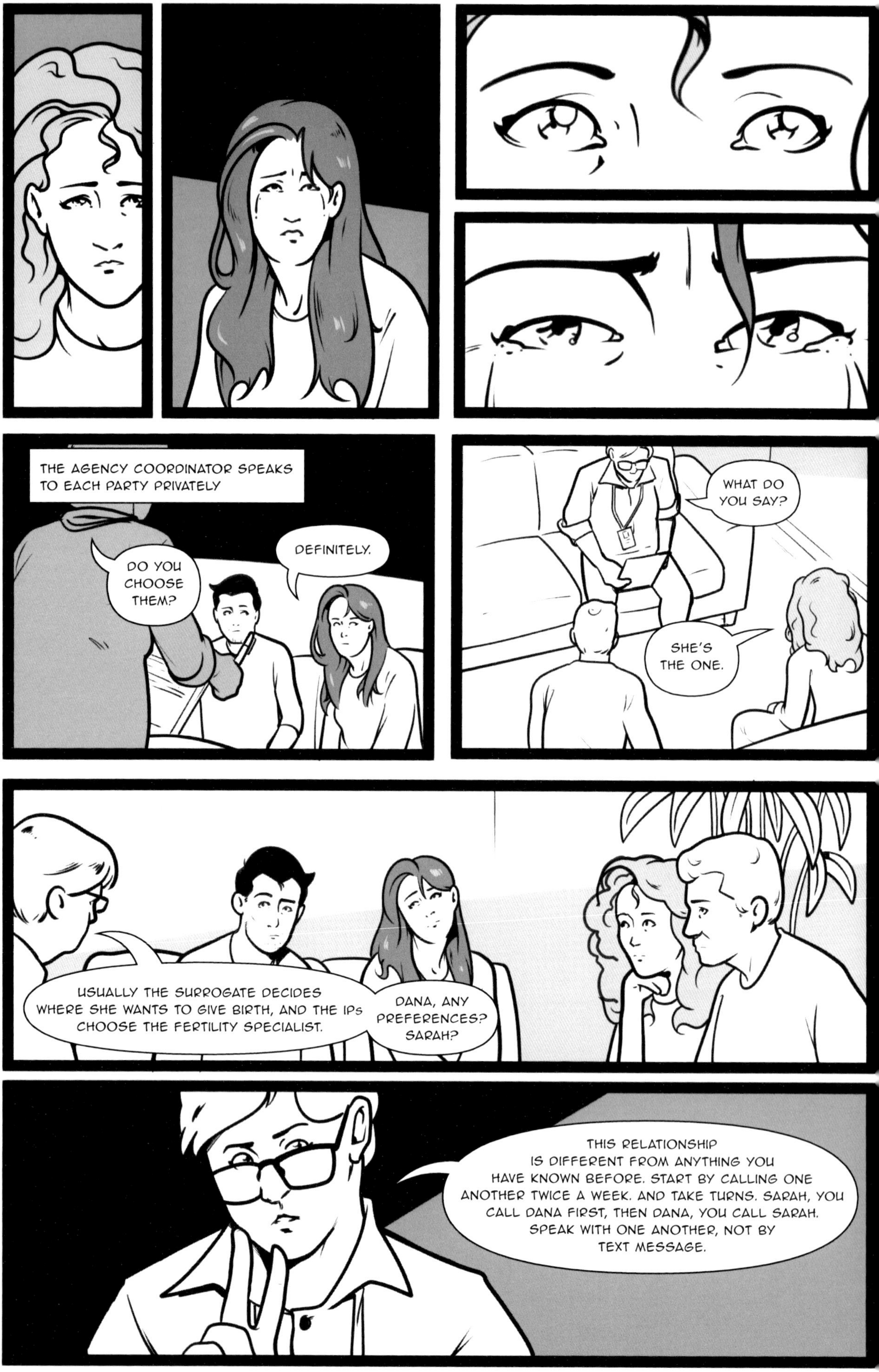
THE AGENCY COORDINATOR SPEAKS TO EACH PARTY PRIVATELY
DO YOU CHOOSE THEM?
DEFINITELY.
WHAT DO YOU SAY?
SHE'S THE ONE.
USUALLY THE SURROGATE DECIDES WHERE SHE WANTS TO GIVE BIRTH, AND THE IPs CHOOSE THE FERTILITY SPECIALIST.
DANA, ANY PREFERENCES? SARAH?
THIS RELATIONSHIP IS DIFFERENT FROM ANYTHING YOU HAVE KNOWN BEFORE. START BY CALLING ONE ANOTHER TWICE A WEEK. AND TAKE TURNS. SARAH, YOU CALL DANA FIRST, THEN DANA, YOU CALL SARAH. SPEAK WITH ONE ANOTHER, NOT BY TEXT MESSAGE.

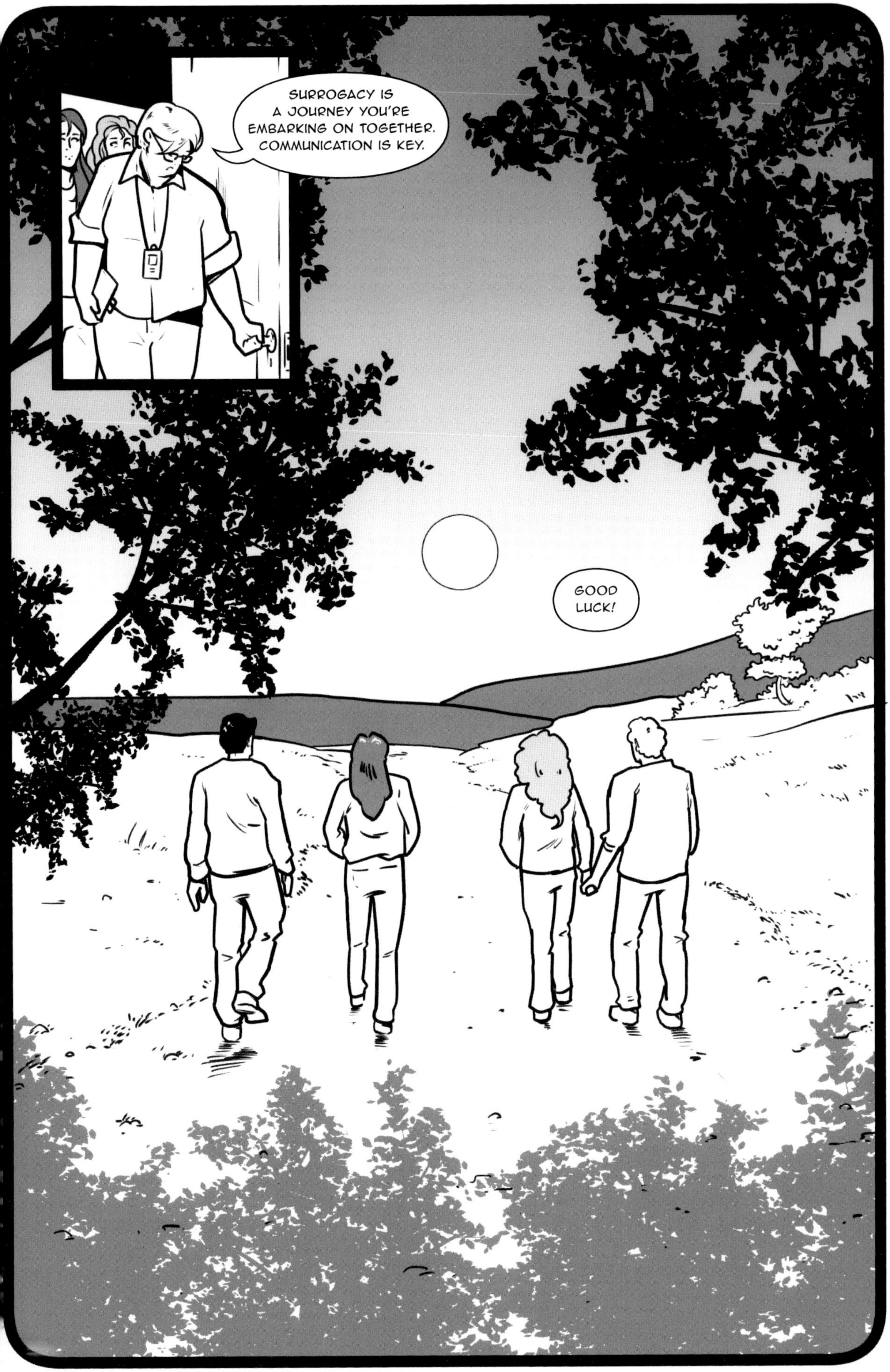
SURROGACY IS A JOURNEY YOU'RE EMBARKING ON TOGETHER. COMMUNICATION IS KEY.
GOOD LUCK!

-CHAPTER 4-
FIRST DATE

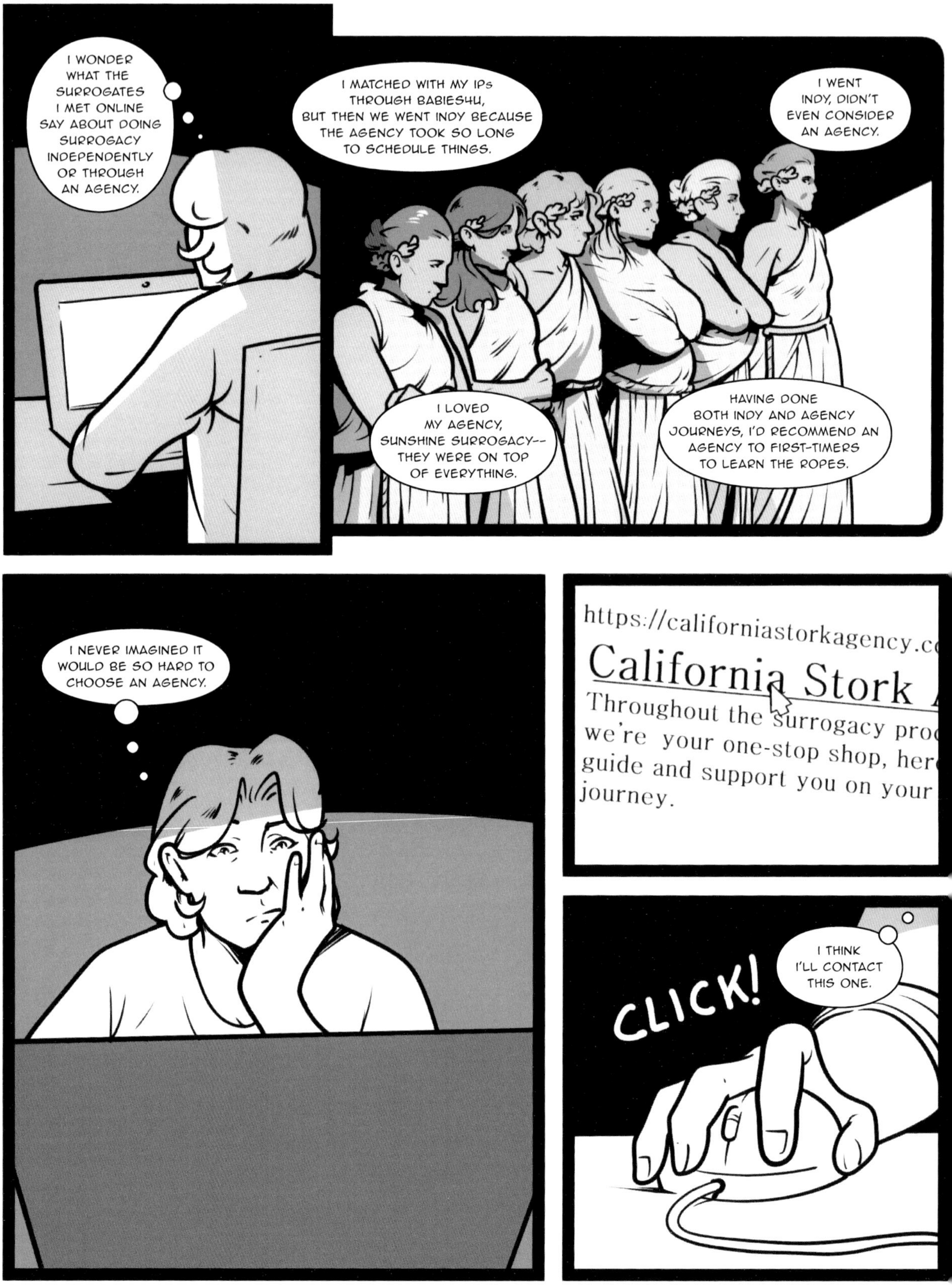

I WONDER WHAT THE SURROGATES I MET ONLINE SAY ABOUT DOING SURROGACY INDEPENDENTLY OR THROUGH AN AGENCY.
I MATCHED WITH MY IPs THROUGH BABIES4U, BUT THEN WE WENT INDY BECAUSE THE AGENCY TOOK SO LONG TO SCHEDULE THINGS.
I WENT INDY, DIDN'T EVEN CONSIDER AN AGENCY.
I LOVED MY AGENCY, SUNSHINE SURROGACY-- THEY WERE ON TOP OF EVERYTHING.
HAVING DONE BOTH INDY AND AGENCY JOURNEYS, I'D RECOMMEND AN AGENCY TO FIRST-TIMERS TO LEARN THE ROPES.
I NEVER IMAGINED IT WOULD BE SO HARD TO CHOOSE AN AGENCY.
https://californiastorkagency.c
California Stork
Throughout the surrogacy pro
we're your one-stop shop, her
guide and support you on your
journey.
CLICK!
I THINK I'LL CONTACT THIS ONE.

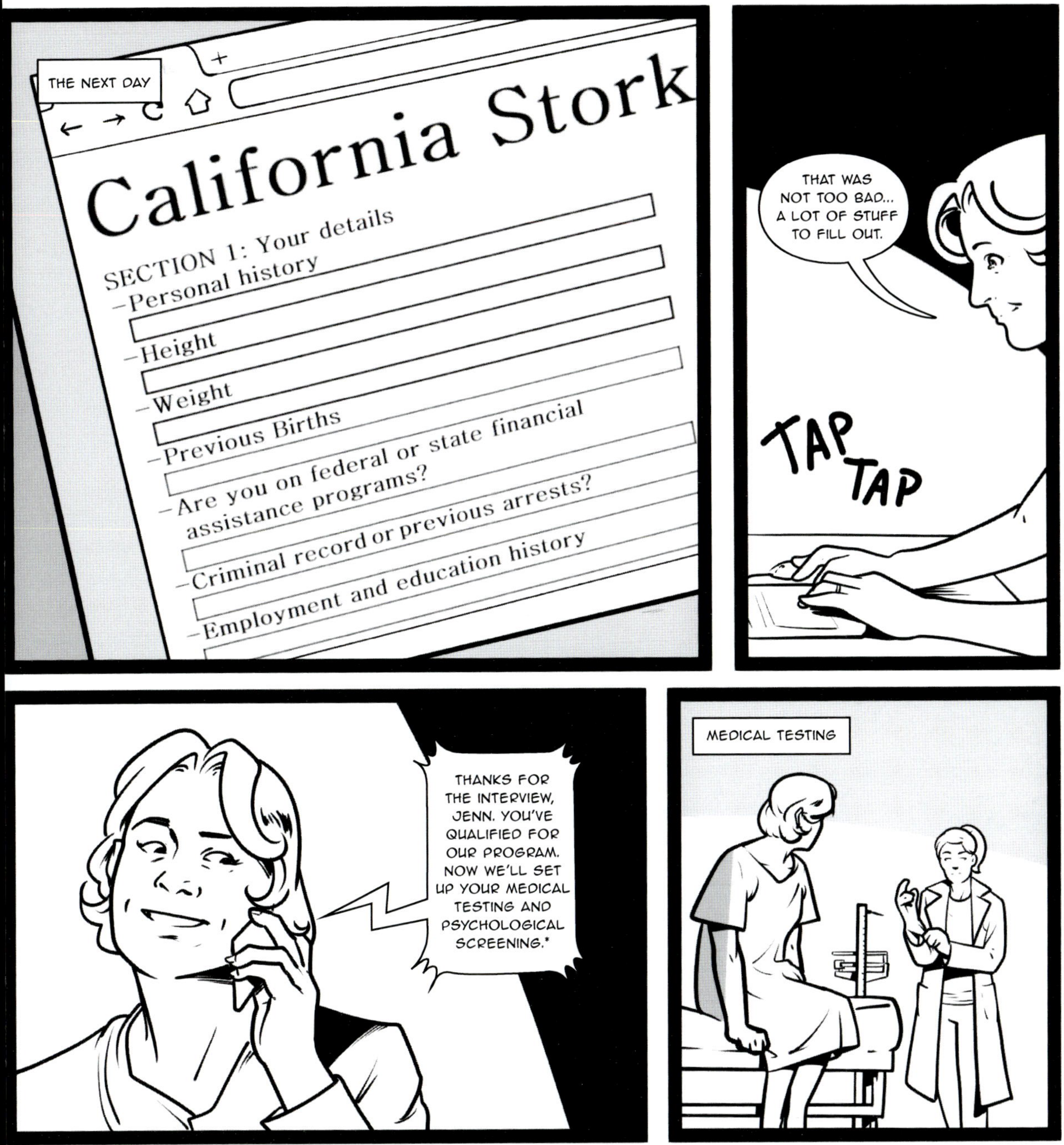
THE NEXT DAY
California Stork
SECTION 1: Your details
–Personal history
–Height
–Weight
–Previous Births
–Are you on federal or state financial assistance programs?
–Criminal record or previous arrests?
–Employment and education history
THAT WAS NOT TOO BAD... A LOT OF STUFF TO FILL OUT.
TAP TAP
THANKS FOR THE INTERVIEW, JENN. YOU'VE QUALIFIED FOR OUR PROGRAM. NOW WE'LL SET UP YOUR MEDICAL TESTING AND PSYCHOLOGICAL SCREENING.*
MEDICAL TESTING

*LEVELS OF SCREENING VARY AMONG US AGENCIES. SOME AGENCIES ONLY SCREEN AFTER A MATCH.

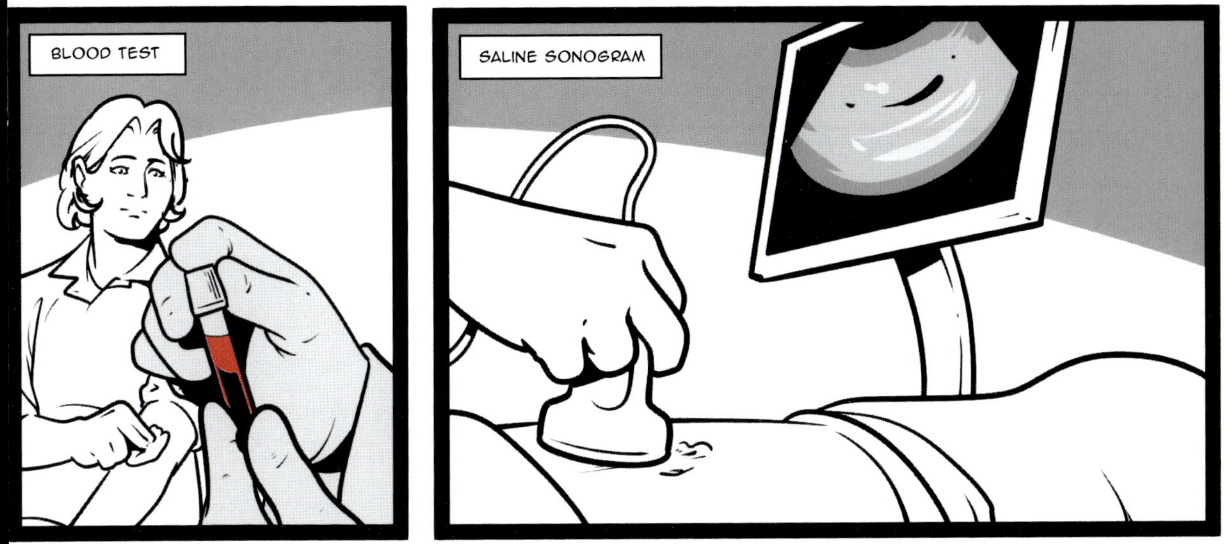
BLOOD TEST
SALINE SONOGRAM

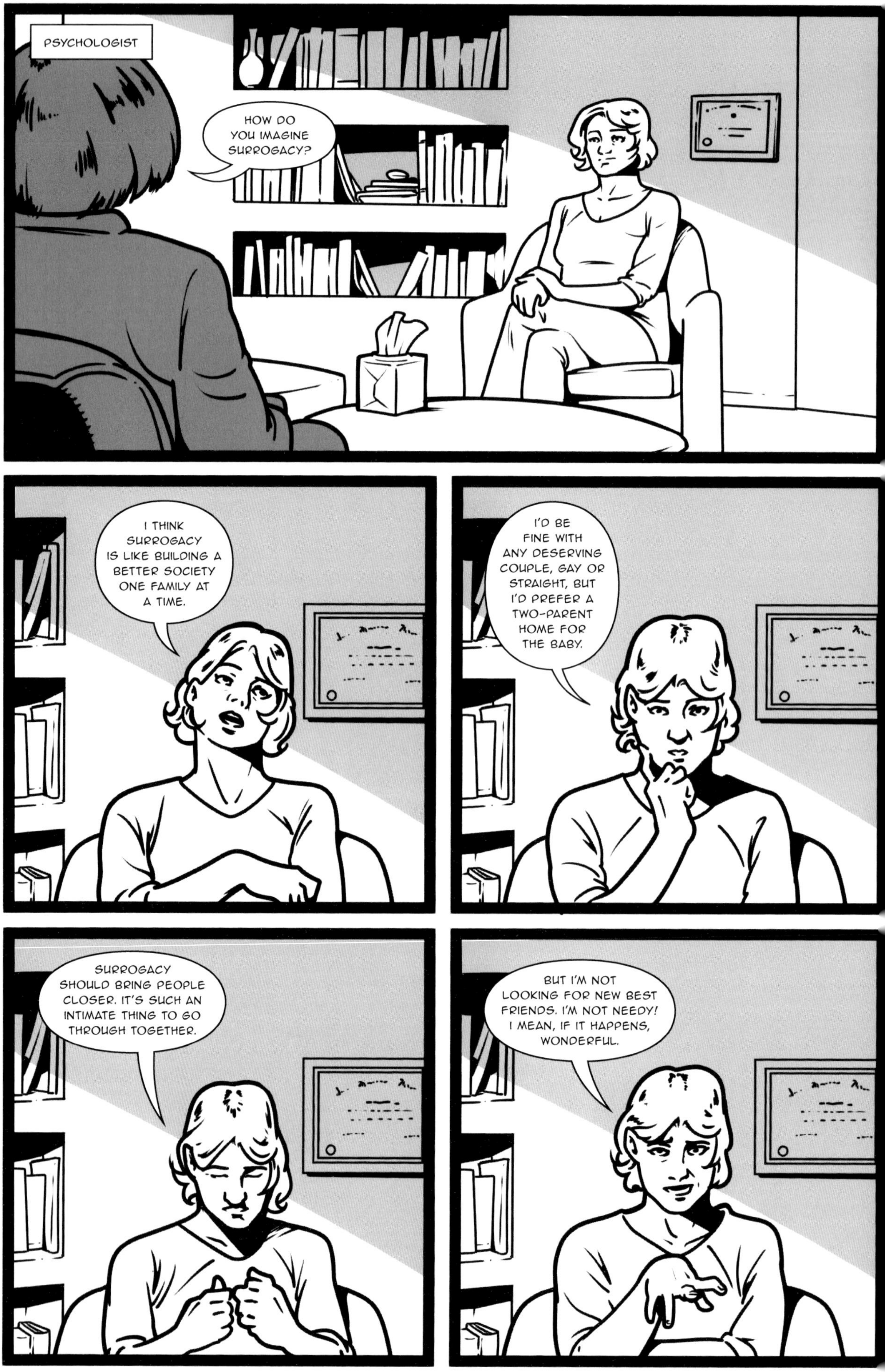
PSYCHOLOGIST
HOW DO YOU IMAGINE SURROGACY?
I THINK SURROGACY IS LIKE BUILDING A BETTER SOCIETY ONE FAMILY AT A TIME.
I'D BE FINE WITH ANY DESERVING COUPLE, GAY OR STRAIGHT, BUT I'D PREFER A TWO-PARENT HOME FOR THE BABY.
SURROGACY SHOULD BRING PEOPLE CLOSER. IT'S SUCH AN INTIMATE THING TO GO THROUGH TOGETHER.
BUT I'M NOT LOOKING FOR NEW BEST FRIENDS. I'M NOT NEEDY! I MEAN, IF IT HAPPENS, WONDERFUL.

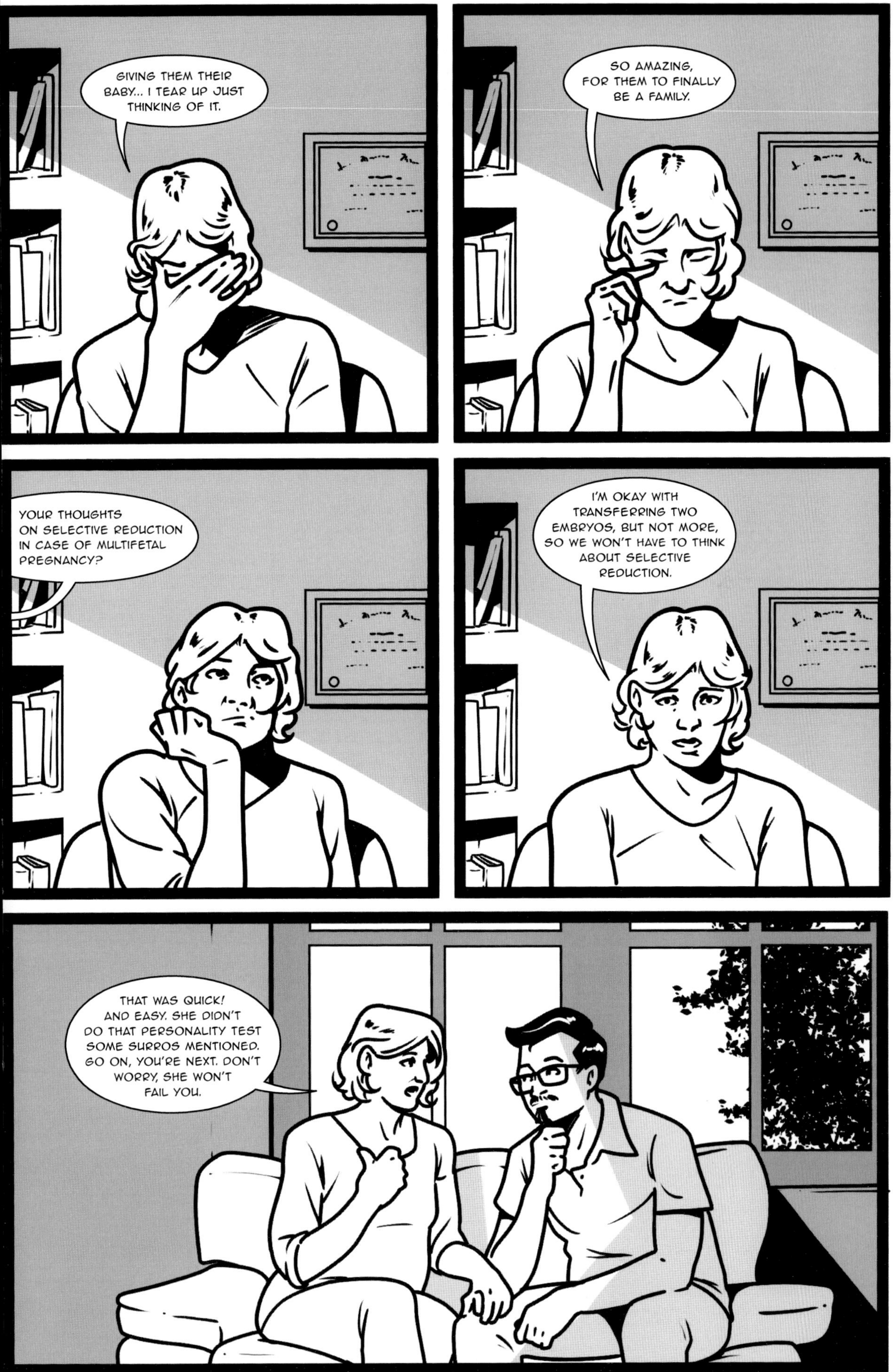
GIVING THEM THEIR BABY... I TEAR UP JUST THINKING OF IT.
SO AMAZING, FOR THEM TO FINALLY BE A FAMILY.
YOUR THOUGHTS ON SELECTIVE REDUCTION IN CASE OF MULTIFETAL PREGNANCY?
I'M OKAY WITH TRANSFERRING TWO EMBRYOS, BUT NOT MORE, SO WE WON'T HAVE TO THINK ABOUT SELECTIVE REDUCTION.
THAT WAS QUICK! AND EASY. SHE DIDN'T DO THAT PERSONALITY TEST SOME SURROS MENTIONED. GO ON, YOU'RE NEXT. DON'T WORRY, SHE WON'T FAIL YOU.

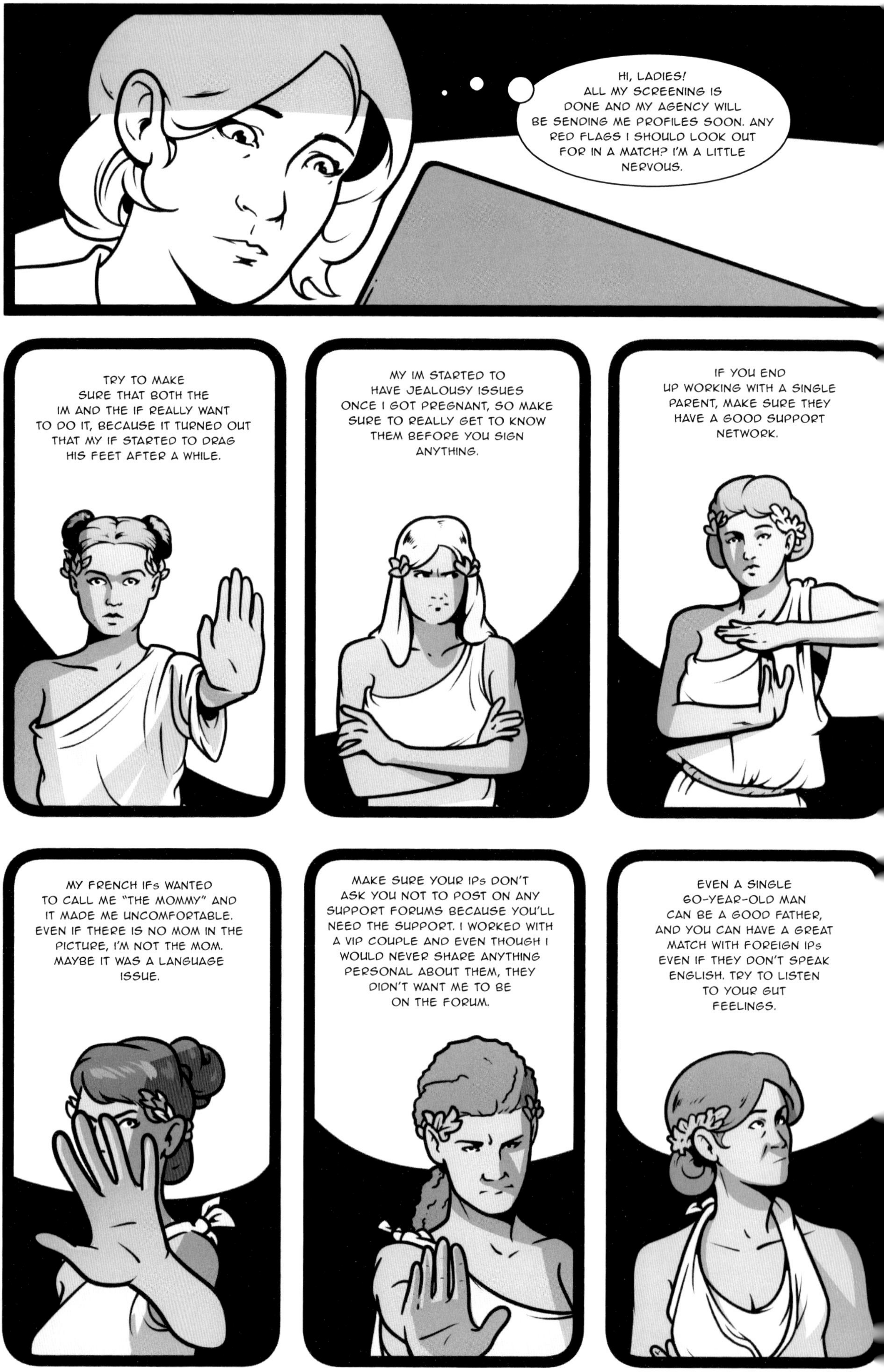
HI, LADIES! ALL MY SCREENING IS DONE AND MY AGENCY WILL BE SENDING ME PROFILES SOON. ANY RED FLAGS I SHOULD LOOK OUT FOR IN A MATCH? I'M A LITTLE NERVOUS.
TRY TO MAKE SURE THAT BOTH THE IM AND THE IF REALLY WANT TO DO IT, BECAUSE IT TURNED OUT THAT MY IF STARTED TO DRAG HIS FEET AFTER A WHILE.
MY IM STARTED TO HAVE JEALOUSY ISSUES ONCE I GOT PREGNANT, SO MAKE SURE TO REALLY GET TO KNOW THEM BEFORE YOU SIGN ANYTHING.
IF YOU END UP WORKING WITH A SINGLE PARENT, MAKE SURE THEY HAVE A GOOD SUPPORT NETWORK.
MY FRENCH IFs WANTED TO CALL ME "THE MOMMY" AND IT MADE ME UNCOMFORTABLE. EVEN IF THERE IS NO MOM IN THE PICTURE, I'M NOT THE MOM. MAYBE IT WAS A LANGUAGE ISSUE.
MAKE SURE YOUR IPs DON'T ASK YOU NOT TO POST ON ANY SUPPORT FORUMS BECAUSE YOU'LL NEED THE SUPPORT. I WORKED WITH A VIP COUPLE AND EVEN THOUGH I WOULD NEVER SHARE ANYTHING PERSONAL ABOUT THEM, THEY DIDN'T WANT ME TO BE ON THE FORUM.
EVEN A SINGLE 60-YEAR-OLD MAN CAN BE A GOOD FATHER, AND YOU CAN HAVE A GREAT MATCH WITH FOREIGN IPs EVEN IF THEY DON'T SPEAK ENGLISH. TRY TO LISTEN TO YOUR GUT FEELINGS.

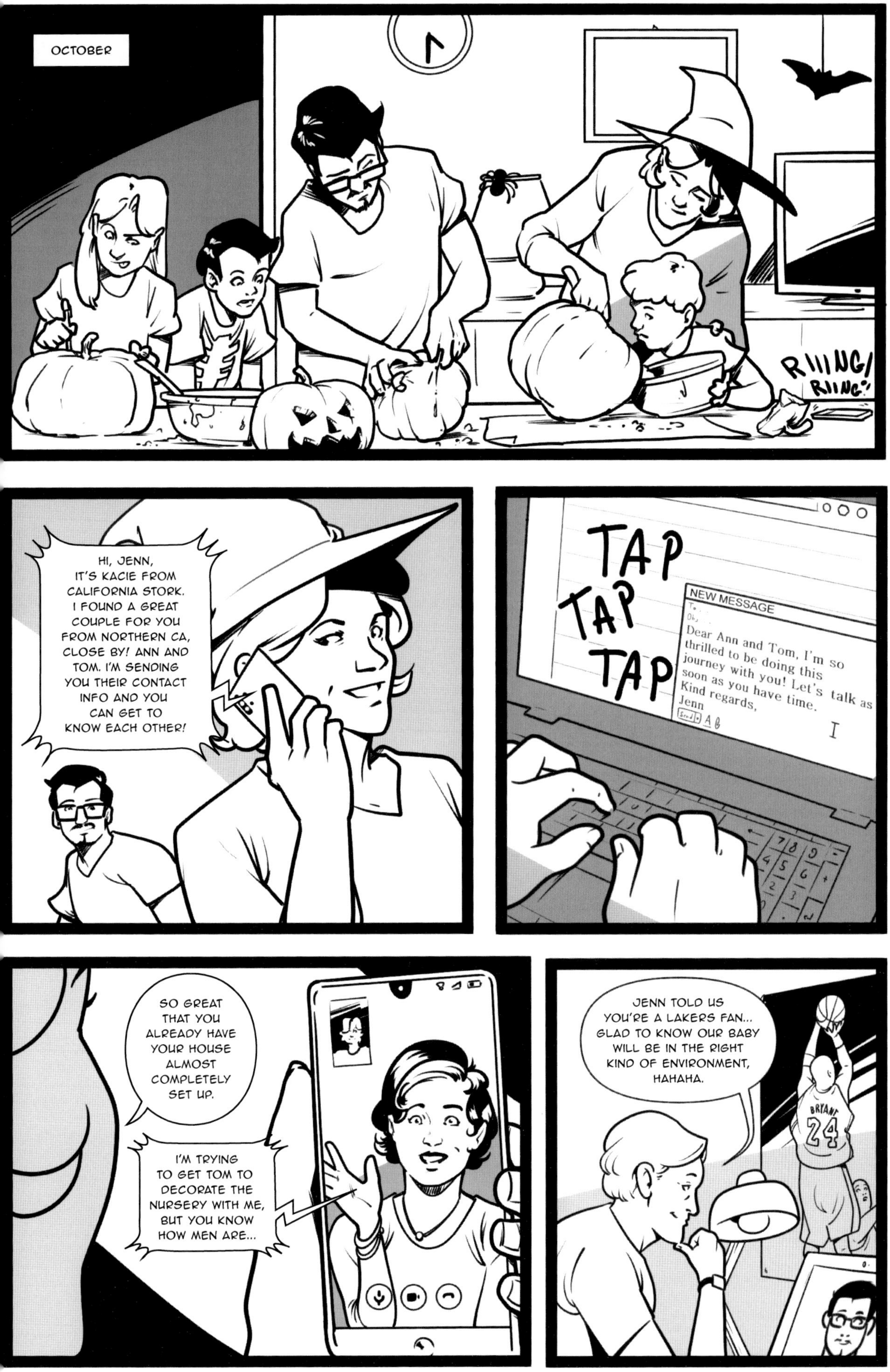
OCTOBER
RIIING! RING!
HI, JENN, IT'S KACIE FROM CALIFORNIA STORK. I FOUND A GREAT COUPLE FOR YOU FROM NORTHERN CA, CLOSE BY! ANN AND TOM. I'M SENDING YOU THEIR CONTACT INFO AND YOU CAN GET TO KNOW EACH OTHER!
TAP TAP TAP
NEW MESSAGE
Dear Ann and Tom, I'm so thrilled to be doing this journey with you! Let's talk as soon as you have time. Kind regards, Jenn
SO GREAT THAT YOU ALREADY HAVE YOUR HOUSE ALMOST COMPLETELY SET UP.
I'M TRYING TO GET TOM TO DECORATE THE NURSERY WITH ME, BUT YOU KNOW HOW MEN ARE...
JENN TOLD US YOU'RE A LAKERS FAN... GLAD TO KNOW OUR BABY WILL BE IN THE RIGHT KIND OF ENVIRONMENT, HAHAHA.
BRYANT 24

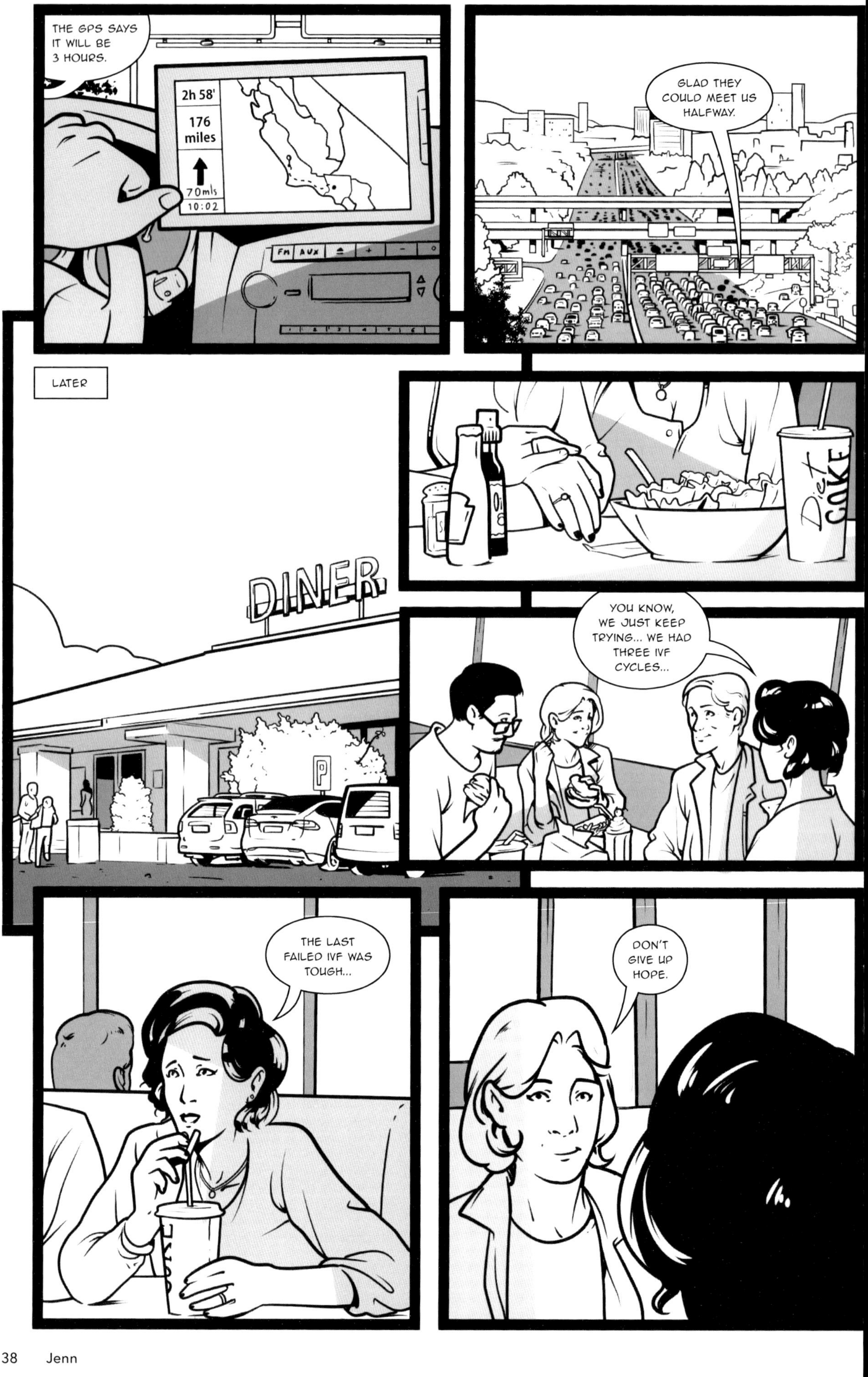
THE GPS SAYS IT WILL BE 3 HOURS.
2h 58'
176 miles
70mls
10:02
FM
AUX
GLAD THEY COULD MEET US HALFWAY.
LATER
DINER
P
Diet COKE
YOU KNOW, WE JUST KEEP TRYING... WE HAD THREE IVF CYCLES...
THE LAST FAILED IVF WAS TOUGH...
DON'T GIVE UP HOPE.

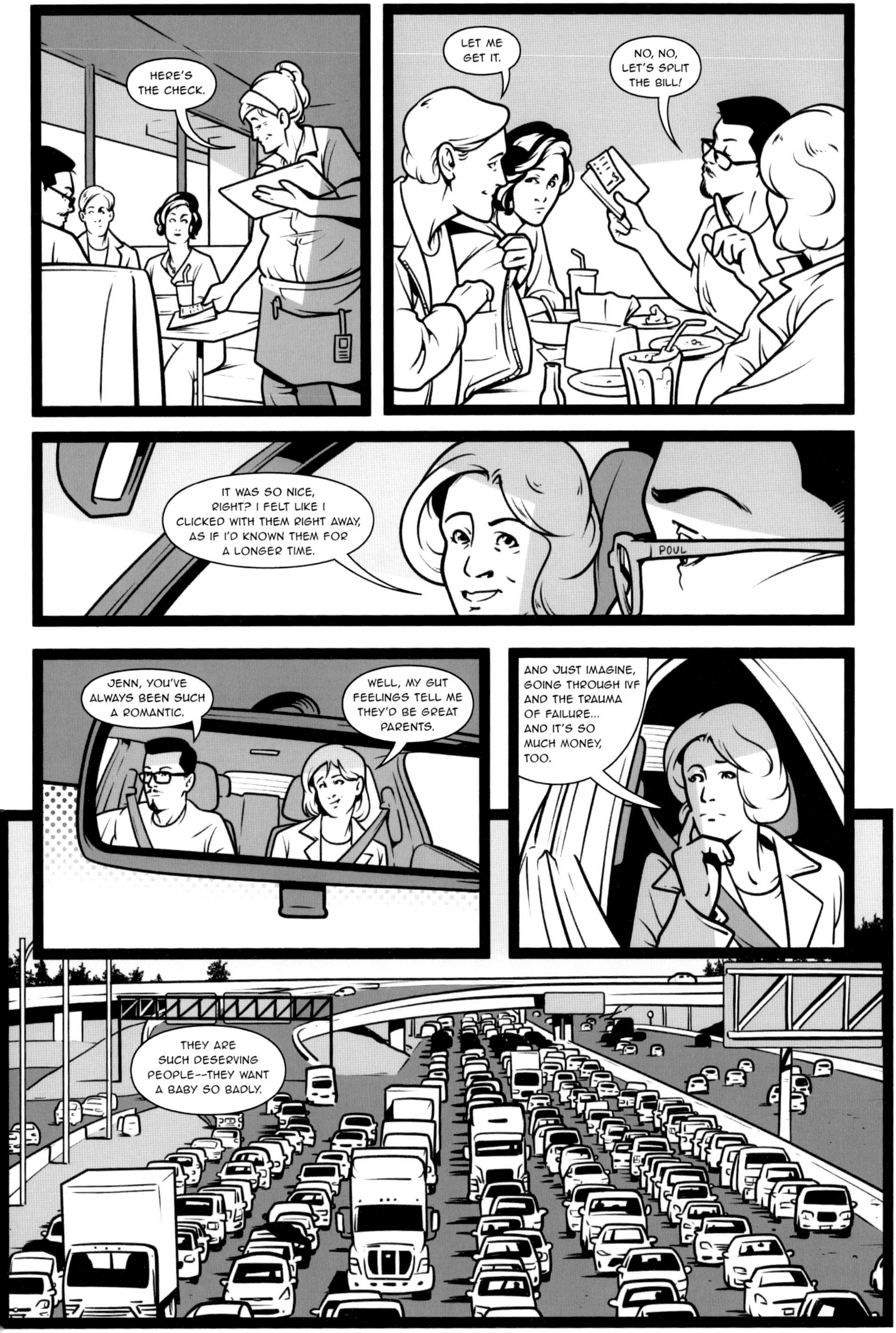
HERE'S THE CHECK.
LET ME GET IT.
NO, NO, LET'S SPLIT THE BILL!
IT WAS SO NICE, RIGHT? I FELT LIKE I CLICKED WITH THEM RIGHT AWAY, AS IF I'D KNOWN THEM FOR A LONGER TIME.
POUL
JENN, YOU'VE ALWAYS BEEN SUCH A ROMANTIC.
WELL, MY GUT FEELINGS TELL ME THEY'D BE GREAT PARENTS.
AND JUST IMAGINE, GOING THROUGH IVF AND THE TRAUMA OF FAILURE... AND IT'S SO MUCH MONEY, TOO.
THEY ARE SUCH DESERVING PEOPLE--THEY WANT A BABY SO BADLY.

INTERLUDE: HENA, SURROGATE IN MUMBAI, INDIA

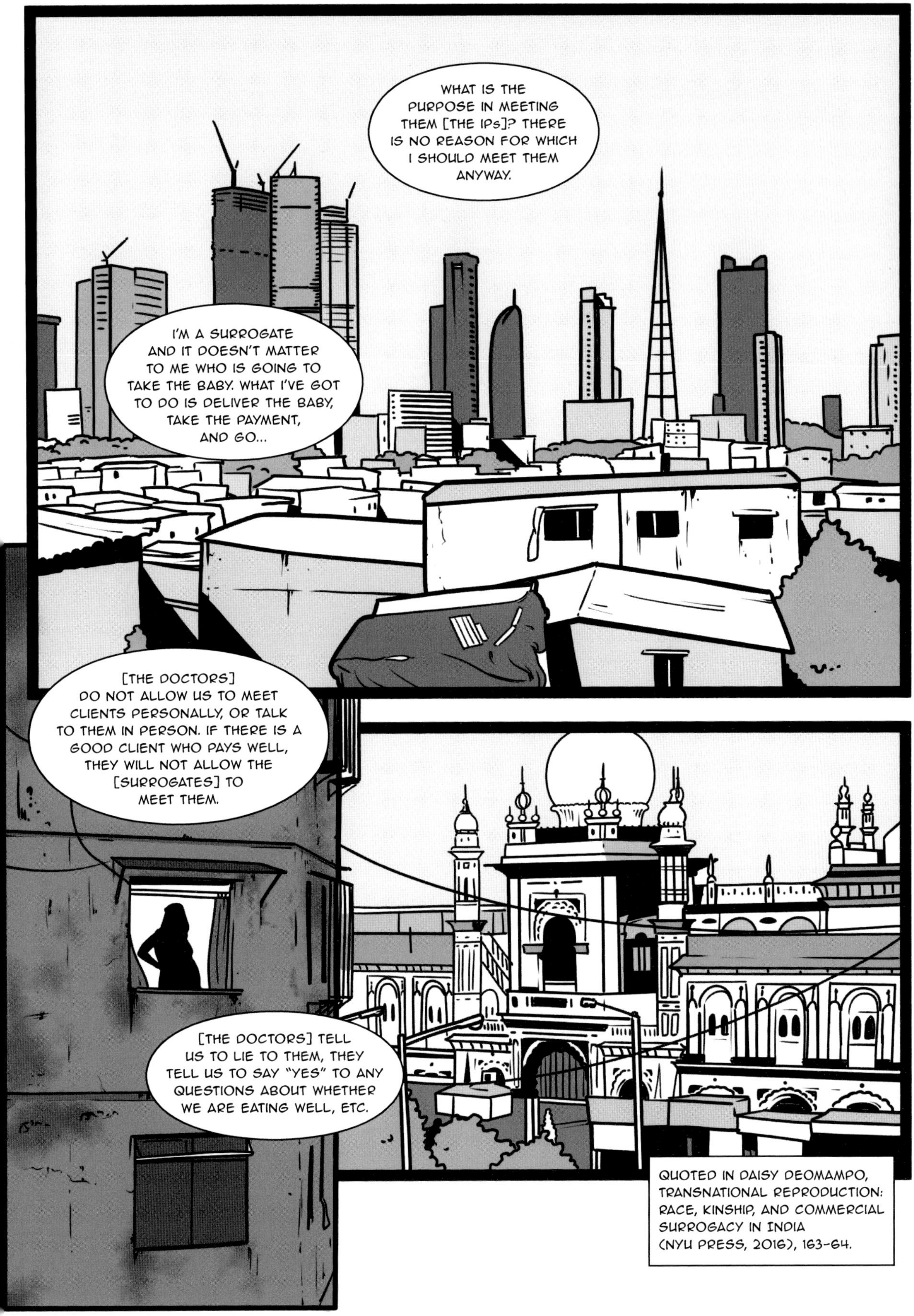
WHAT IS THE PURPOSE IN MEETING THEM [THE IPs]? THERE IS NO REASON FOR WHICH I SHOULD MEET THEM ANYWAY.
I'M A SURROGATE AND IT DOESN'T MATTER TO ME WHO IS GOING TO TAKE THE BABY. WHAT I'VE GOT TO DO IS DELIVER THE BABY, TAKE THE PAYMENT, AND GO...
[THE DOCTORS] DO NOT ALLOW US TO MEET CLIENTS PERSONALLY, OR TALK TO THEM IN PERSON. IF THERE IS A GOOD CLIENT WHO PAYS WELL, THEY WILL NOT ALLOW THE [SURROGATES] TO MEET THEM.
[THE DOCTORS] TELL US TO LIE TO THEM, THEY TELL US TO SAY "YES" TO ANY QUESTIONS ABOUT WHETHER WE ARE EATING WELL, ETC.
QUOTED IN DAISY DEOMAMPO, TRANSNATIONAL REPRODUCTION: RACE, KINSHIP, AND COMMERCIAL SURROGACY IN INDIA (NYU PRESS, 2016), 163–64.

-CHAPTER 5-
WEIGHING THE RISKS

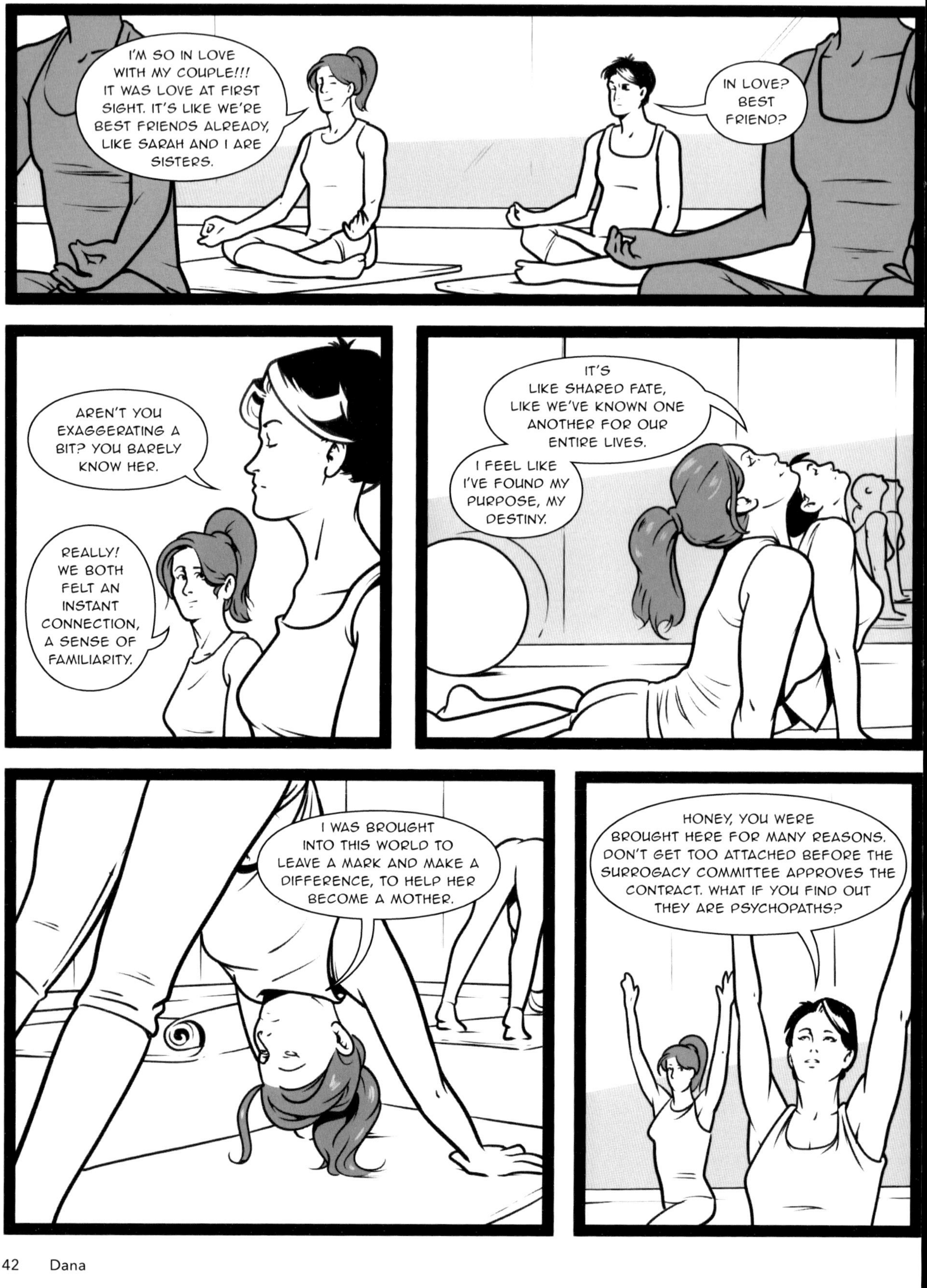
I'M SO IN LOVE WITH MY COUPLE!!! IT WAS LOVE AT FIRST SIGHT. IT'S LIKE WE'RE BEST FRIENDS ALREADY, LIKE SARAH AND I ARE SISTERS.
IN LOVE? BEST FRIEND?
AREN'T YOU EXAGGERATING A BIT? YOU BARELY KNOW HER.
REALLY! WE BOTH FELT AN INSTANT CONNECTION, A SENSE OF FAMILIARITY.
IT'S LIKE SHARED FATE, LIKE WE'VE KNOWN ONE ANOTHER FOR OUR ENTIRE LIVES.
I FEEL LIKE I'VE FOUND MY PURPOSE, MY DESTINY.
I WAS BROUGHT INTO THIS WORLD TO LEAVE A MARK AND MAKE A DIFFERENCE, TO HELP HER BECOME A MOTHER.
HONEY, YOU WERE BROUGHT HERE FOR MANY REASONS. DON'T GET TOO ATTACHED BEFORE THE SURROGACY COMMITTEE APPROVES THE CONTRACT. WHAT IF YOU FIND OUT THEY ARE PSYCHOPATHS?

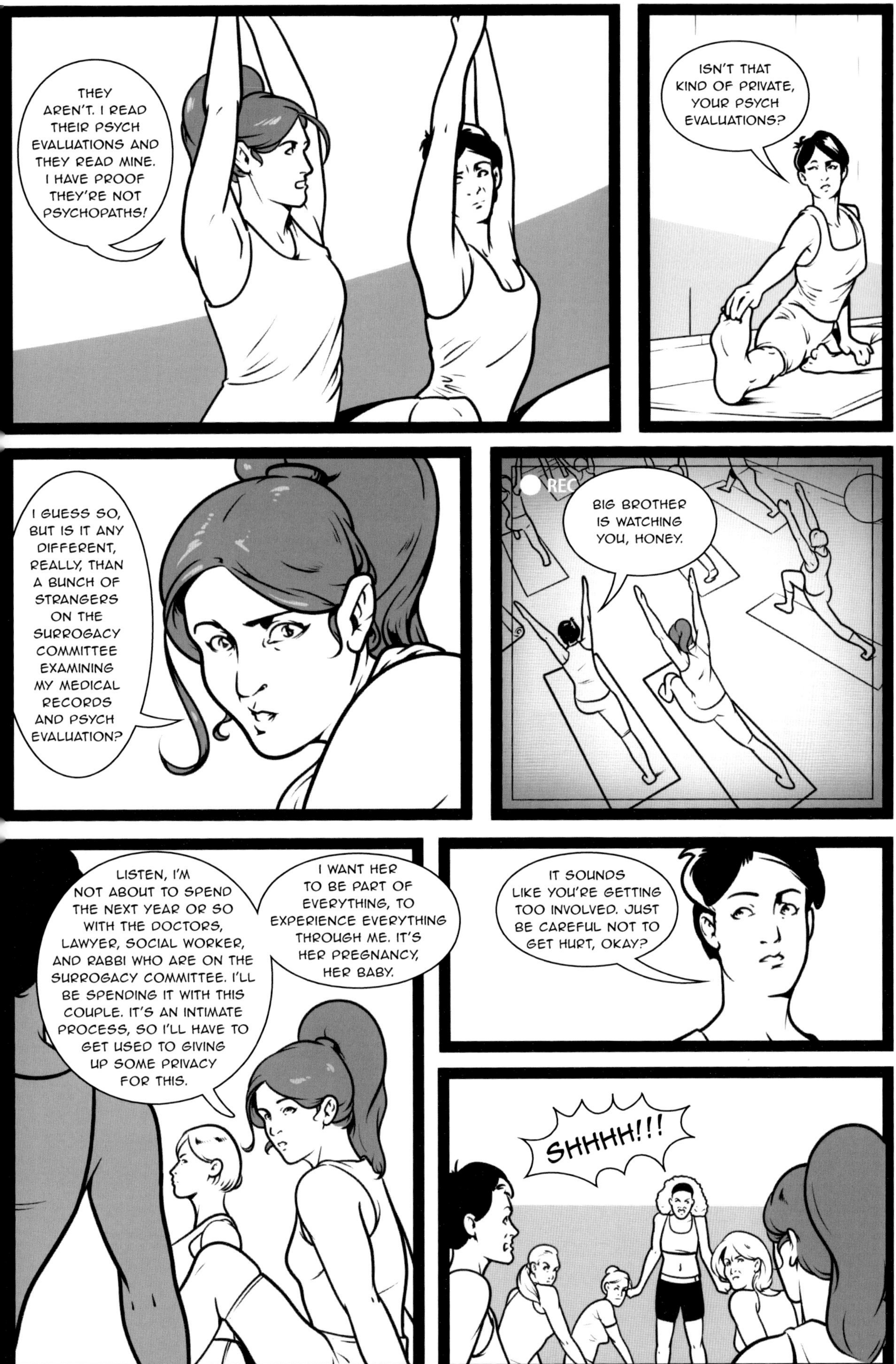
THEY AREN'T. I READ THEIR PSYCH EVALUATIONS AND THEY READ MINE. I HAVE PROOF THEY'RE NOT PSYCHOPATHS!
ISN'T THAT KIND OF PRIVATE, YOUR PSYCH EVALUATIONS?
I GUESS SO, BUT IS IT ANY DIFFERENT, REALLY, THAN A BUNCH OF STRANGERS ON THE SURROGACY COMMITTEE EXAMINING MY MEDICAL RECORDS AND PSYCH EVALUATION?
REC
BIG BROTHER IS WATCHING YOU, HONEY.
LISTEN, I'M NOT ABOUT TO SPEND THE NEXT YEAR OR SO WITH THE DOCTORS, LAWYER, SOCIAL WORKER, AND RABBI WHO ARE ON THE SURROGACY COMMITTEE. I'LL BE SPENDING IT WITH THIS COUPLE. IT'S AN INTIMATE PROCESS, SO I'LL HAVE TO GET USED TO GIVING UP SOME PRIVACY FOR THIS.
I WANT HER TO BE PART OF EVERYTHING, TO EXPERIENCE EVERYTHING THROUGH ME. IT'S HER PREGNANCY, HER BABY.
IT SOUNDS LIKE YOU'RE GETTING TOO INVOLVED. JUST BE CAREFUL NOT TO GET HURT, OKAY?
SHHHH!!!

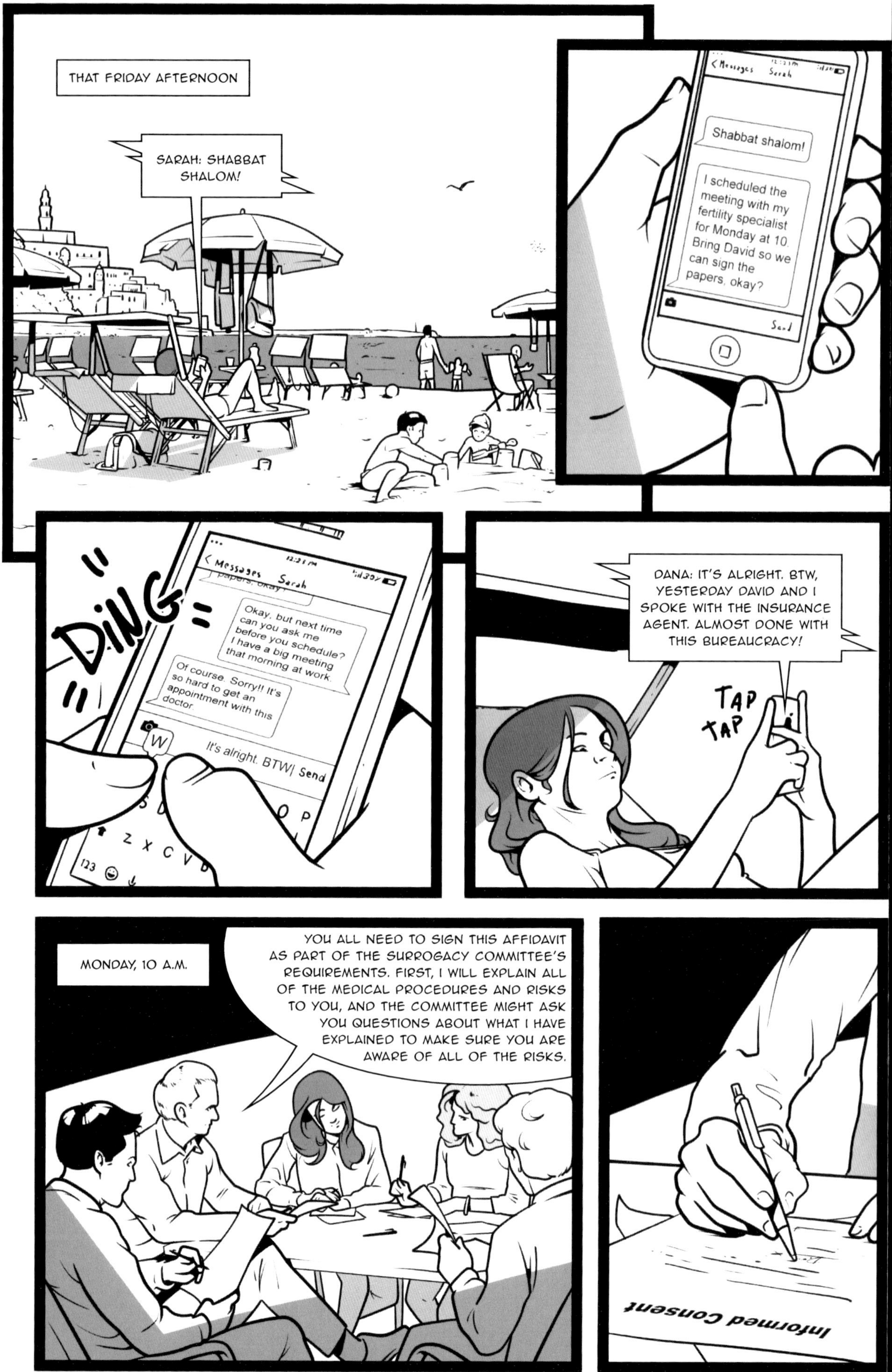
THAT FRIDAY AFTERNOON
SARAH: SHABBAT SHALOM!
Shabbat shalom!
I scheduled the meeting with my fertility specialist for Monday at 10. Bring David so we can sign the papers, okay?
DING
Okay, but next time can you ask me before you schedule? I have a big meeting that morning at work.
Of course. Sorry!! It's so hard to get an appointment with this doctor.
It's alright. BTW| Send
DANA: IT'S ALRIGHT. BTW, YESTERDAY DAVID AND I SPOKE WITH THE INSURANCE AGENT. ALMOST DONE WITH THIS BUREAUCRACY!
TAP TAP
MONDAY, 10 A.M.
YOU ALL NEED TO SIGN THIS AFFIDAVIT AS PART OF THE SURROGACY COMMITTEE'S REQUIREMENTS. FIRST, I WILL EXPLAIN ALL OF THE MEDICAL PROCEDURES AND RISKS TO YOU, AND THE COMMITTEE MIGHT ASK YOU QUESTIONS ABOUT WHAT I HAVE EXPLAINED TO MAKE SURE YOU ARE AWARE OF ALL OF THE RISKS.
Informed Consent

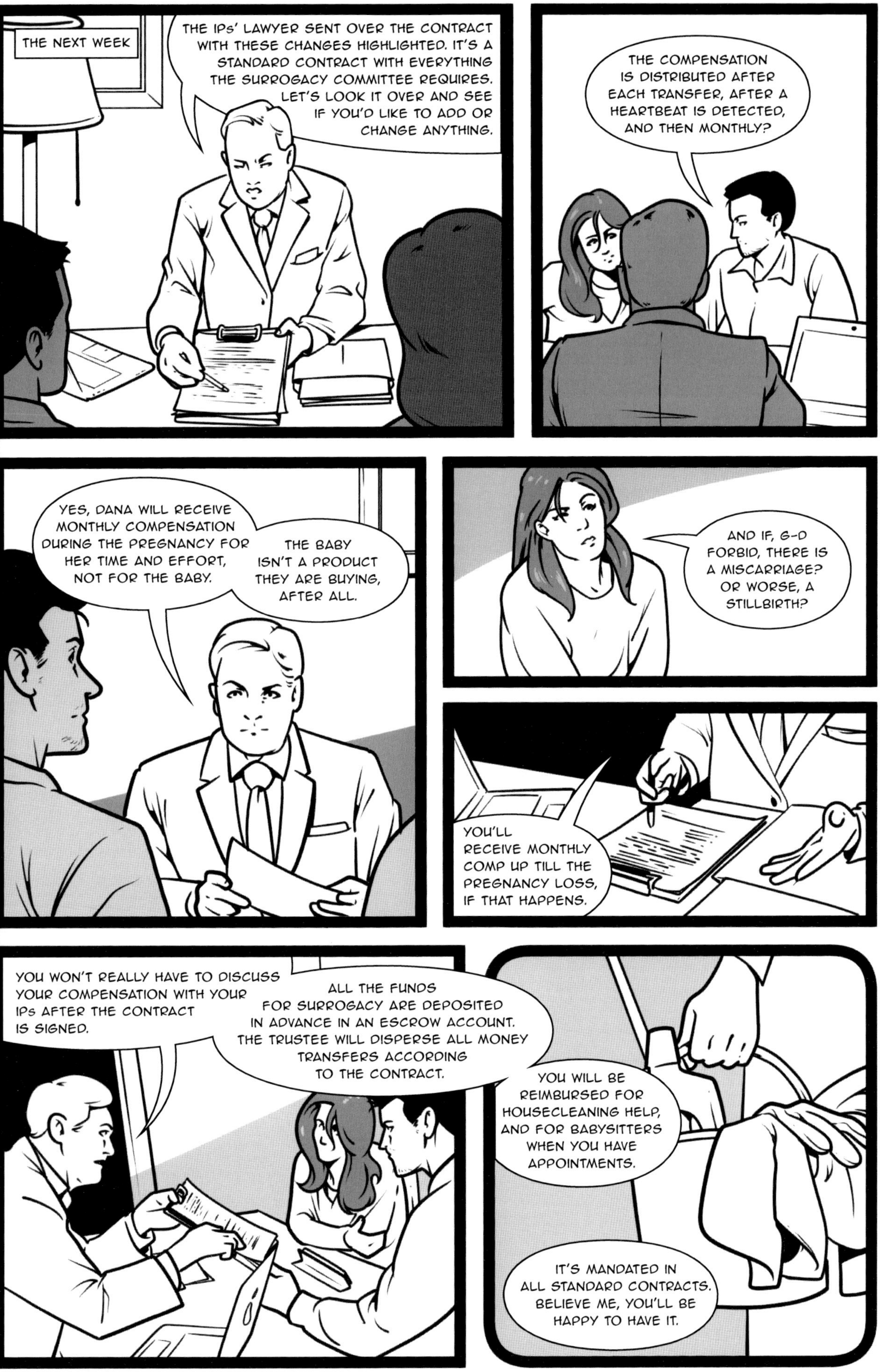
THE NEXT WEEK
THE IPs' LAWYER SENT OVER THE CONTRACT WITH THESE CHANGES HIGHLIGHTED. IT'S A STANDARD CONTRACT WITH EVERYTHING THE SURROGACY COMMITTEE REQUIRES. LET'S LOOK IT OVER AND SEE IF YOU'D LIKE TO ADD OR CHANGE ANYTHING.
THE COMPENSATION IS DISTRIBUTED AFTER EACH TRANSFER, AFTER A HEARTBEAT IS DETECTED, AND THEN MONTHLY?
YES, DANA WILL RECEIVE MONTHLY COMPENSATION DURING THE PREGNANCY FOR HER TIME AND EFFORT, NOT FOR THE BABY.
THE BABY ISN'T A PRODUCT THEY ARE BUYING, AFTER ALL.
AND IF, G-D FORBID, THERE IS A MISCARRIAGE? OR WORSE, A STILLBIRTH?
YOU'LL RECEIVE MONTHLY COMP UP TILL THE PREGNANCY LOSS, IF THAT HAPPENS.
YOU WON'T REALLY HAVE TO DISCUSS YOUR COMPENSATION WITH YOUR IPs AFTER THE CONTRACT IS SIGNED.
ALL THE FUNDS FOR SURROGACY ARE DEPOSITED IN ADVANCE IN AN ESCROW ACCOUNT. THE TRUSTEE WILL DISPERSE ALL MONEY TRANSFERS ACCORDING TO THE CONTRACT.
YOU WILL BE REIMBURSED FOR HOUSECLEANING HELP, AND FOR BABYSITTERS WHEN YOU HAVE APPOINTMENTS.
IT'S MANDATED IN ALL STANDARD CONTRACTS. BELIEVE ME, YOU'LL BE HAPPY TO HAVE IT.

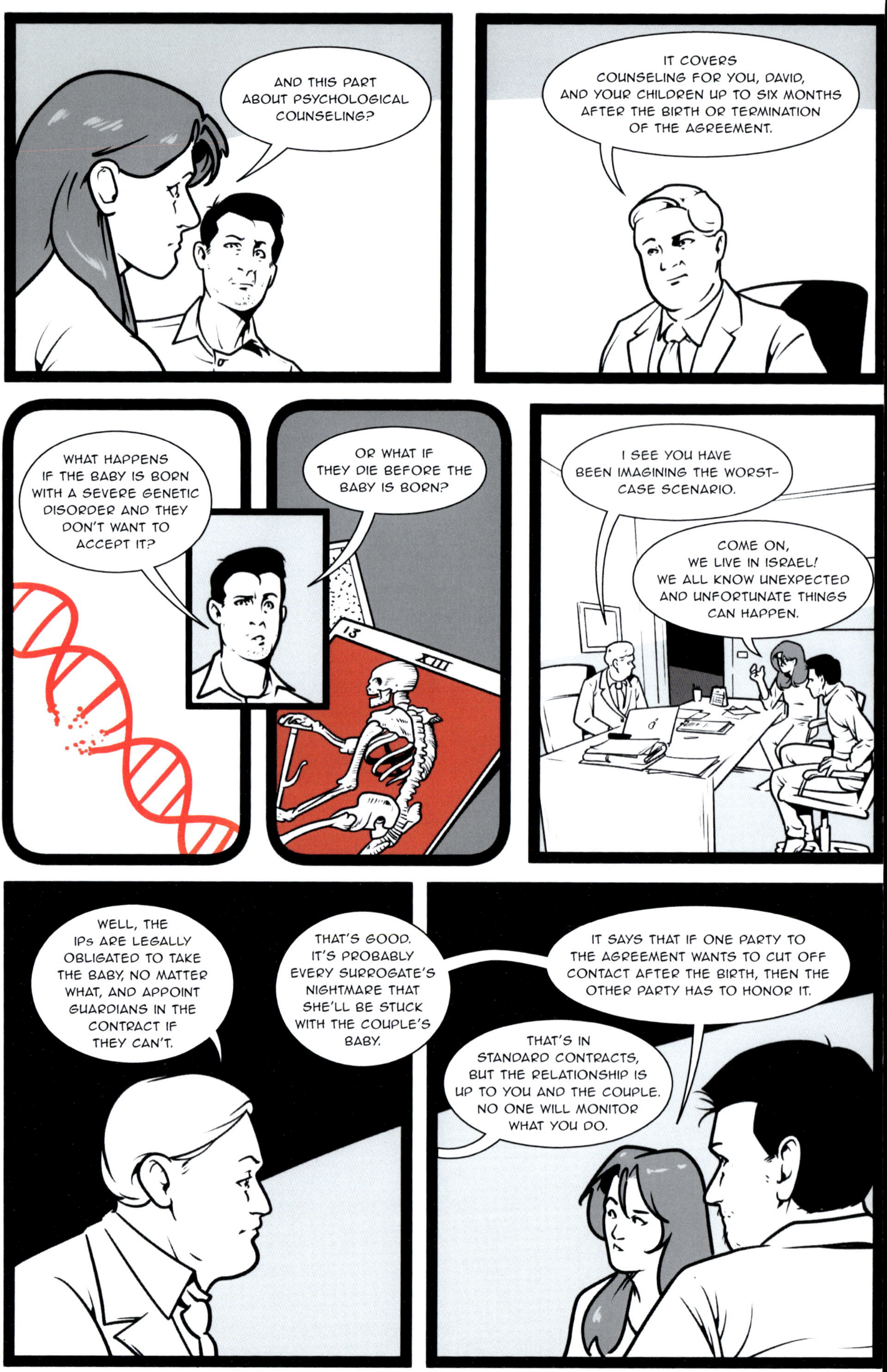
AND THIS PART ABOUT PSYCHOLOGICAL COUNSELING?
IT COVERS COUNSELING FOR YOU, DAVID, AND YOUR CHILDREN UP TO SIX MONTHS AFTER THE BIRTH OR TERMINATION OF THE AGREEMENT.
WHAT HAPPENS IF THE BABY IS BORN WITH A SEVERE GENETIC DISORDER AND THEY DON'T WANT TO ACCEPT IT?
OR WHAT IF THEY DIE BEFORE THE BABY IS BORN?
13
XIII
I SEE YOU HAVE BEEN IMAGINING THE WORST-CASE SCENARIO.
COME ON, WE LIVE IN ISRAEL! WE ALL KNOW UNEXPECTED AND UNFORTUNATE THINGS CAN HAPPEN.
WELL, THE IPs ARE LEGALLY OBLIGATED TO TAKE THE BABY, NO MATTER WHAT, AND APPOINT GUARDIANS IN THE CONTRACT IF THEY CAN'T.
THAT'S GOOD. IT'S PROBABLY EVERY SURROGATE'S NIGHTMARE THAT SHE'LL BE STUCK WITH THE COUPLE'S BABY.
IT SAYS THAT IF ONE PARTY TO THE AGREEMENT WANTS TO CUT OFF CONTACT AFTER THE BIRTH, THEN THE OTHER PARTY HAS TO HONOR IT.
THAT'S IN STANDARD CONTRACTS, BUT THE RELATIONSHIP IS UP TO YOU AND THE COUPLE. NO ONE WILL MONITOR WHAT YOU DO.

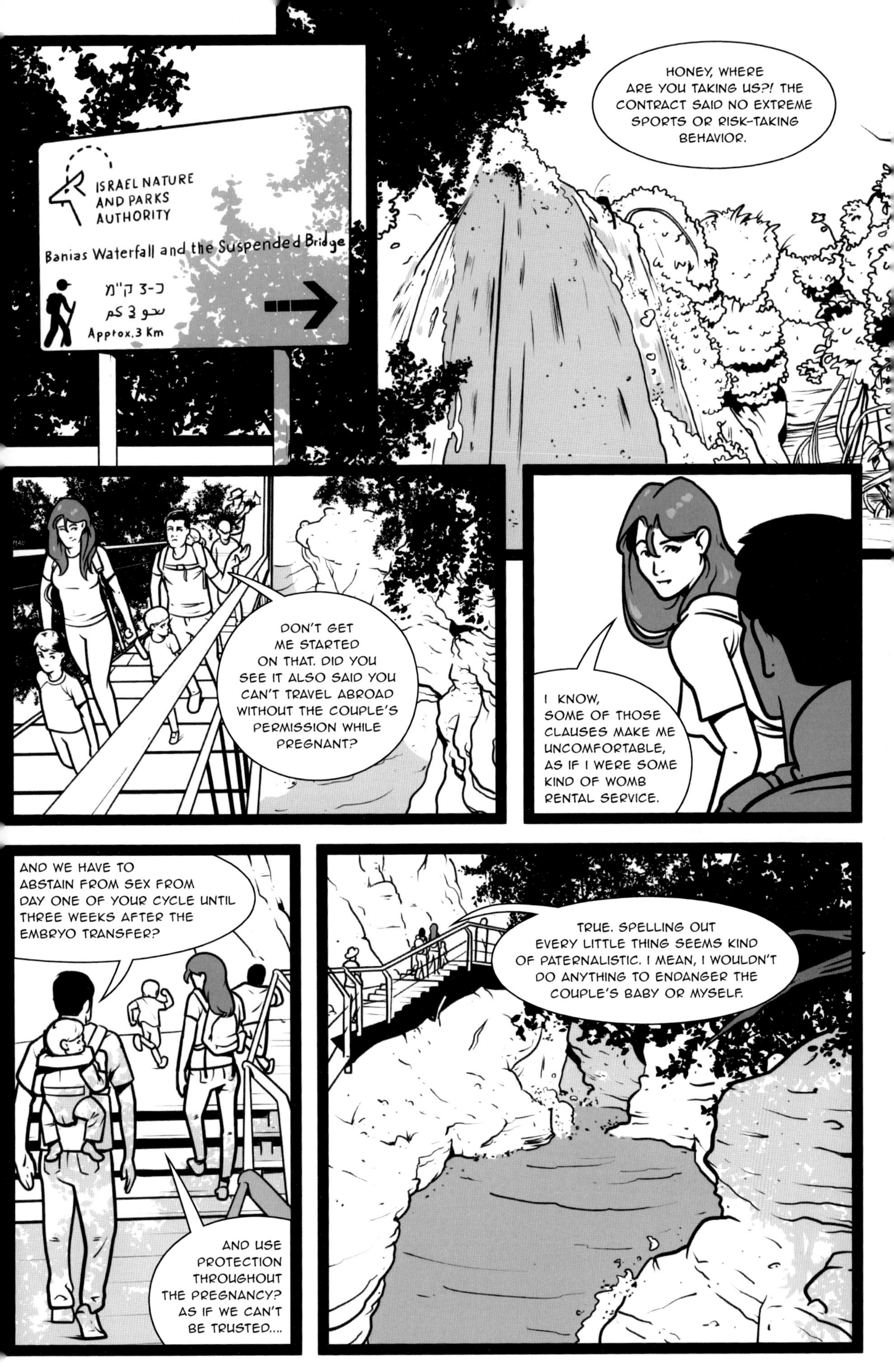
ISRAEL NATURE AND PARKS AUTHORITY
Banias Waterfall and the Suspended Bridge
כ-3 ק"מ
نحو 3 كم
Approx. 3 Km
HONEY, WHERE ARE YOU TAKING US?! THE CONTRACT SAID NO EXTREME SPORTS OR RISK-TAKING BEHAVIOR.
DON'T GET ME STARTED ON THAT. DID YOU SEE IT ALSO SAID YOU CAN'T TRAVEL ABROAD WITHOUT THE COUPLE'S PERMISSION WHILE PREGNANT?
I KNOW, SOME OF THOSE CLAUSES MAKE ME UNCOMFORTABLE, AS IF I WERE SOME KIND OF WOMB RENTAL SERVICE.
AND WE HAVE TO ABSTAIN FROM SEX FROM DAY ONE OF YOUR CYCLE UNTIL THREE WEEKS AFTER THE EMBRYO TRANSFER?
AND USE PROTECTION THROUGHOUT THE PREGNANCY? AS IF WE CAN'T BE TRUSTED....
TRUE. SPELLING OUT EVERY LITTLE THING SEEMS KIND OF PATERNALISTIC. I MEAN, I WOULDN'T DO ANYTHING TO ENDANGER THE COUPLE'S BABY OR MYSELF.

-CHAPTER 6-
CONTRACT

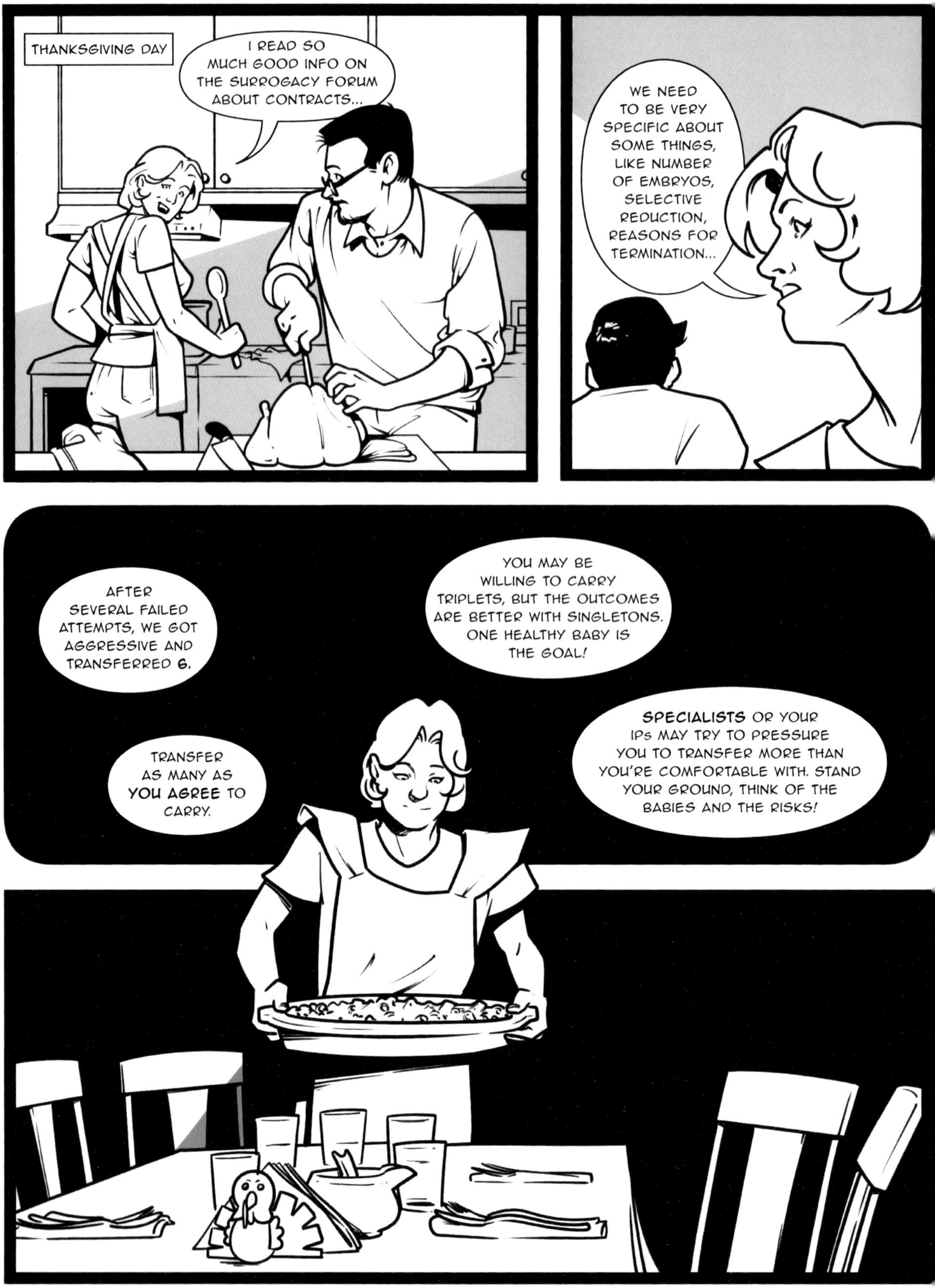
THANKSGIVING DAY
I READ SO MUCH GOOD INFO ON THE SURROGACY FORUM ABOUT CONTRACTS...
WE NEED TO BE VERY SPECIFIC ABOUT SOME THINGS, LIKE NUMBER OF EMBRYOS, SELECTIVE REDUCTION, REASONS FOR TERMINATION...
AFTER SEVERAL FAILED ATTEMPTS, WE GOT AGGRESSIVE AND TRANSFERRED 6.
YOU MAY BE WILLING TO CARRY TRIPLETS, BUT THE OUTCOMES ARE BETTER WITH SINGLETONS. ONE HEALTHY BABY IS THE GOAL!
TRANSFER AS MANY AS YOU AGREE TO CARRY.
SPECIALISTS OR YOUR IPs MAY TRY TO PRESSURE YOU TO TRANSFER MORE THAN YOU'RE COMFORTABLE WITH. STAND YOUR GROUND, THINK OF THE BABIES AND THE RISKS!

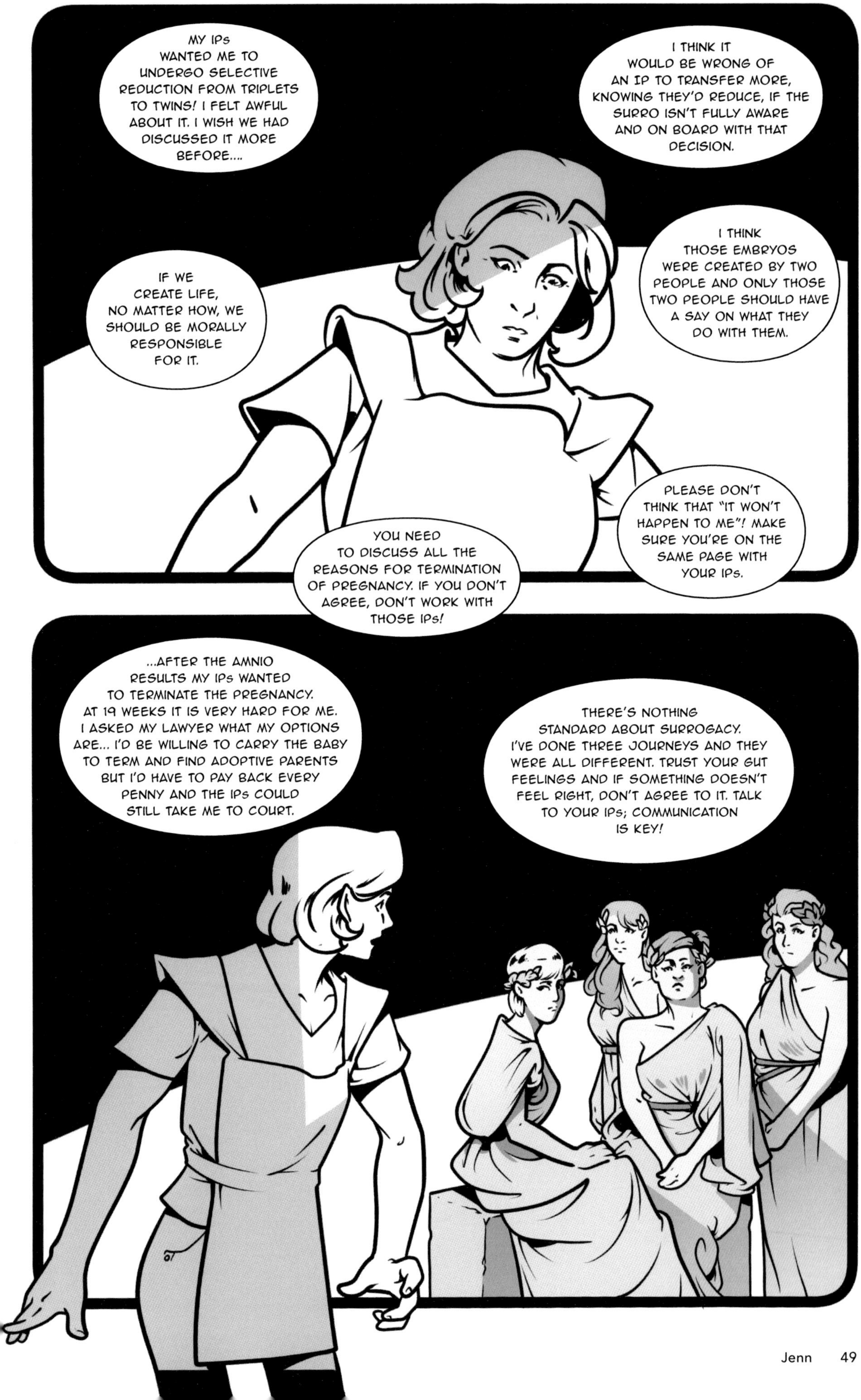
MY IPs WANTED ME TO UNDERGO SELECTIVE REDUCTION FROM TRIPLETS TO TWINS! I FELT AWFUL ABOUT IT. I WISH WE HAD DISCUSSED IT MORE BEFORE....
I THINK IT WOULD BE WRONG OF AN IP TO TRANSFER MORE, KNOWING THEY'D REDUCE, IF THE SURRO ISN'T FULLY AWARE AND ON BOARD WITH THAT DECISION.
IF WE CREATE LIFE, NO MATTER HOW, WE SHOULD BE MORALLY RESPONSIBLE FOR IT.
I THINK THOSE EMBRYOS WERE CREATED BY TWO PEOPLE AND ONLY THOSE TWO PEOPLE SHOULD HAVE A SAY ON WHAT THEY DO WITH THEM.
YOU NEED TO DISCUSS ALL THE REASONS FOR TERMINATION OF PREGNANCY. IF YOU DON'T AGREE, DON'T WORK WITH THOSE IPs!
PLEASE DON'T THINK THAT "IT WON'T HAPPEN TO ME"! MAKE SURE YOU'RE ON THE SAME PAGE WITH YOUR IPs.
...AFTER THE AMNIO RESULTS MY IPs WANTED TO TERMINATE THE PREGNANCY. AT 19 WEEKS IT IS VERY HARD FOR ME. I ASKED MY LAWYER WHAT MY OPTIONS ARE... I'D BE WILLING TO CARRY THE BABY TO TERM AND FIND ADOPTIVE PARENTS BUT I'D HAVE TO PAY BACK EVERY PENNY AND THE IPs COULD STILL TAKE ME TO COURT.
THERE'S NOTHING STANDARD ABOUT SURROGACY. I'VE DONE THREE JOURNEYS AND THEY WERE ALL DIFFERENT. TRUST YOUR GUT FEELINGS AND IF SOMETHING DOESN'T FEEL RIGHT, DON'T AGREE TO IT. TALK TO YOUR IPs; COMMUNICATION IS KEY!

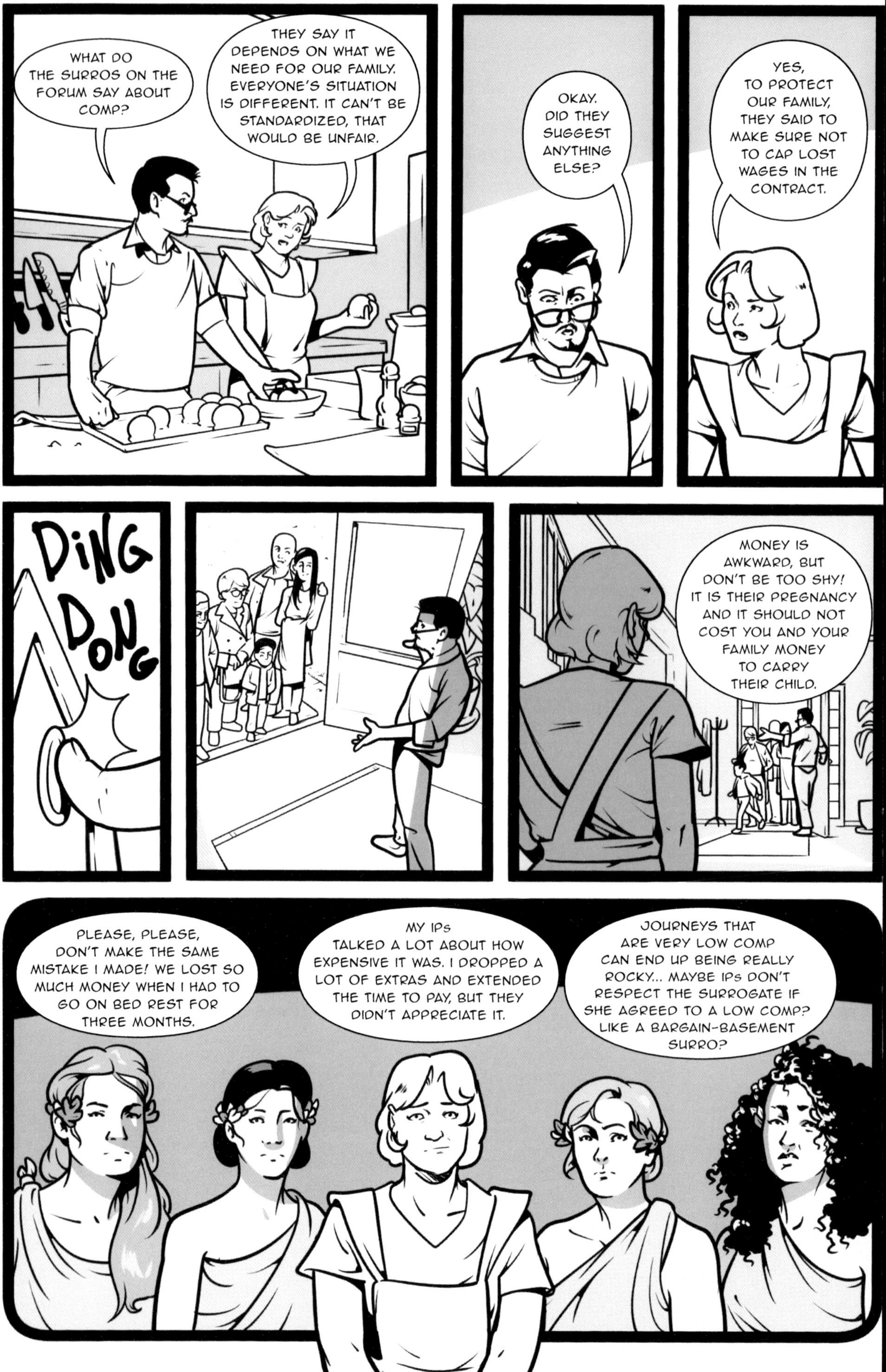
WHAT DO THE SURROS ON THE FORUM SAY ABOUT COMP?
THEY SAY IT DEPENDS ON WHAT WE NEED FOR OUR FAMILY. EVERYONE'S SITUATION IS DIFFERENT. IT CAN'T BE STANDARDIZED, THAT WOULD BE UNFAIR.
OKAY. DID THEY SUGGEST ANYTHING ELSE?
YES, TO PROTECT OUR FAMILY, THEY SAID TO MAKE SURE NOT TO CAP LOST WAGES IN THE CONTRACT.
DING DONG
MONEY IS AWKWARD, BUT DON'T BE TOO SHY! IT IS THEIR PREGNANCY AND IT SHOULD NOT COST YOU AND YOUR FAMILY MONEY TO CARRY THEIR CHILD.
PLEASE, PLEASE, DON'T MAKE THE SAME MISTAKE I MADE! WE LOST SO MUCH MONEY WHEN I HAD TO GO ON BED REST FOR THREE MONTHS.
MY IPs TALKED A LOT ABOUT HOW EXPENSIVE IT WAS. I DROPPED A LOT OF EXTRAS AND EXTENDED THE TIME TO PAY, BUT THEY DIDN'T APPRECIATE IT.
JOURNEYS THAT ARE VERY LOW COMP CAN END UP BEING REALLY ROCKY... MAYBE IPs DON'T RESPECT THE SURROGATE IF SHE AGREED TO A LOW COMP? LIKE A BARGAIN-BASEMENT SURRO?

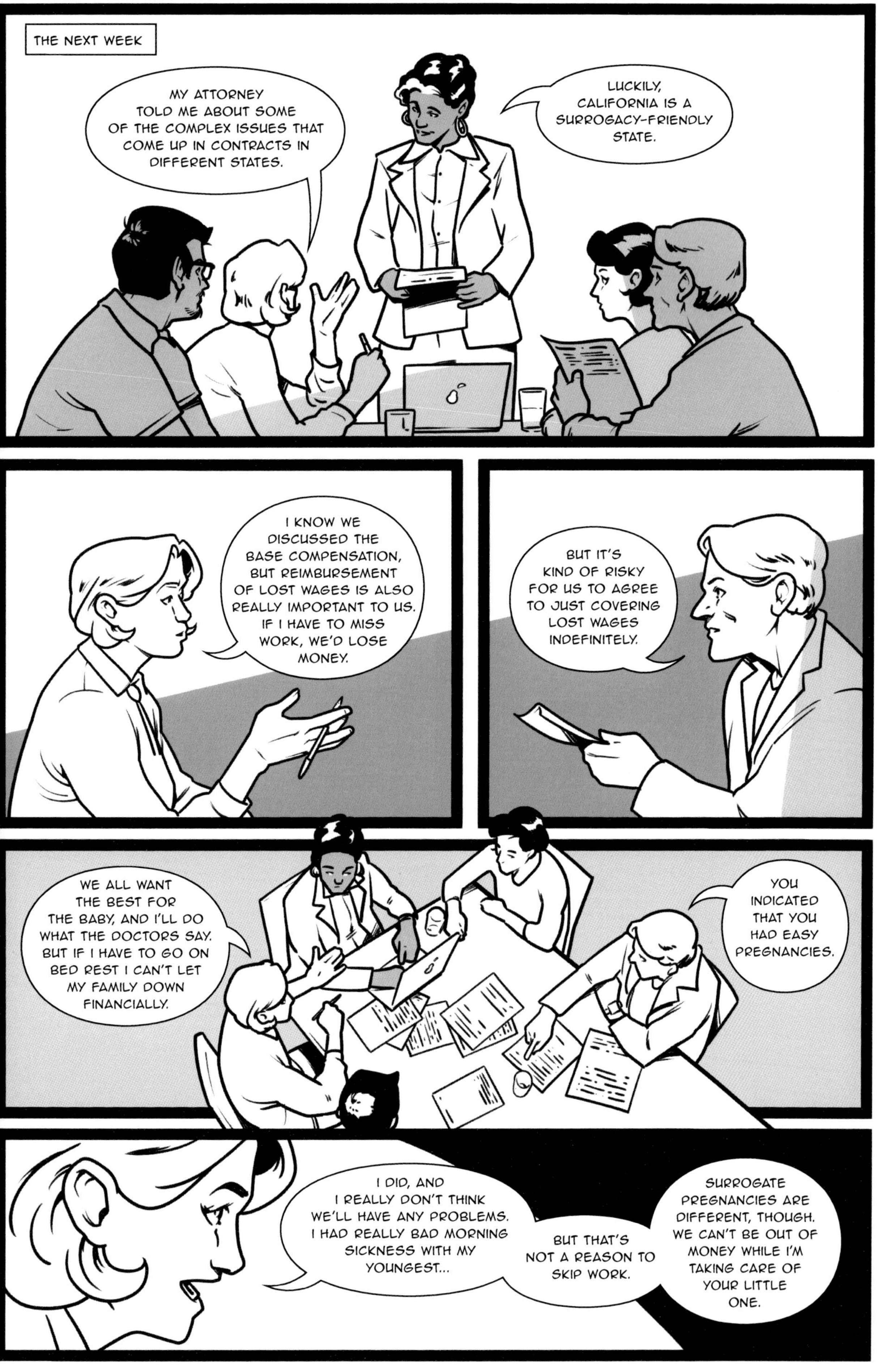
THE NEXT WEEK
MY ATTORNEY TOLD ME ABOUT SOME OF THE COMPLEX ISSUES THAT COME UP IN CONTRACTS IN DIFFERENT STATES.
LUCKILY, CALIFORNIA IS A SURROGACY-FRIENDLY STATE.
I KNOW WE DISCUSSED THE BASE COMPENSATION, BUT REIMBURSEMENT OF LOST WAGES IS ALSO REALLY IMPORTANT TO US. IF I HAVE TO MISS WORK, WE'D LOSE MONEY.
BUT IT'S KIND OF RISKY FOR US TO AGREE TO JUST COVERING LOST WAGES INDEFINITELY.
WE ALL WANT THE BEST FOR THE BABY, AND I'LL DO WHAT THE DOCTORS SAY. BUT IF I HAVE TO GO ON BED REST I CAN'T LET MY FAMILY DOWN FINANCIALLY.
YOU INDICATED THAT YOU HAD EASY PREGNANCIES.
I DID, AND I REALLY DON'T THINK WE'LL HAVE ANY PROBLEMS. I HAD REALLY BAD MORNING SICKNESS WITH MY YOUNGEST...
BUT THAT'S NOT A REASON TO SKIP WORK.
SURROGATE PREGNANCIES ARE DIFFERENT, THOUGH. WE CAN'T BE OUT OF MONEY WHILE I'M TAKING CARE OF YOUR LITTLE ONE.

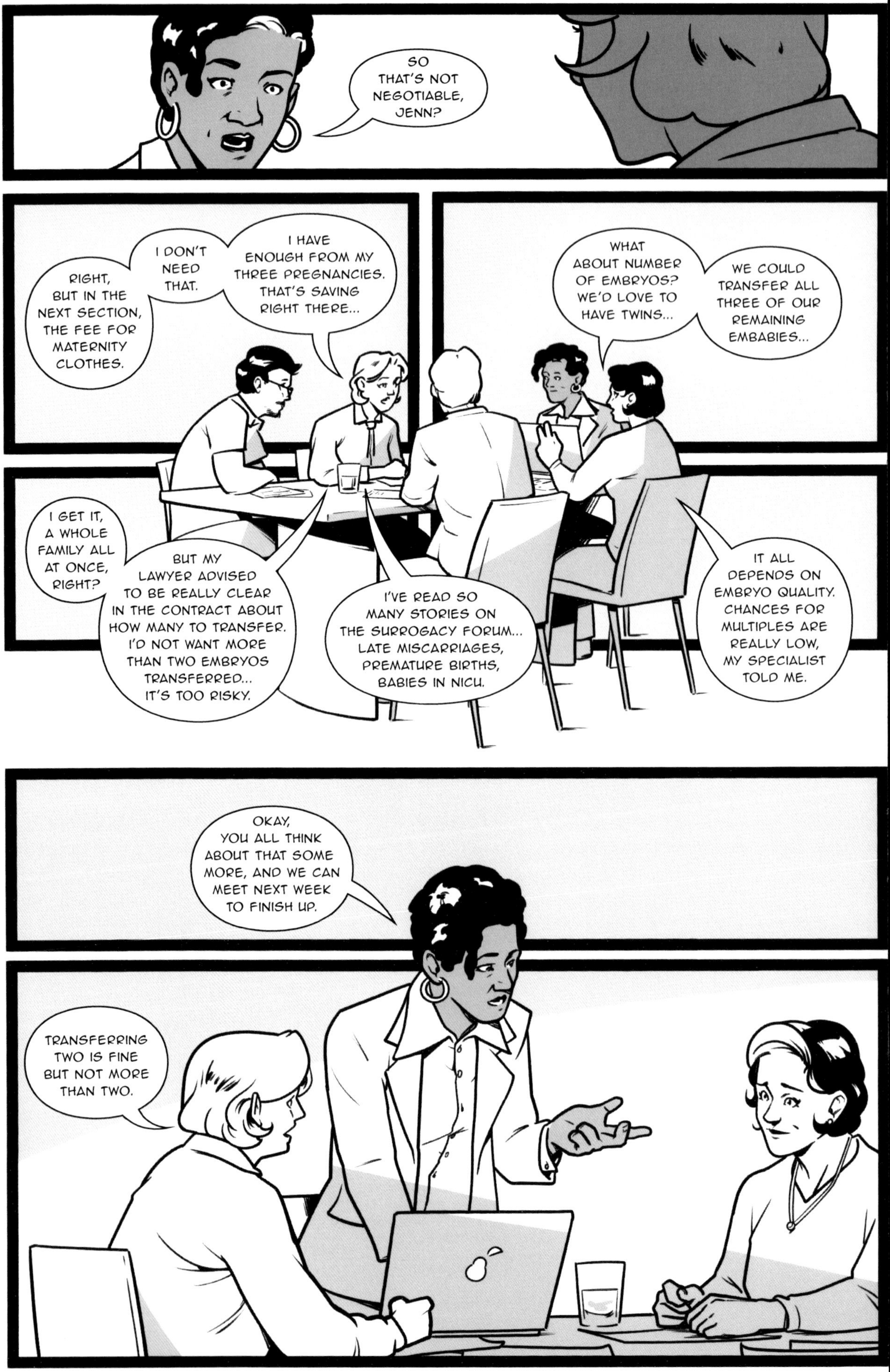
SO THAT'S NOT NEGOTIABLE, JENN?
RIGHT, BUT IN THE NEXT SECTION, THE FEE FOR MATERNITY CLOTHES.
I DON'T NEED THAT.
I HAVE ENOUGH FROM MY THREE PREGNANCIES. THAT'S SAVING RIGHT THERE...
WHAT ABOUT NUMBER OF EMBRYOS? WE'D LOVE TO HAVE TWINS...
WE COULD TRANSFER ALL THREE OF OUR REMAINING EMBABIES...
I GET IT, A WHOLE FAMILY ALL AT ONCE, RIGHT?
BUT MY LAWYER ADVISED TO BE REALLY CLEAR IN THE CONTRACT ABOUT HOW MANY TO TRANSFER. I'D NOT WANT MORE THAN TWO EMBRYOS TRANSFERRED... IT'S TOO RISKY.
I'VE READ SO MANY STORIES ON THE SURROGACY FORUM... LATE MISCARRIAGES, PREMATURE BIRTHS, BABIES IN NICU.
IT ALL DEPENDS ON EMBRYO QUALITY. CHANCES FOR MULTIPLES ARE REALLY LOW, MY SPECIALIST TOLD ME.
OKAY, YOU ALL THINK ABOUT THAT SOME MORE, AND WE CAN MEET NEXT WEEK TO FINISH UP.
TRANSFERRING TWO IS FINE BUT NOT MORE THAN TWO.

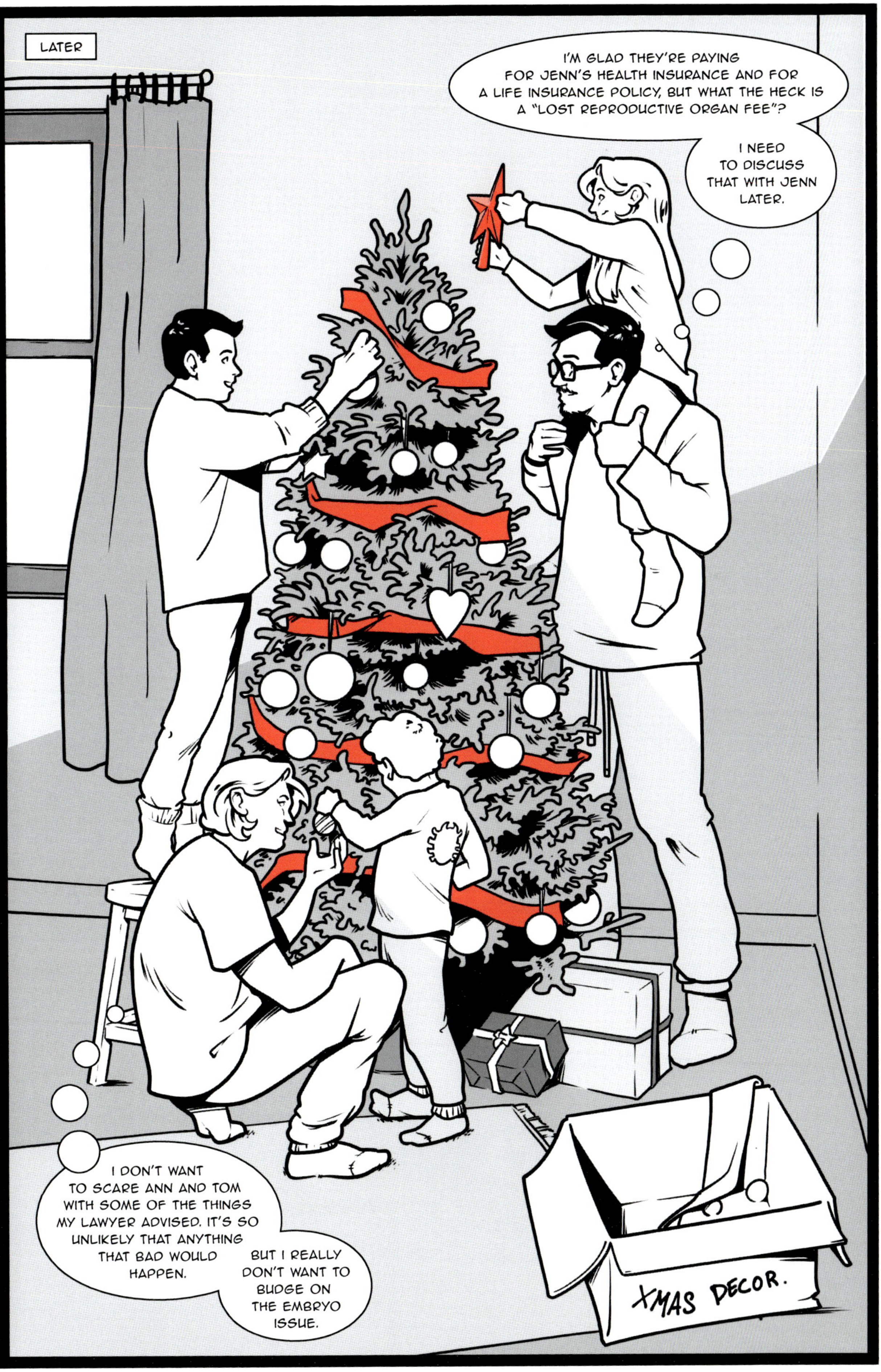
LATER
I'M GLAD THEY'RE PAYING FOR JENN'S HEALTH INSURANCE AND FOR A LIFE INSURANCE POLICY, BUT WHAT THE HECK IS A "LOST REPRODUCTIVE ORGAN FEE"?
I NEED TO DISCUSS THAT WITH JENN LATER.
I DON'T WANT TO SCARE ANN AND TOM WITH SOME OF THE THINGS MY LAWYER ADVISED. IT'S SO UNLIKELY THAT ANYTHING THAT BAD WOULD HAPPEN.
BUT I REALLY DON'T WANT TO BUDGE ON THE EMBRYO ISSUE.
XMAS DECOR.

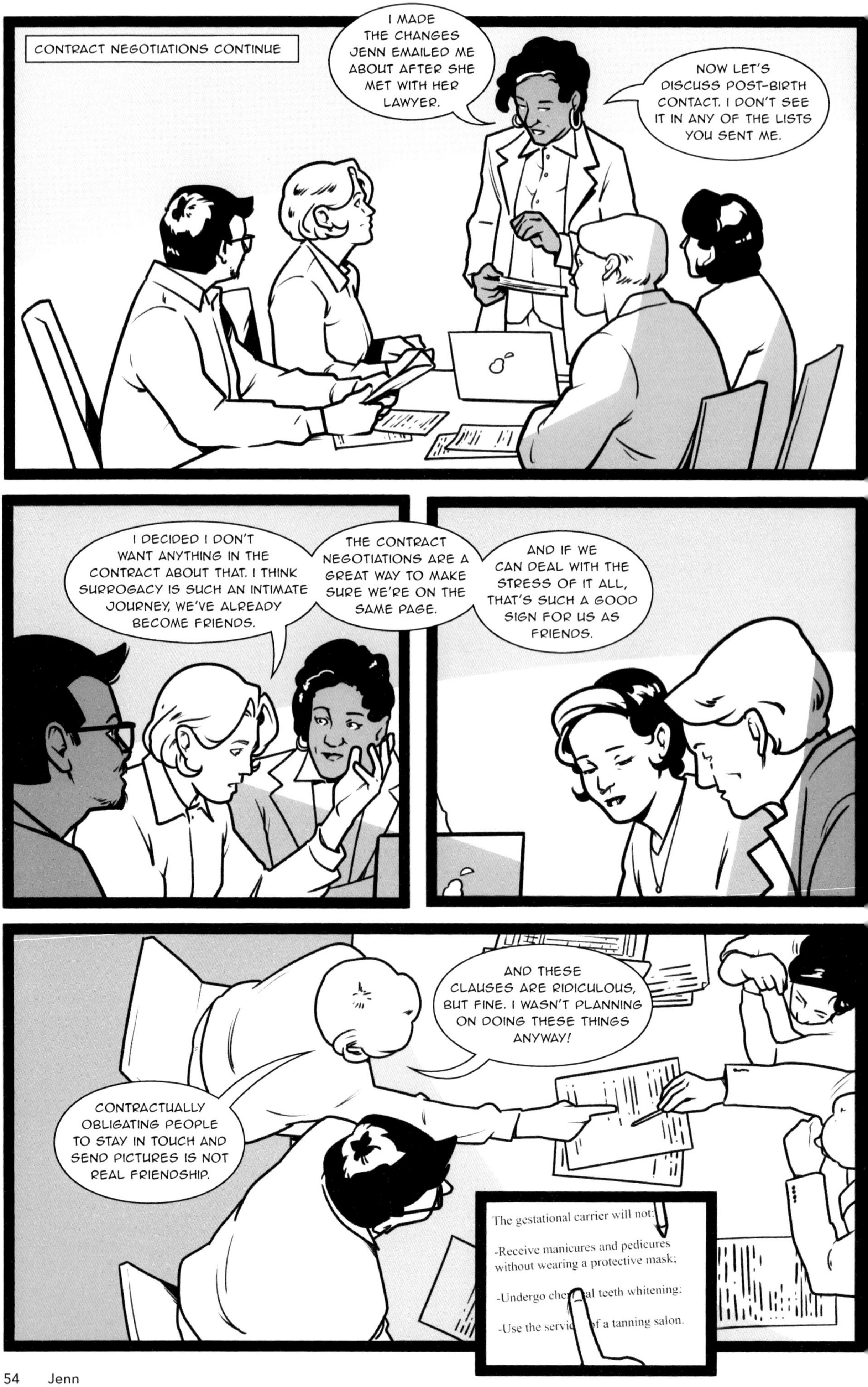
CONTRACT NEGOTIATIONS CONTINUE
I MADE THE CHANGES JENN EMAILED ME ABOUT AFTER SHE MET WITH HER LAWYER.
NOW LET'S DISCUSS POST-BIRTH CONTACT. I DON'T SEE IT IN ANY OF THE LISTS YOU SENT ME.
I DECIDED I DON'T WANT ANYTHING IN THE CONTRACT ABOUT THAT. I THINK SURROGACY IS SUCH AN INTIMATE JOURNEY, WE'VE ALREADY BECOME FRIENDS.
THE CONTRACT NEGOTIATIONS ARE A GREAT WAY TO MAKE SURE WE'RE ON THE SAME PAGE.
AND IF WE CAN DEAL WITH THE STRESS OF IT ALL, THAT'S SUCH A GOOD SIGN FOR US AS FRIENDS.
AND THESE CLAUSES ARE RIDICULOUS, BUT FINE. I WASN'T PLANNING ON DOING THESE THINGS ANYWAY!
CONTRACTUALLY OBLIGATING PEOPLE TO STAY IN TOUCH AND SEND PICTURES IS NOT REAL FRIENDSHIP.
The gestational carrier will not:
-Receive manicures and pedicures without wearing a protective mask;
-Undergo che al teeth whitening;
-Use the servic f a tanning salon.

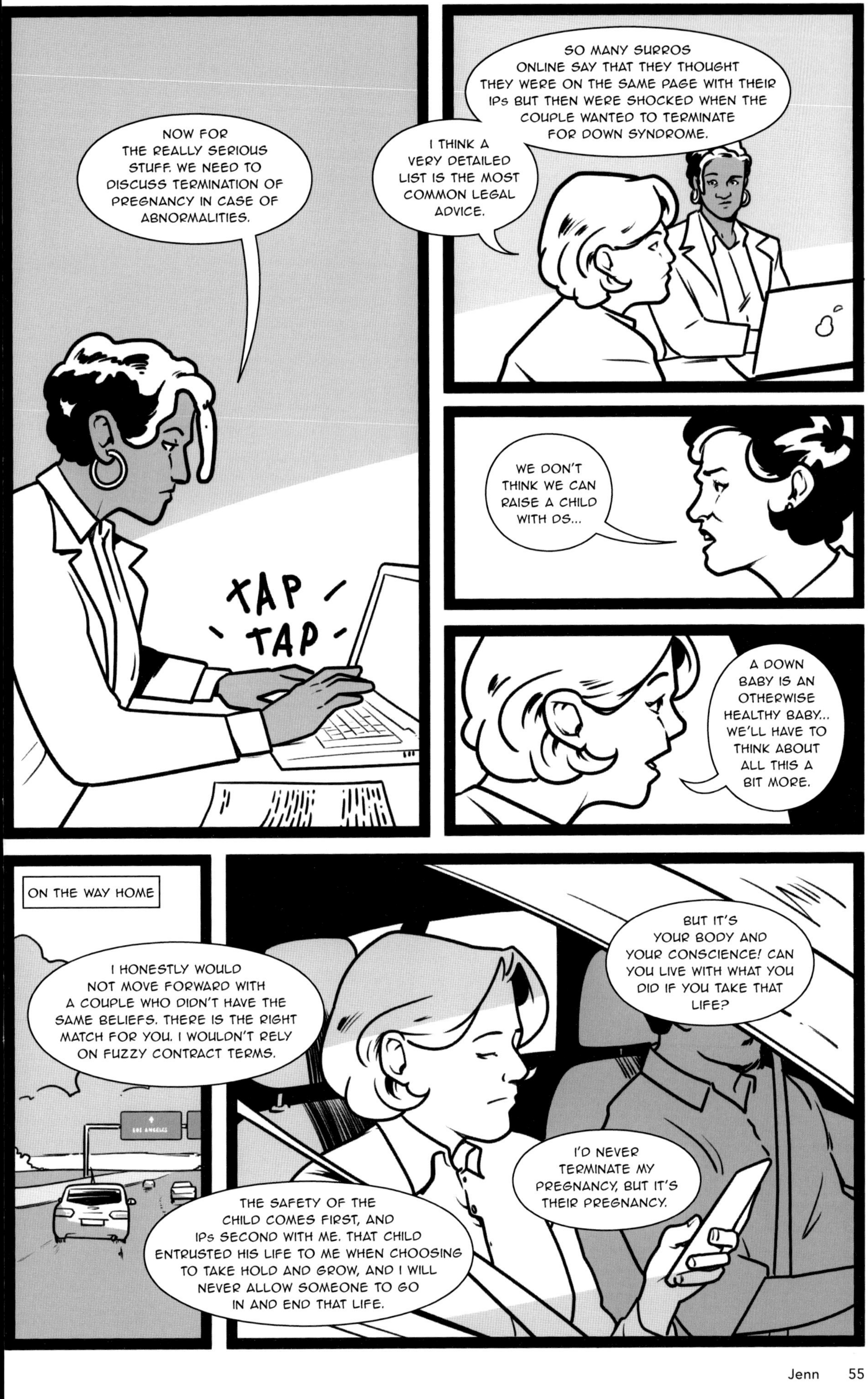
NOW FOR THE REALLY SERIOUS STUFF. WE NEED TO DISCUSS TERMINATION OF PREGNANCY IN CASE OF ABNORMALITIES.
TAP TAP
SO MANY SURROS ONLINE SAY THAT THEY THOUGHT THEY WERE ON THE SAME PAGE WITH THEIR IPs BUT THEN WERE SHOCKED WHEN THE COUPLE WANTED TO TERMINATE FOR DOWN SYNDROME.
I THINK A VERY DETAILED LIST IS THE MOST COMMON LEGAL ADVICE.
WE DON'T THINK WE CAN RAISE A CHILD WITH DS...
A DOWN BABY IS AN OTHERWISE HEALTHY BABY... WE'LL HAVE TO THINK ABOUT ALL THIS A BIT MORE.
ON THE WAY HOME
I HONESTLY WOULD NOT MOVE FORWARD WITH A COUPLE WHO DIDN'T HAVE THE SAME BELIEFS. THERE IS THE RIGHT MATCH FOR YOU. I WOULDN'T RELY ON FUZZY CONTRACT TERMS.
BUT IT'S YOUR BODY AND YOUR CONSCIENCE! CAN YOU LIVE WITH WHAT YOU DID IF YOU TAKE THAT LIFE?
I'D NEVER TERMINATE MY PREGNANCY, BUT IT'S THEIR PREGNANCY.
THE SAFETY OF THE CHILD COMES FIRST, AND IPs SECOND WITH ME. THAT CHILD ENTRUSTED HIS LIFE TO ME WHEN CHOOSING TO TAKE HOLD AND GROW, AND I WILL NEVER ALLOW SOMEONE TO GO IN AND END THAT LIFE.

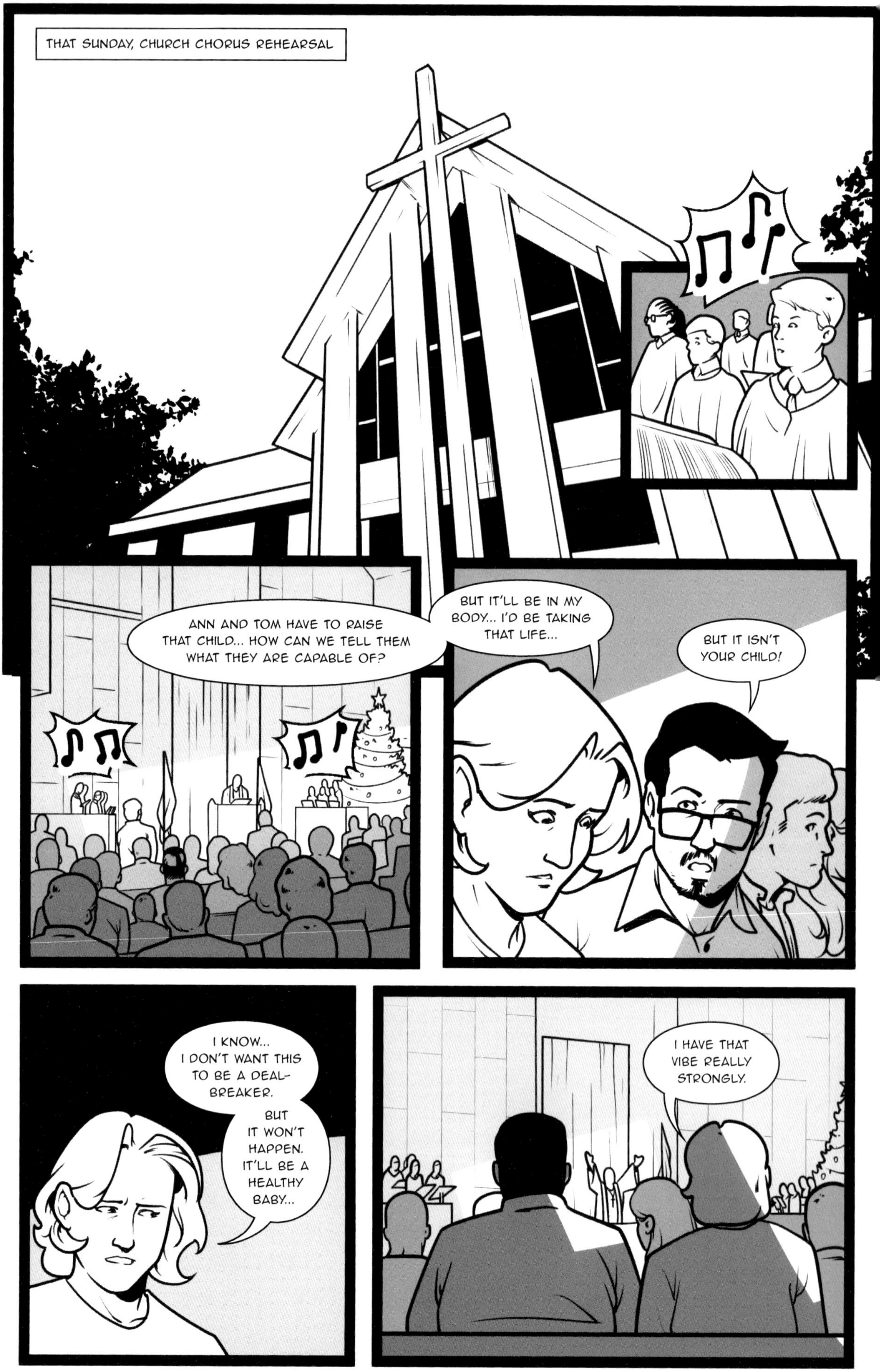
THAT SUNDAY, CHURCH CHORUS REHEARSAL
ANN AND TOM HAVE TO RAISE THAT CHILD... HOW CAN WE TELL THEM WHAT THEY ARE CAPABLE OF?
BUT IT'LL BE IN MY BODY... I'D BE TAKING THAT LIFE...
BUT IT ISN'T YOUR CHILD!
I KNOW... I DON'T WANT THIS TO BE A DEAL-BREAKER.
BUT IT WON'T HAPPEN. IT'LL BE A HEALTHY BABY...
I HAVE THAT VIBE REALLY STRONGLY.

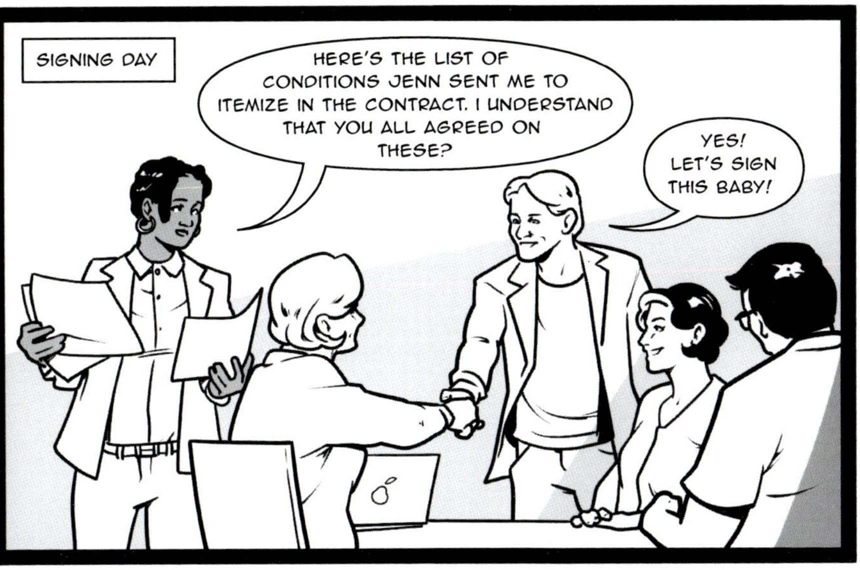
SIGNING DAY
HERE'S THE LIST OF CONDITIONS JENN SENT ME TO ITEMIZE IN THE CONTRACT. I UNDERSTAND THAT YOU ALL AGREED ON THESE?
YES! LET'S SIGN THIS BABY!

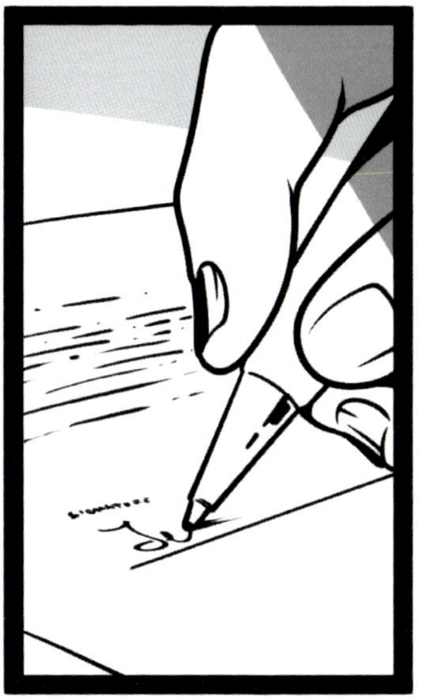

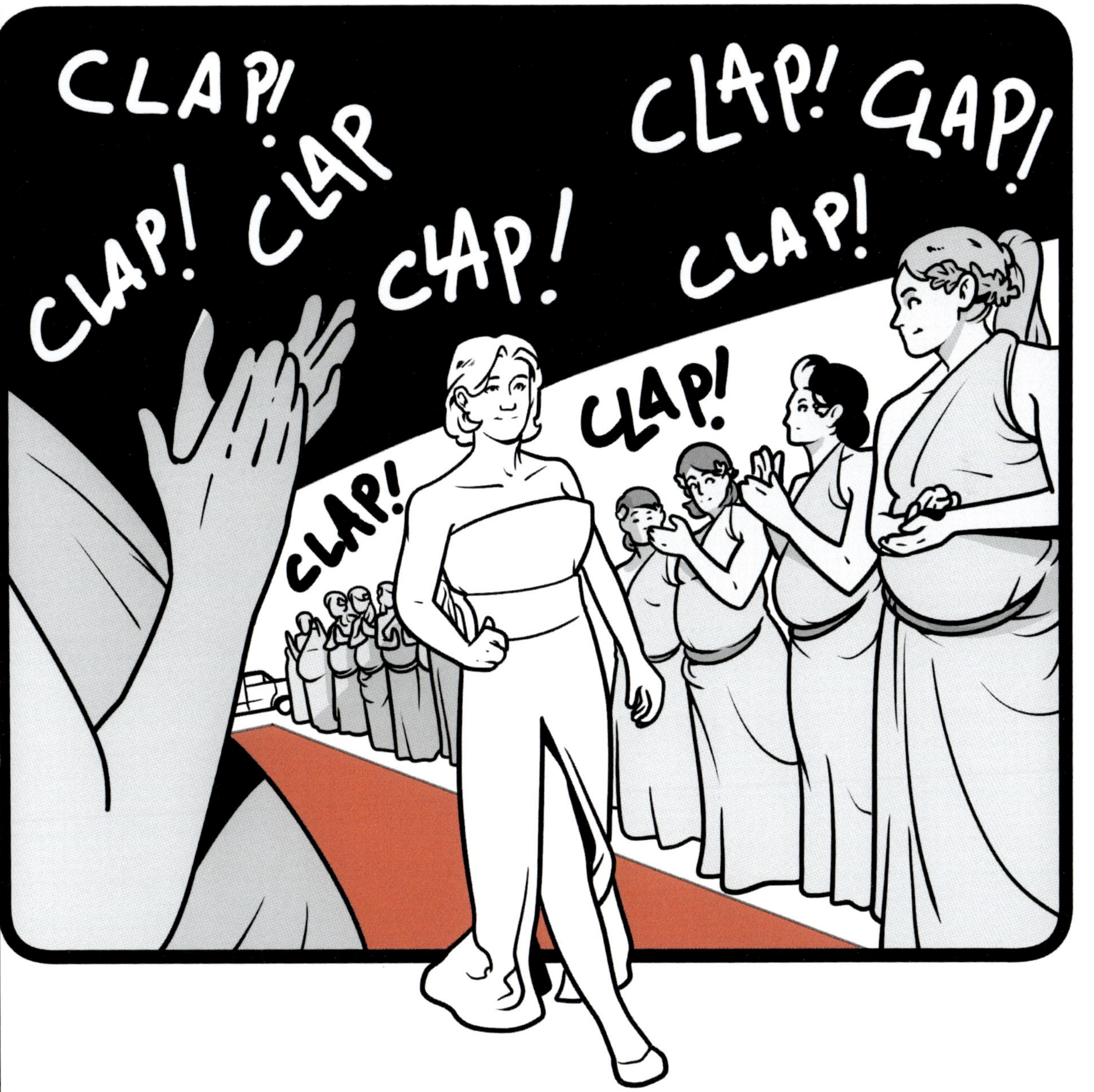
CLAP!
CLAP! CLAP
CLAP!
CLAP! CLAP!
CLAP!
CLAP!
CLAP!

INTERLUDE: GABRIELA, SURROGATE FROM MOLDOVA

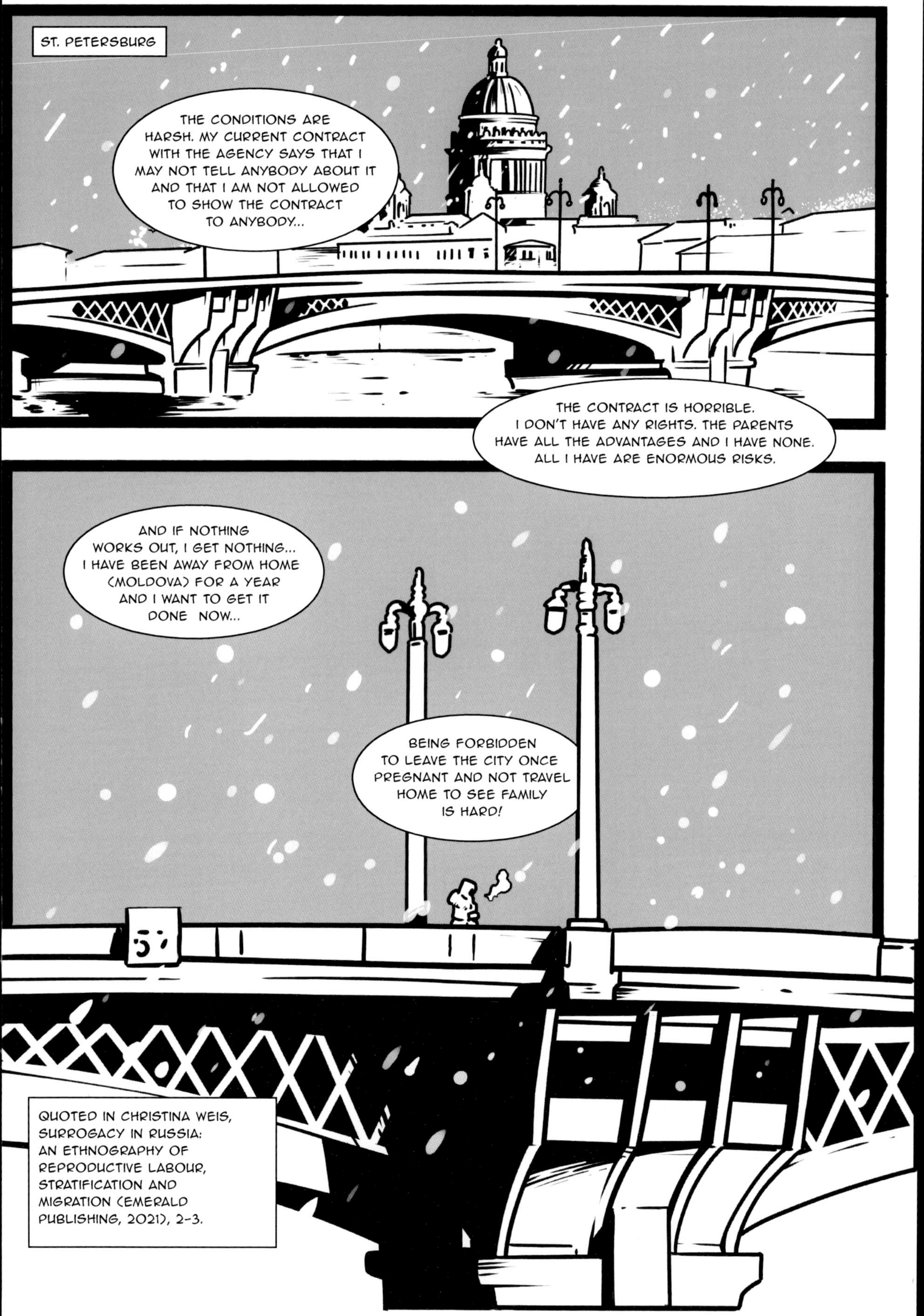
ST. PETERSBURG
THE CONDITIONS ARE HARSH. MY CURRENT CONTRACT WITH THE AGENCY SAYS THAT I MAY NOT TELL ANYBODY ABOUT IT AND THAT I AM NOT ALLOWED TO SHOW THE CONTRACT TO ANYBODY...
THE CONTRACT IS HORRIBLE. I DON'T HAVE ANY RIGHTS. THE PARENTS HAVE ALL THE ADVANTAGES AND I HAVE NONE. ALL I HAVE ARE ENORMOUS RISKS.
AND IF NOTHING WORKS OUT, I GET NOTHING... I HAVE BEEN AWAY FROM HOME (MOLDOVA) FOR A YEAR AND I WANT TO GET IT DONE NOW...
BEING FORBIDDEN TO LEAVE THE CITY ONCE PREGNANT AND NOT TRAVEL HOME TO SEE FAMILY IS HARD!

QUOTED IN CHRISTINA WEIS, SURROGACY IN RUSSIA: AN ETHNOGRAPHY OF REPRODUCTIVE LABOUR, STRATIFICATION AND MIGRATION (EMERALD PUBLISHING, 2021), 2–3.

-CHAPTER 7-
THE STATE

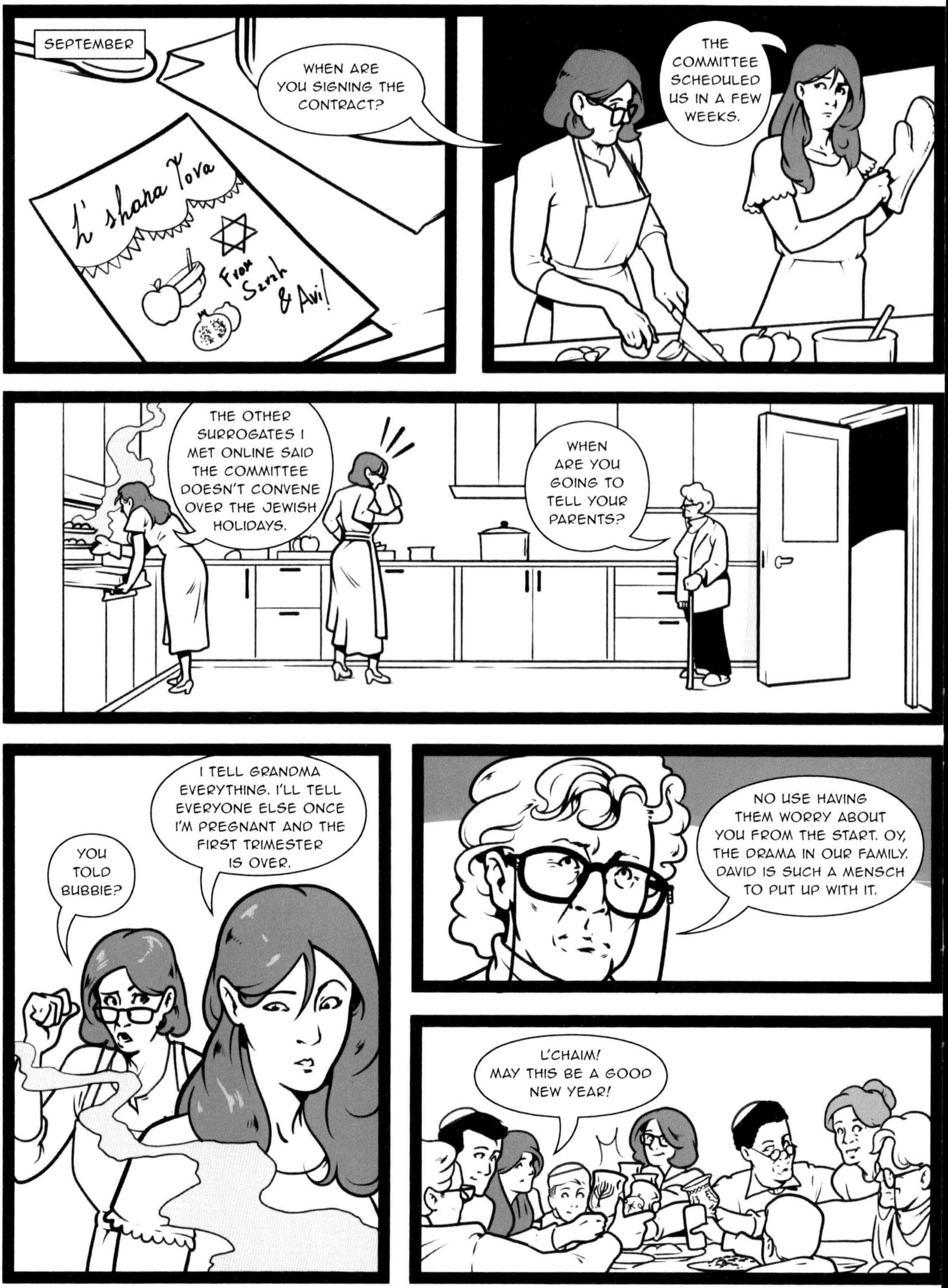
SEPTEMBER
L'shana Tova
From Sarah & Avi!
WHEN ARE YOU SIGNING THE CONTRACT?
THE COMMITTEE SCHEDULED US IN A FEW WEEKS.
THE OTHER SURROGATES I MET ONLINE SAID THE COMMITTEE DOESN'T CONVENE OVER THE JEWISH HOLIDAYS.
WHEN ARE YOU GOING TO TELL YOUR PARENTS?
YOU TOLD BUBBIE?
I TELL GRANDMA EVERYTHING. I'LL TELL EVERYONE ELSE ONCE I'M PREGNANT AND THE FIRST TRIMESTER IS OVER.
NO USE HAVING THEM WORRY ABOUT YOU FROM THE START. OY, THE DRAMA IN OUR FAMILY. DAVID IS SUCH A MENSCH TO PUT UP WITH IT.
L'CHAIM! MAY THIS BE A GOOD NEW YEAR!

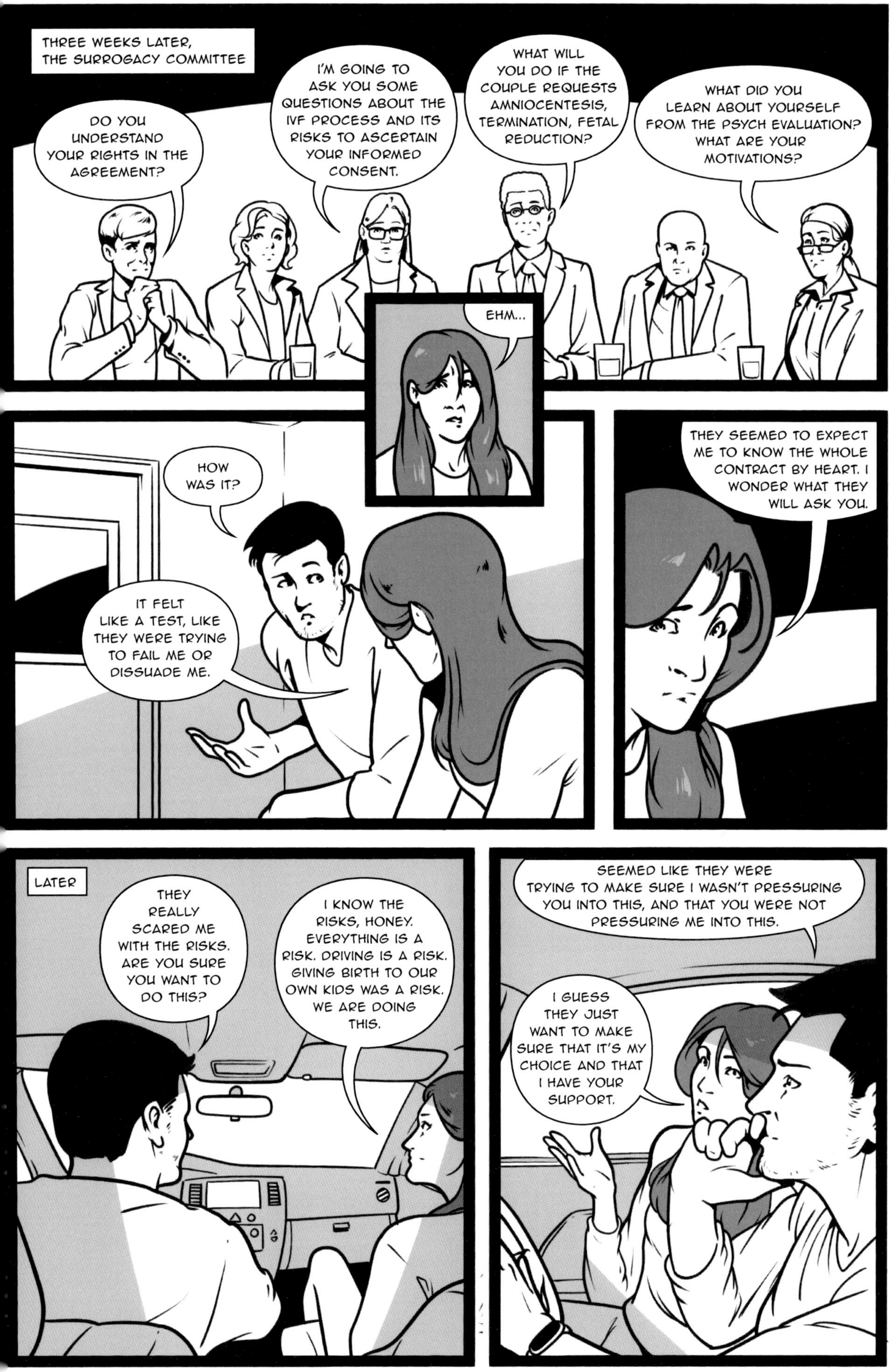
THREE WEEKS LATER, THE SURROGACY COMMITTEE
DO YOU UNDERSTAND YOUR RIGHTS IN THE AGREEMENT?
I'M GOING TO ASK YOU SOME QUESTIONS ABOUT THE IVF PROCESS AND ITS RISKS TO ASCERTAIN YOUR INFORMED CONSENT.
WHAT WILL YOU DO IF THE COUPLE REQUESTS AMNIOCENTESIS, TERMINATION, FETAL REDUCTION?
WHAT DID YOU LEARN ABOUT YOURSELF FROM THE PSYCH EVALUATION? WHAT ARE YOUR MOTIVATIONS?
EHM...
HOW WAS IT?
IT FELT LIKE A TEST, LIKE THEY WERE TRYING TO FAIL ME OR DISSUADE ME.
THEY SEEMED TO EXPECT ME TO KNOW THE WHOLE CONTRACT BY HEART. I WONDER WHAT THEY WILL ASK YOU.
LATER
THEY REALLY SCARED ME WITH THE RISKS. ARE YOU SURE YOU WANT TO DO THIS?
I KNOW THE RISKS, HONEY. EVERYTHING IS A RISK. DRIVING IS A RISK. GIVING BIRTH TO OUR OWN KIDS WAS A RISK. WE ARE DOING THIS.
SEEMED LIKE THEY WERE TRYING TO MAKE SURE I WASN'T PRESSURING YOU INTO THIS, AND THAT YOU WERE NOT PRESSURING ME INTO THIS.
I GUESS THEY JUST WANT TO MAKE SURE THAT IT'S MY CHOICE AND THAT I HAVE YOUR SUPPORT.

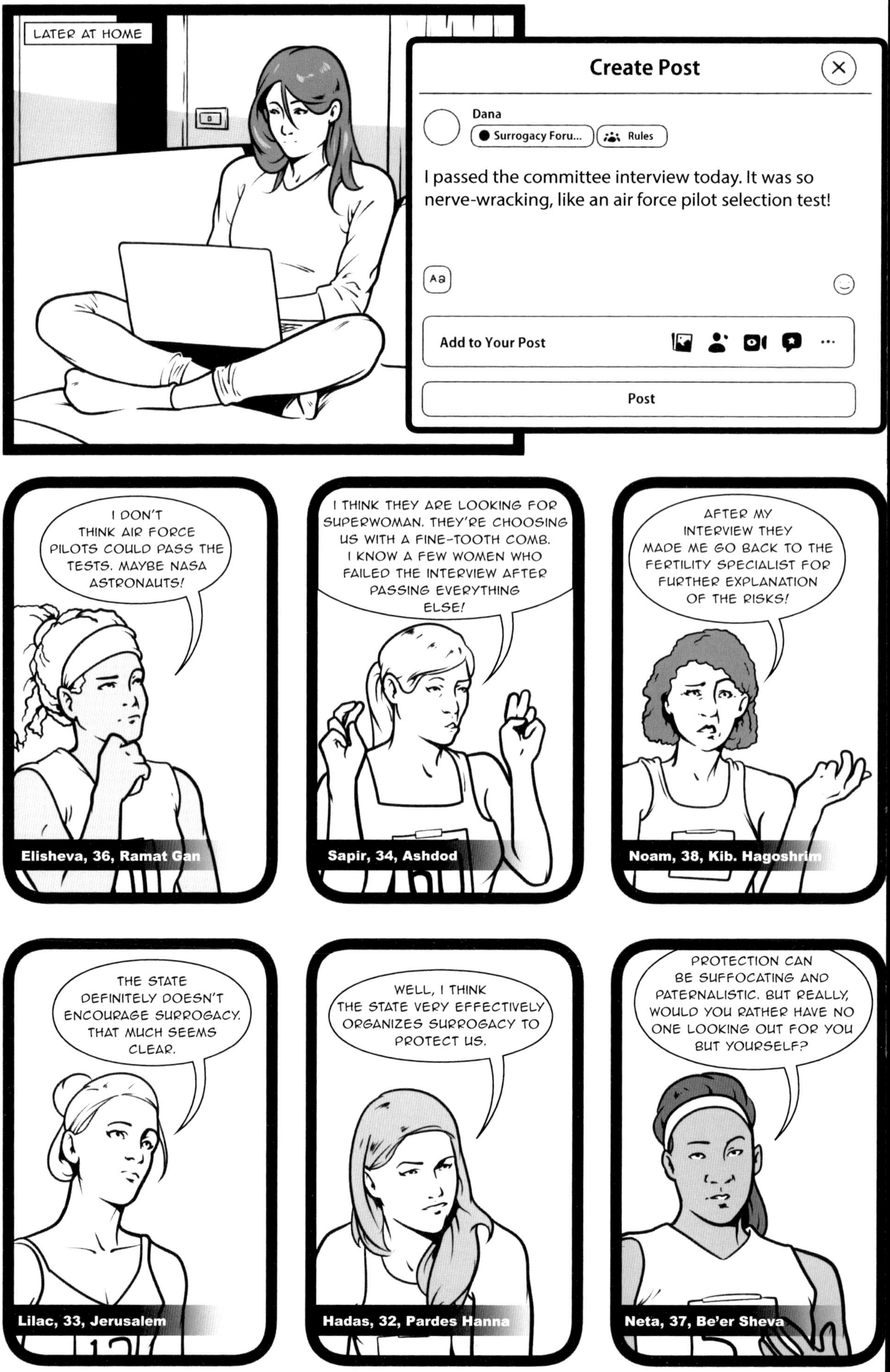
LATER AT HOME
Create Post
Dana
Surrogacy Foru...
Rules
I passed the committee interview today. It was so nerve-wracking, like an air force pilot selection test!
Add to Your Post
Post
I DON'T THINK AIR FORCE PILOTS COULD PASS THE TESTS. MAYBE NASA ASTRONAUTS!
Elisheva, 36, Ramat Gan
I THINK THEY ARE LOOKING FOR SUPERWOMAN. THEY'RE CHOOSING US WITH A FINE-TOOTH COMB. I KNOW A FEW WOMEN WHO FAILED THE INTERVIEW AFTER PASSING EVERYTHING ELSE!
Sapir, 34, Ashdod
AFTER MY INTERVIEW THEY MADE ME GO BACK TO THE FERTILITY SPECIALIST FOR FURTHER EXPLANATION OF THE RISKS!
Noam, 38, Kib. Hagoshrim
THE STATE DEFINITELY DOESN'T ENCOURAGE SURROGACY. THAT MUCH SEEMS CLEAR.
Lilac, 33, Jerusalem
WELL, I THINK THE STATE VERY EFFECTIVELY ORGANIZES SURROGACY TO PROTECT US.
Hadas, 32, Pardes Hanna
PROTECTION CAN BE SUFFOCATING AND PATERNALISTIC. BUT REALLY, WOULD YOU RATHER HAVE NO ONE LOOKING OUT FOR YOU BUT YOURSELF?
Neta, 37, Be'er Sheva

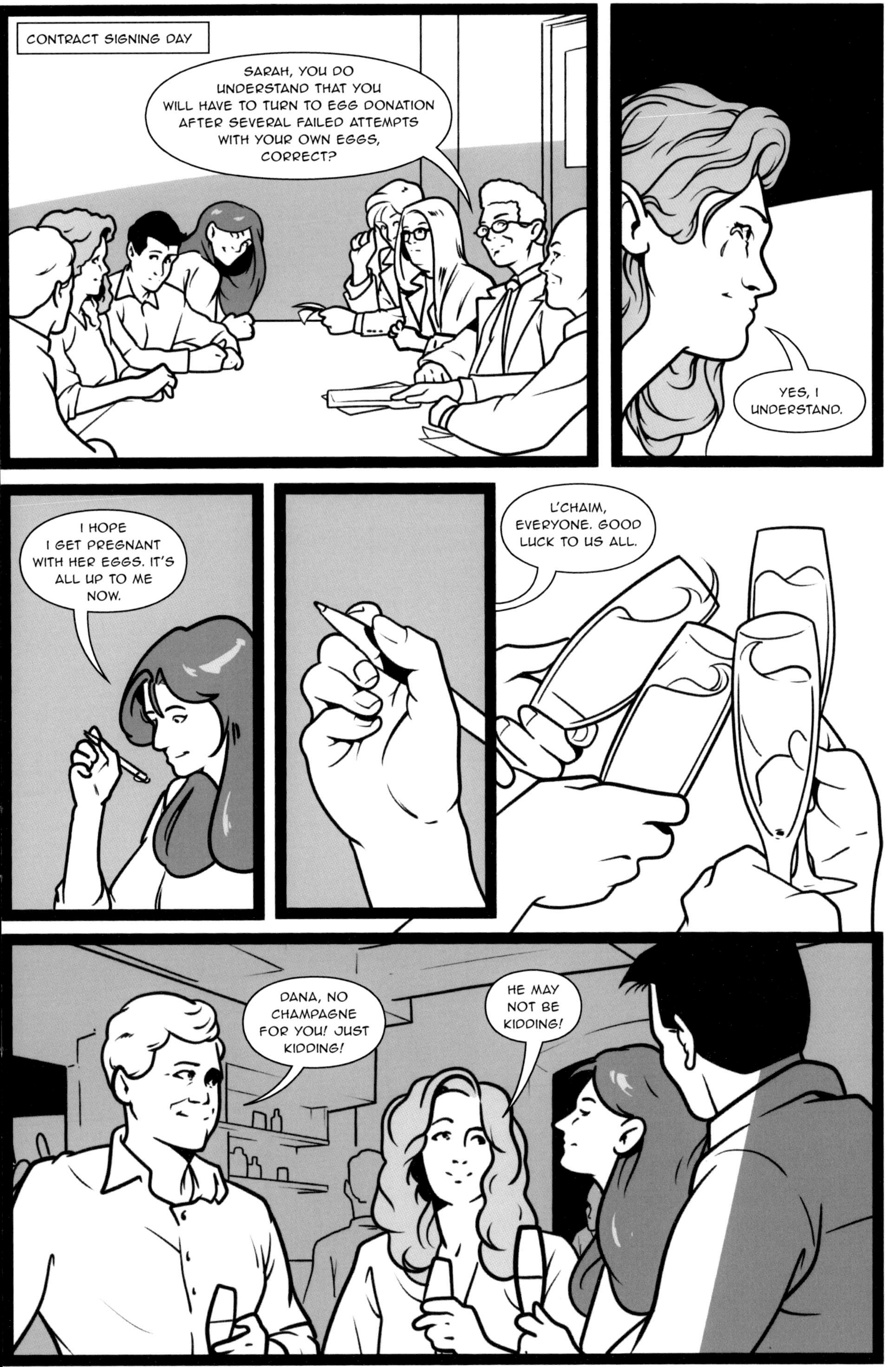
CONTRACT SIGNING DAY
SARAH, YOU DO UNDERSTAND THAT YOU WILL HAVE TO TURN TO EGG DONATION AFTER SEVERAL FAILED ATTEMPTS WITH YOUR OWN EGGS, CORRECT?
YES, I UNDERSTAND.
I HOPE I GET PREGNANT WITH HER EGGS. IT'S ALL UP TO ME NOW.
L'CHAIM, EVERYONE. GOOD LUCK TO US ALL.
DANA, NO CHAMPAGNE FOR YOU! JUST KIDDING!
HE MAY NOT BE KIDDING!

-CHAPTER 8-
TRANSFER

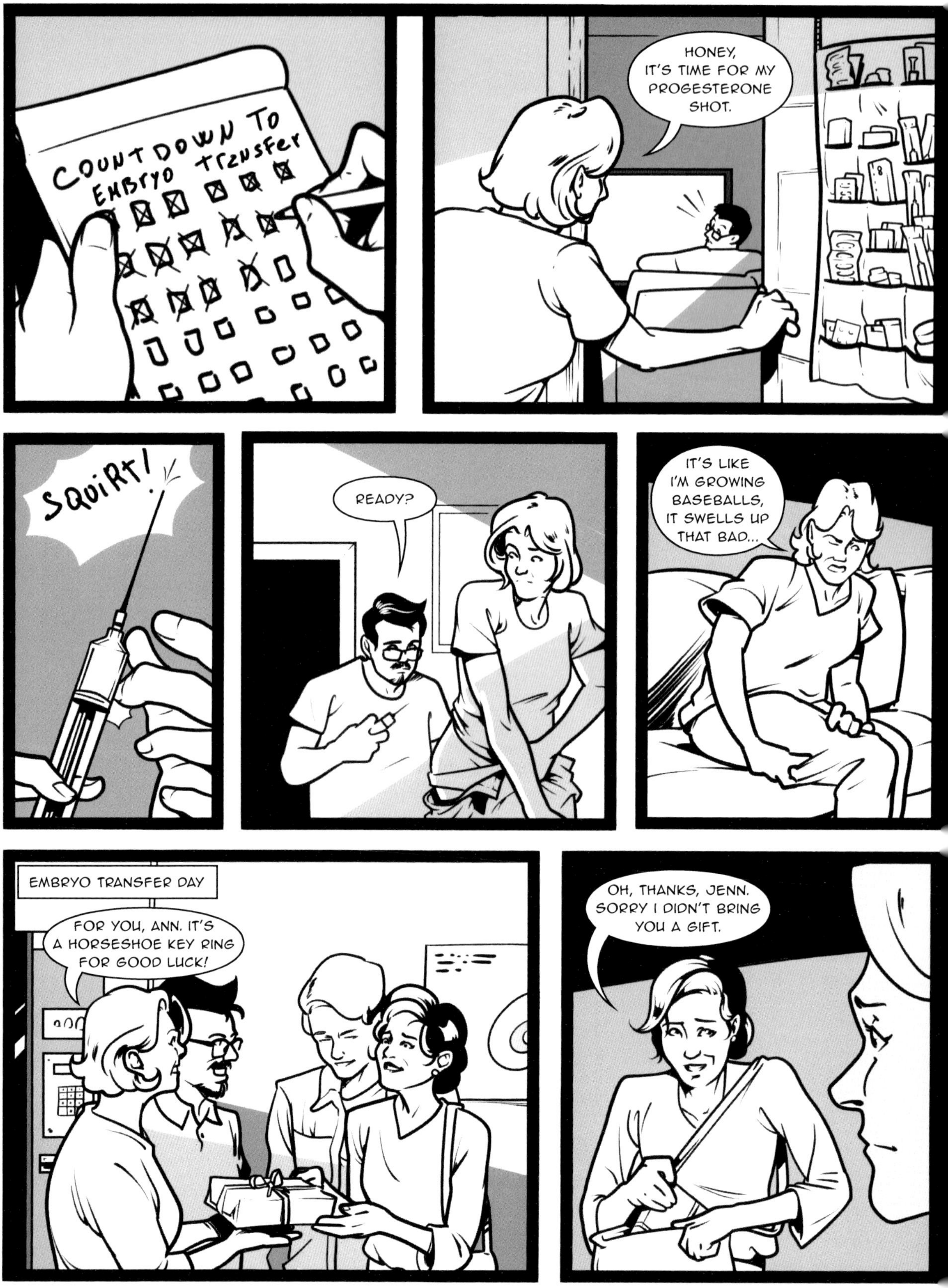
COUNTDOWN TO
EMBRYO TRANSFER
HONEY, IT'S TIME FOR MY PROGESTERONE SHOT.
SQUIRT!
READY?
IT'S LIKE I'M GROWING BASEBALLS, IT SWELLS UP THAT BAD...
EMBRYO TRANSFER DAY
FOR YOU, ANN. IT'S A HORSESHOE KEY RING FOR GOOD LUCK!
OH, THANKS, JENN. SORRY I DIDN'T BRING YOU A GIFT.

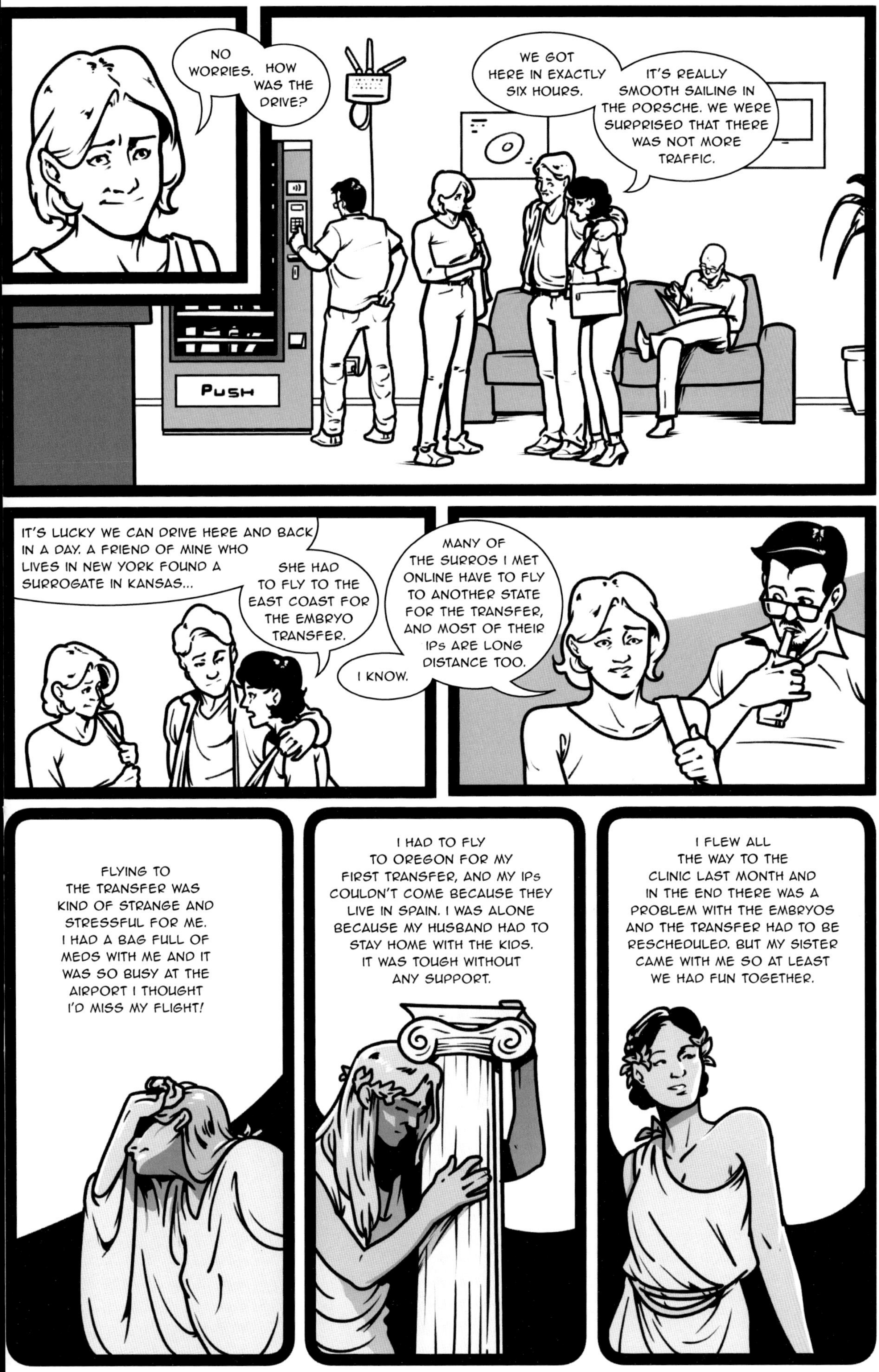
NO WORRIES. HOW WAS THE DRIVE?
WE GOT HERE IN EXACTLY SIX HOURS.
IT'S REALLY SMOOTH SAILING IN THE PORSCHE. WE WERE SURPRISED THAT THERE WAS NOT MORE TRAFFIC.
PUSH
IT'S LUCKY WE CAN DRIVE HERE AND BACK IN A DAY. A FRIEND OF MINE WHO LIVES IN NEW YORK FOUND A SURROGATE IN KANSAS...
SHE HAD TO FLY TO THE EAST COAST FOR THE EMBRYO TRANSFER.
I KNOW.
MANY OF THE SURROS I MET ONLINE HAVE TO FLY TO ANOTHER STATE FOR THE TRANSFER, AND MOST OF THEIR IPs ARE LONG DISTANCE TOO.
FLYING TO THE TRANSFER WAS KIND OF STRANGE AND STRESSFUL FOR ME. I HAD A BAG FULL OF MEDS WITH ME AND IT WAS SO BUSY AT THE AIRPORT I THOUGHT I'D MISS MY FLIGHT!
I HAD TO FLY TO OREGON FOR MY FIRST TRANSFER, AND MY IPs COULDN'T COME BECAUSE THEY LIVE IN SPAIN. I WAS ALONE BECAUSE MY HUSBAND HAD TO STAY HOME WITH THE KIDS. IT WAS TOUGH WITHOUT ANY SUPPORT.
I FLEW ALL THE WAY TO THE CLINIC LAST MONTH AND IN THE END THERE WAS A PROBLEM WITH THE EMBRYOS AND THE TRANSFER HAD TO BE RESCHEDULED. BUT MY SISTER CAME WITH ME SO AT LEAST WE HAD FUN TOGETHER.

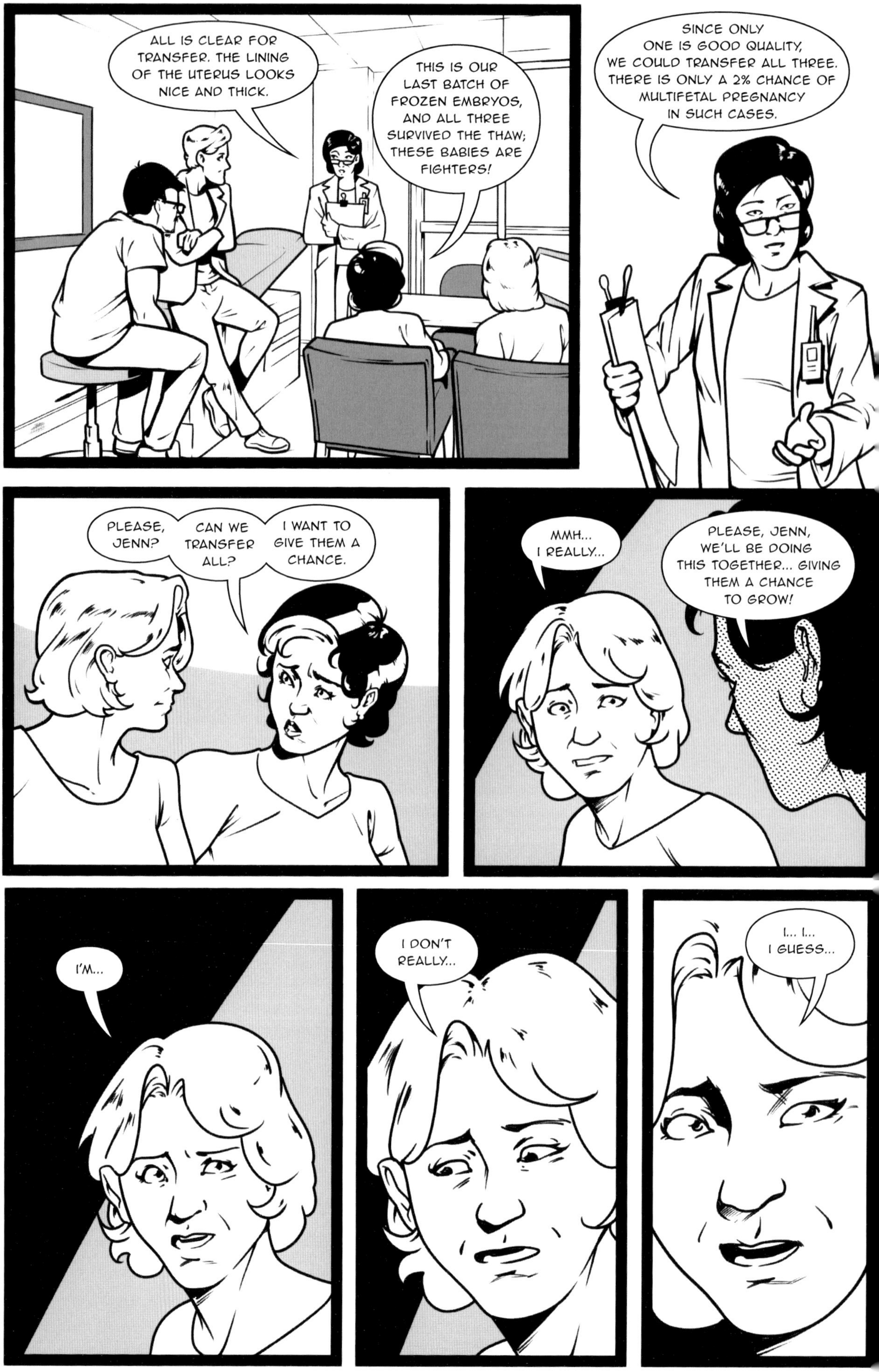
ALL IS CLEAR FOR TRANSFER. THE LINING OF THE UTERUS LOOKS NICE AND THICK.
THIS IS OUR LAST BATCH OF FROZEN EMBRYOS, AND ALL THREE SURVIVED THE THAW; THESE BABIES ARE FIGHTERS!
SINCE ONLY ONE IS GOOD QUALITY, WE COULD TRANSFER ALL THREE. THERE IS ONLY A 2% CHANCE OF MULTIFETAL PREGNANCY IN SUCH CASES.
PLEASE, JENN?
CAN WE TRANSFER ALL?
I WANT TO GIVE THEM A CHANCE.
MMH... I REALLY...
PLEASE, JENN, WE'LL BE DOING THIS TOGETHER... GIVING THEM A CHANCE TO GROW!
I'M...
I DON'T REALLY...
I... I... I GUESS...

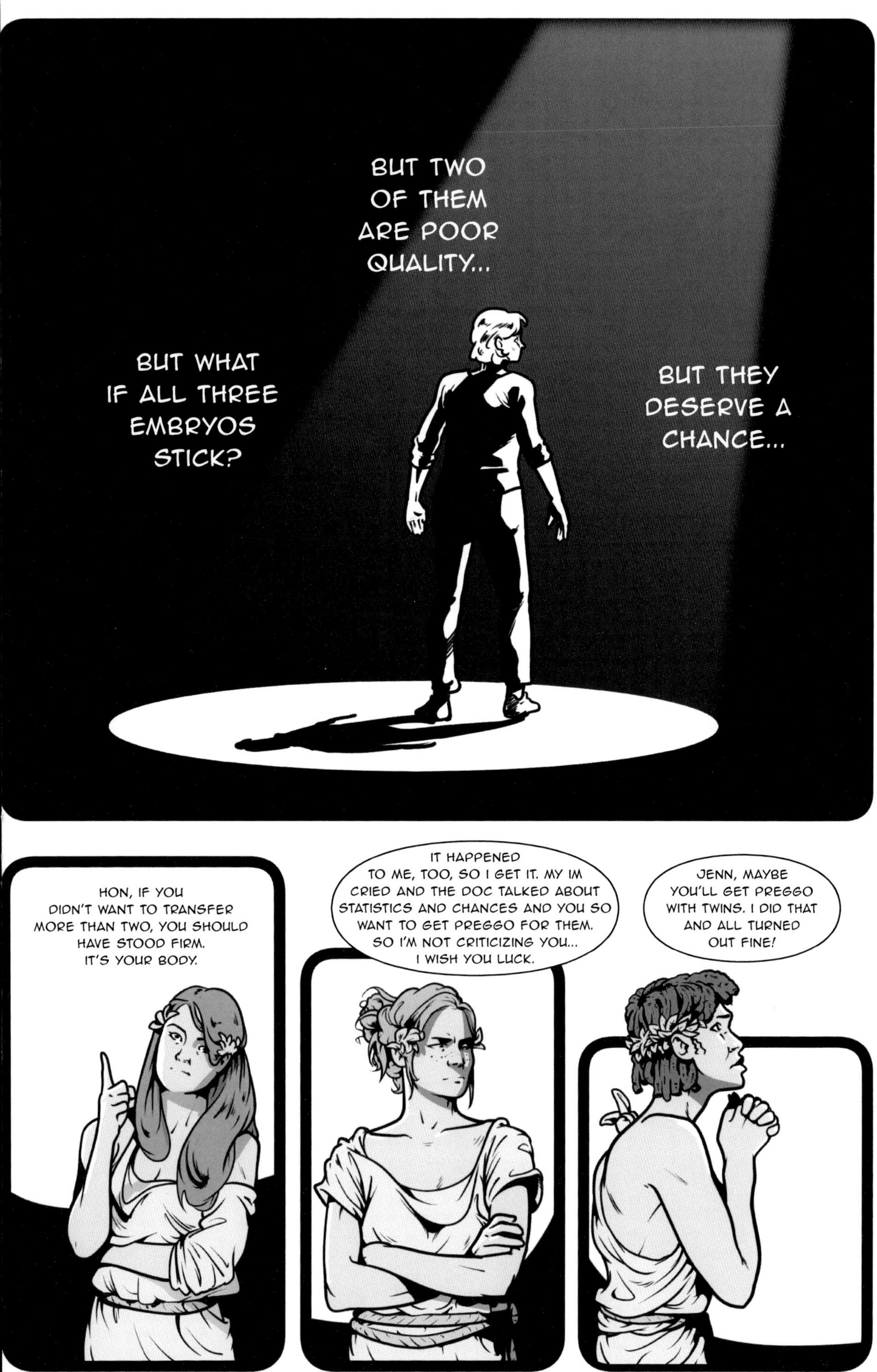
BUT TWO OF THEM ARE POOR QUALITY...
BUT WHAT IF ALL THREE EMBRYOS STICK?
BUT THEY DESERVE A CHANCE...
HON, IF YOU DIDN'T WANT TO TRANSFER MORE THAN TWO, YOU SHOULD HAVE STOOD FIRM. IT'S YOUR BODY.
IT HAPPENED TO ME, TOO, SO I GET IT. MY IM CRIED AND THE DOC TALKED ABOUT STATISTICS AND CHANCES AND YOU SO WANT TO GET PREGGO FOR THEM. SO I'M NOT CRITICIZING YOU... I WISH YOU LUCK.
JENN, MAYBE YOU'LL GET PREGGO WITH TWINS. I DID THAT AND ALL TURNED OUT FINE!

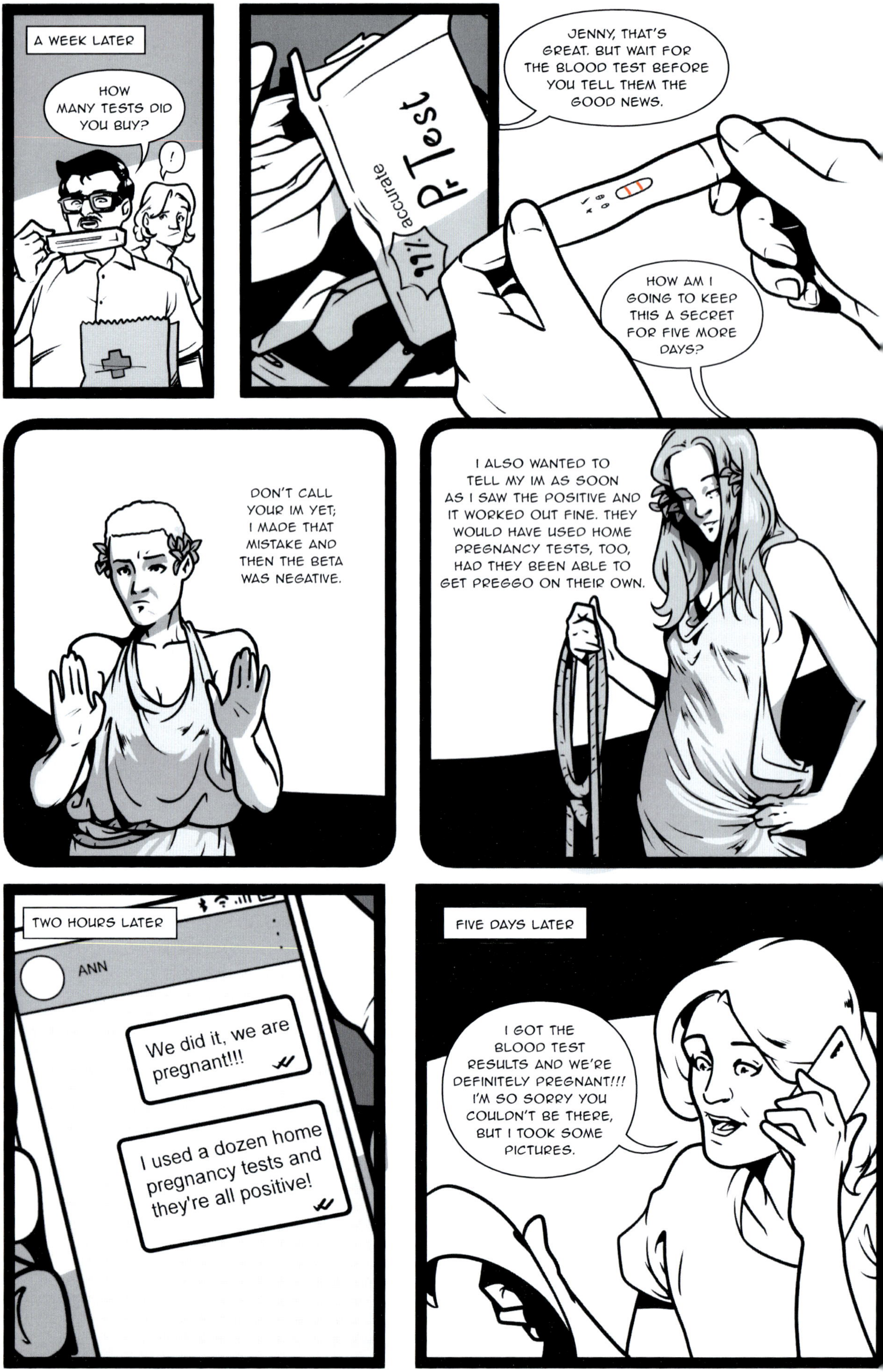
A WEEK LATER
HOW MANY TESTS DID YOU BUY?
!
accurate
Pr Test
99%
JENNY, THAT'S GREAT. BUT WAIT FOR THE BLOOD TEST BEFORE YOU TELL THEM THE GOOD NEWS.
HOW AM I GOING TO KEEP THIS A SECRET FOR FIVE MORE DAYS?
DON'T CALL YOUR IM YET; I MADE THAT MISTAKE AND THEN THE BETA WAS NEGATIVE.
I ALSO WANTED TO TELL MY IM AS SOON AS I SAW THE POSITIVE AND IT WORKED OUT FINE. THEY WOULD HAVE USED HOME PREGNANCY TESTS, TOO, HAD THEY BEEN ABLE TO GET PREGGO ON THEIR OWN.
TWO HOURS LATER
ANN
We did it, we are pregnant!!!
I used a dozen home pregnancy tests and they're all positive!
FIVE DAYS LATER
I GOT THE BLOOD TEST RESULTS AND WE'RE DEFINITELY PREGNANT!!! I'M SO SORRY YOU COULDN'T BE THERE, BUT I TOOK SOME PICTURES.

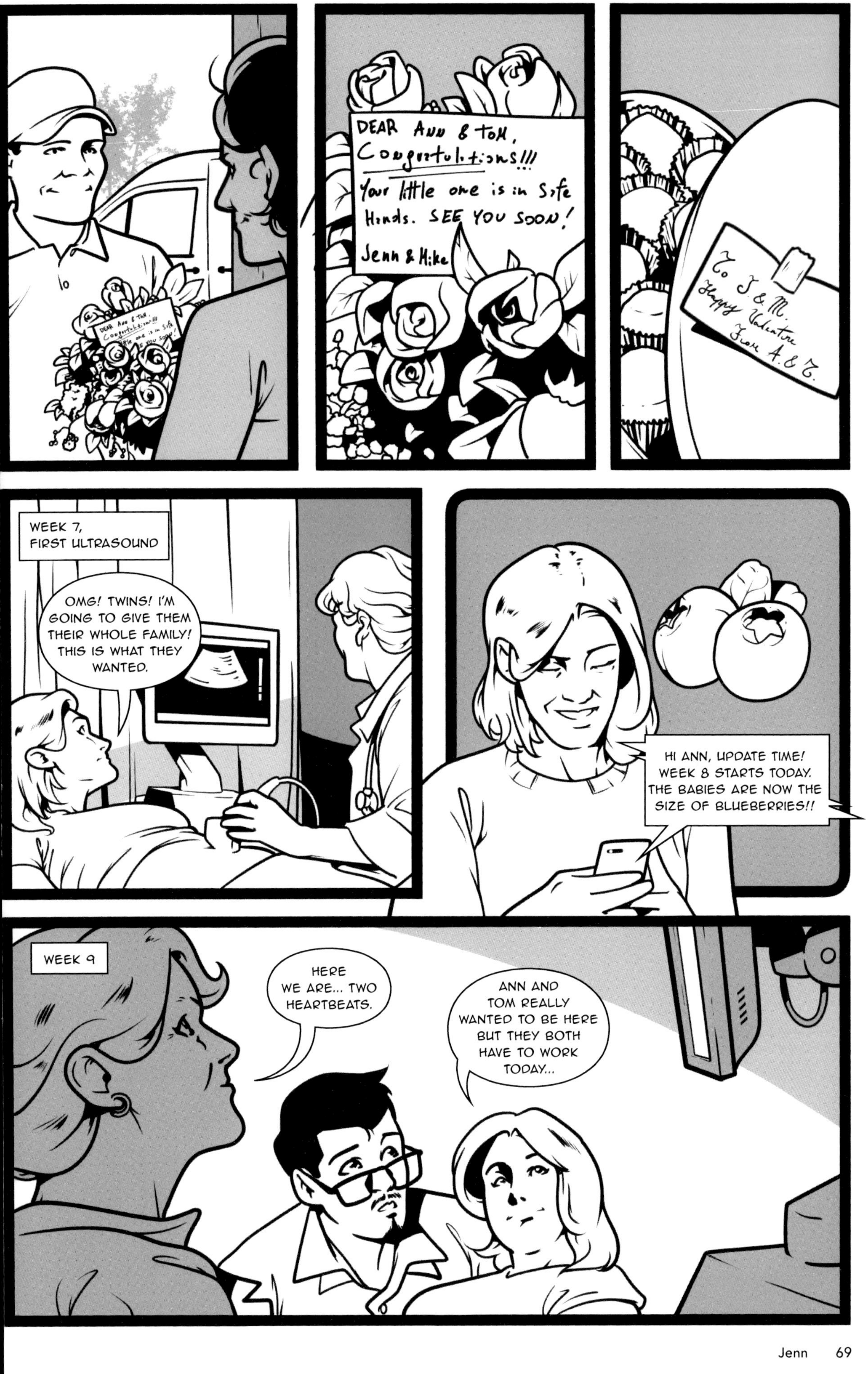
DEAR Ann & Tom,
Congratulations!!!
Your little one is in Safe Hands. SEE YOU SOON!
Jenn & Mike
To J & M.
Happy Valentine
From A & T.
WEEK 7, FIRST ULTRASOUND
OMG! TWINS! I'M GOING TO GIVE THEM THEIR WHOLE FAMILY! THIS IS WHAT THEY WANTED.
HI ANN, UPDATE TIME! WEEK 8 STARTS TODAY. THE BABIES ARE NOW THE SIZE OF BLUEBERRIES!!
WEEK 9
HERE WE ARE... TWO HEARTBEATS.
ANN AND TOM REALLY WANTED TO BE HERE BUT THEY BOTH HAVE TO WORK TODAY...

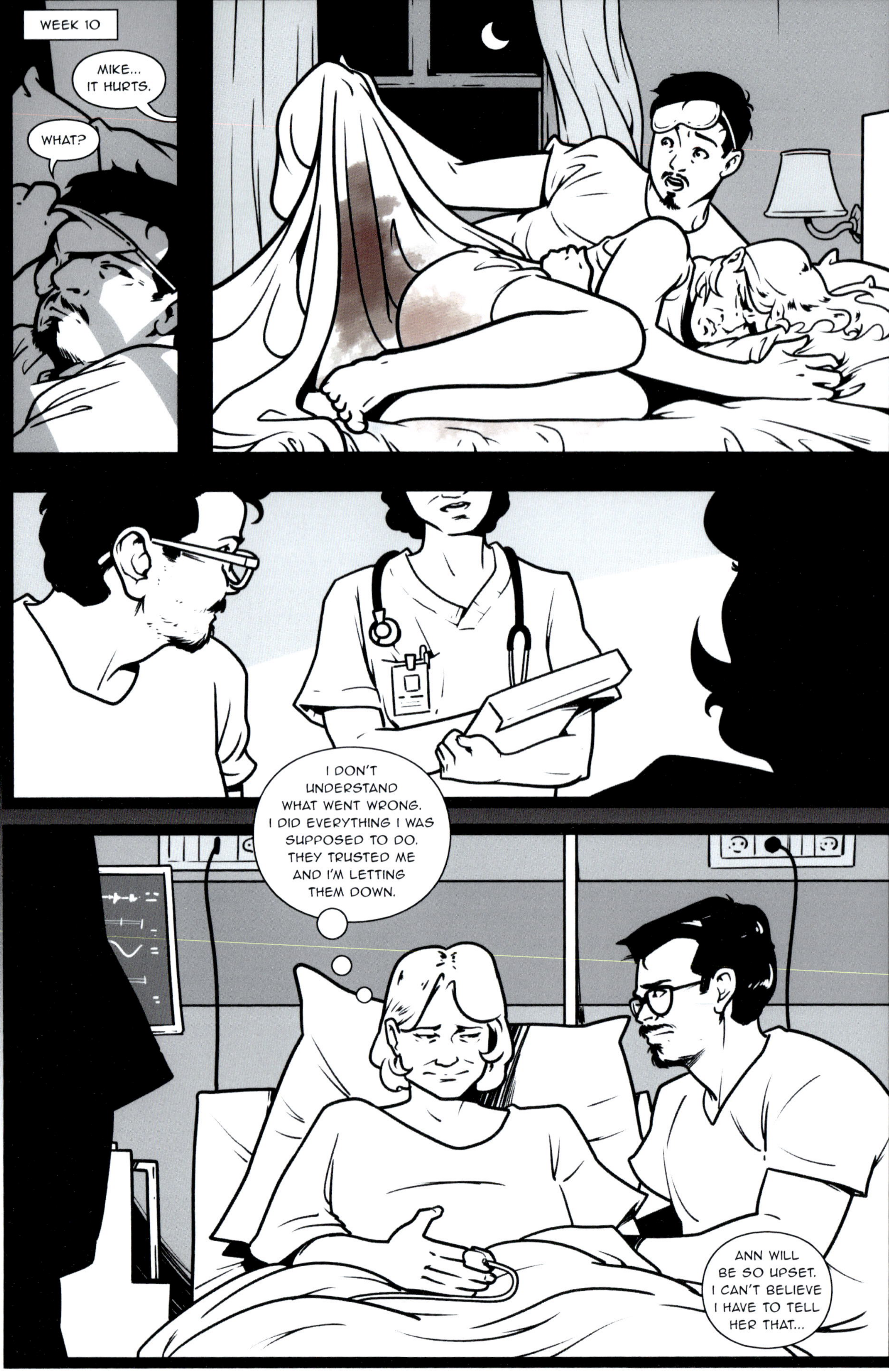
WEEK 10
MIKE... IT HURTS.
WHAT?
I DON'T UNDERSTAND WHAT WENT WRONG. I DID EVERYTHING I WAS SUPPOSED TO DO. THEY TRUSTED ME AND I'M LETTING THEM DOWN.
ANN WILL BE SO UPSET. I CAN'T BELIEVE I HAVE TO TELL HER THAT...

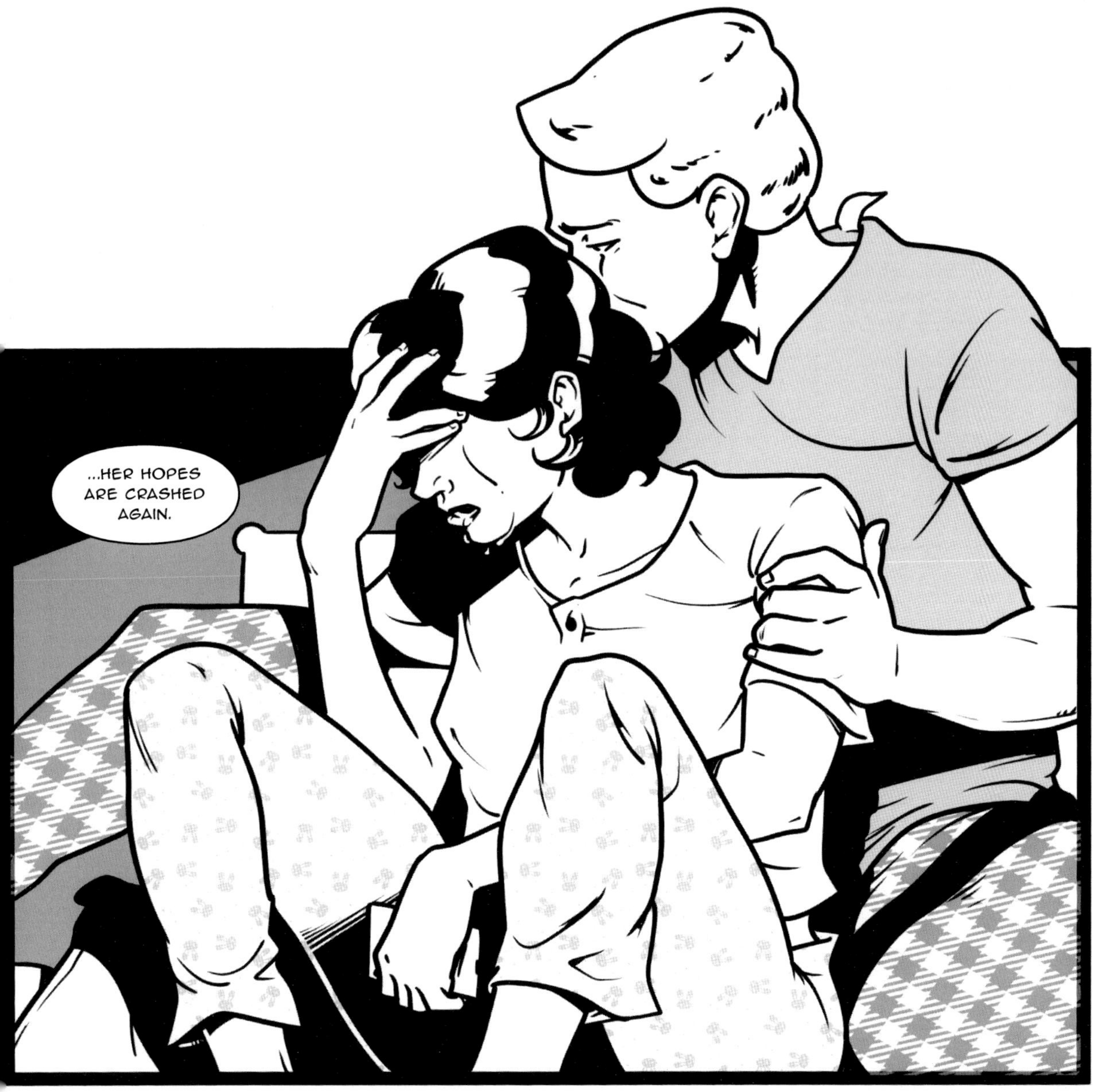
...HER HOPES ARE CRASHED AGAIN.

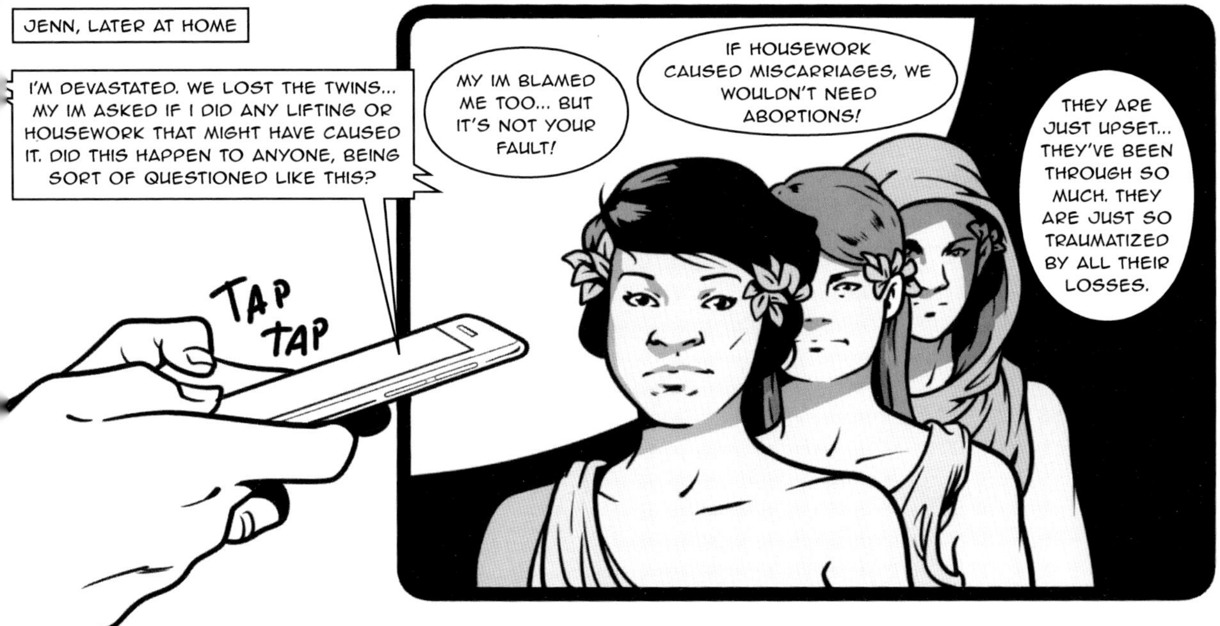
JENN, LATER AT HOME
I'M DEVASTATED. WE LOST THE TWINS... MY IM ASKED IF I DID ANY LIFTING OR HOUSEWORK THAT MIGHT HAVE CAUSED IT. DID THIS HAPPEN TO ANYONE, BEING SORT OF QUESTIONED LIKE THIS?
TAP TAP
MY IM BLAMED ME TOO... BUT IT'S NOT YOUR FAULT!
IF HOUSEWORK CAUSED MISCARRIAGES, WE WOULDN'T NEED ABORTIONS!
THEY ARE JUST UPSET... THEY'VE BEEN THROUGH SO MUCH. THEY ARE JUST SO TRAUMATIZED BY ALL THEIR LOSSES.

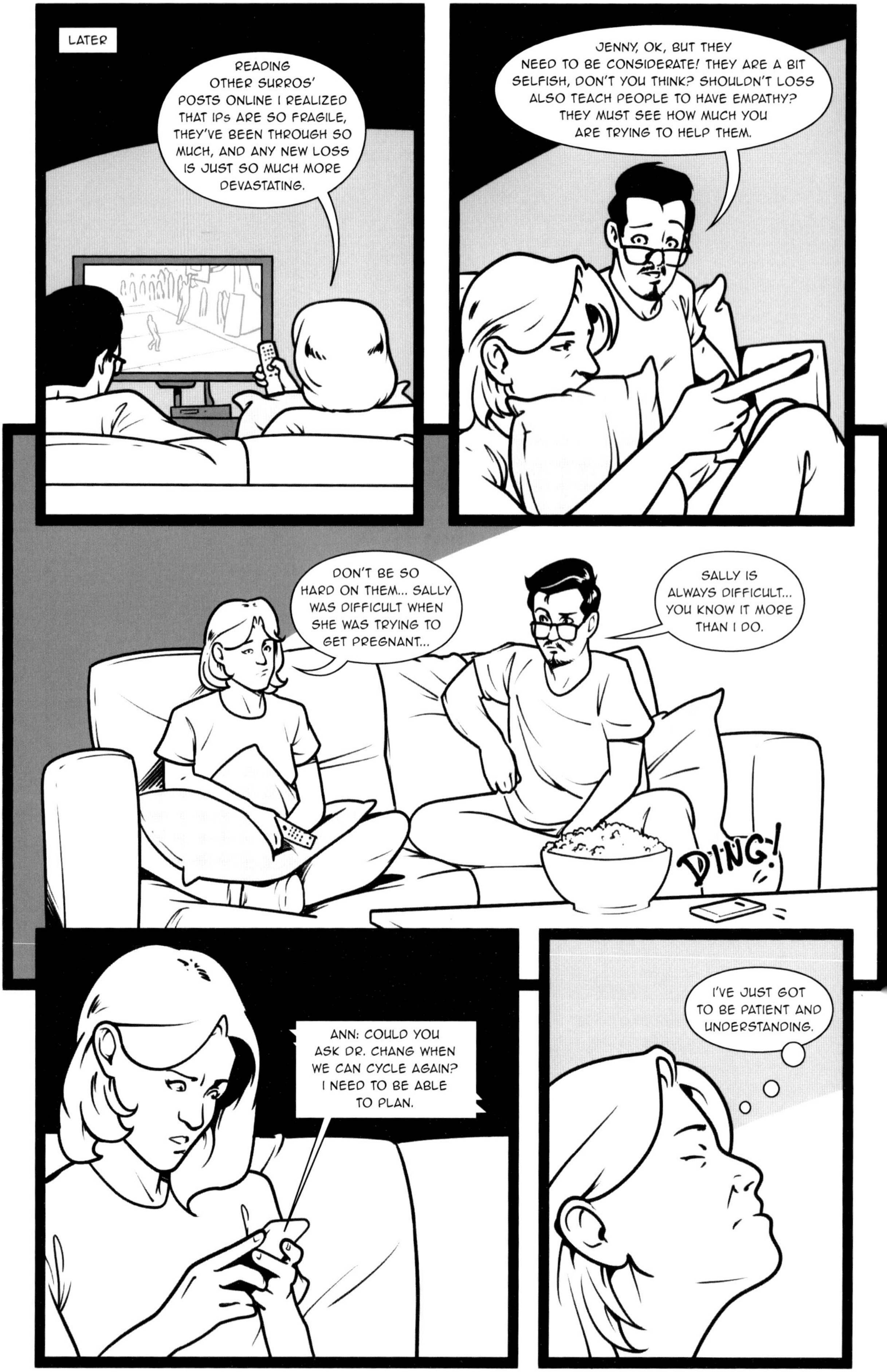
LATER
READING OTHER SURROS' POSTS ONLINE I REALIZED THAT IPs ARE SO FRAGILE, THEY'VE BEEN THROUGH SO MUCH, AND ANY NEW LOSS IS JUST SO MUCH MORE DEVASTATING.
JENNY, OK, BUT THEY NEED TO BE CONSIDERATE! THEY ARE A BIT SELFISH, DON'T YOU THINK? SHOULDN'T LOSS ALSO TEACH PEOPLE TO HAVE EMPATHY? THEY MUST SEE HOW MUCH YOU ARE TRYING TO HELP THEM.
DON'T BE SO HARD ON THEM... SALLY WAS DIFFICULT WHEN SHE WAS TRYING TO GET PREGNANT...
SALLY IS ALWAYS DIFFICULT... YOU KNOW IT MORE THAN I DO.
DING!
ANN: COULD YOU ASK DR. CHANG WHEN WE CAN CYCLE AGAIN? I NEED TO BE ABLE TO PLAN.
I'VE JUST GOT TO BE PATIENT AND UNDERSTANDING.

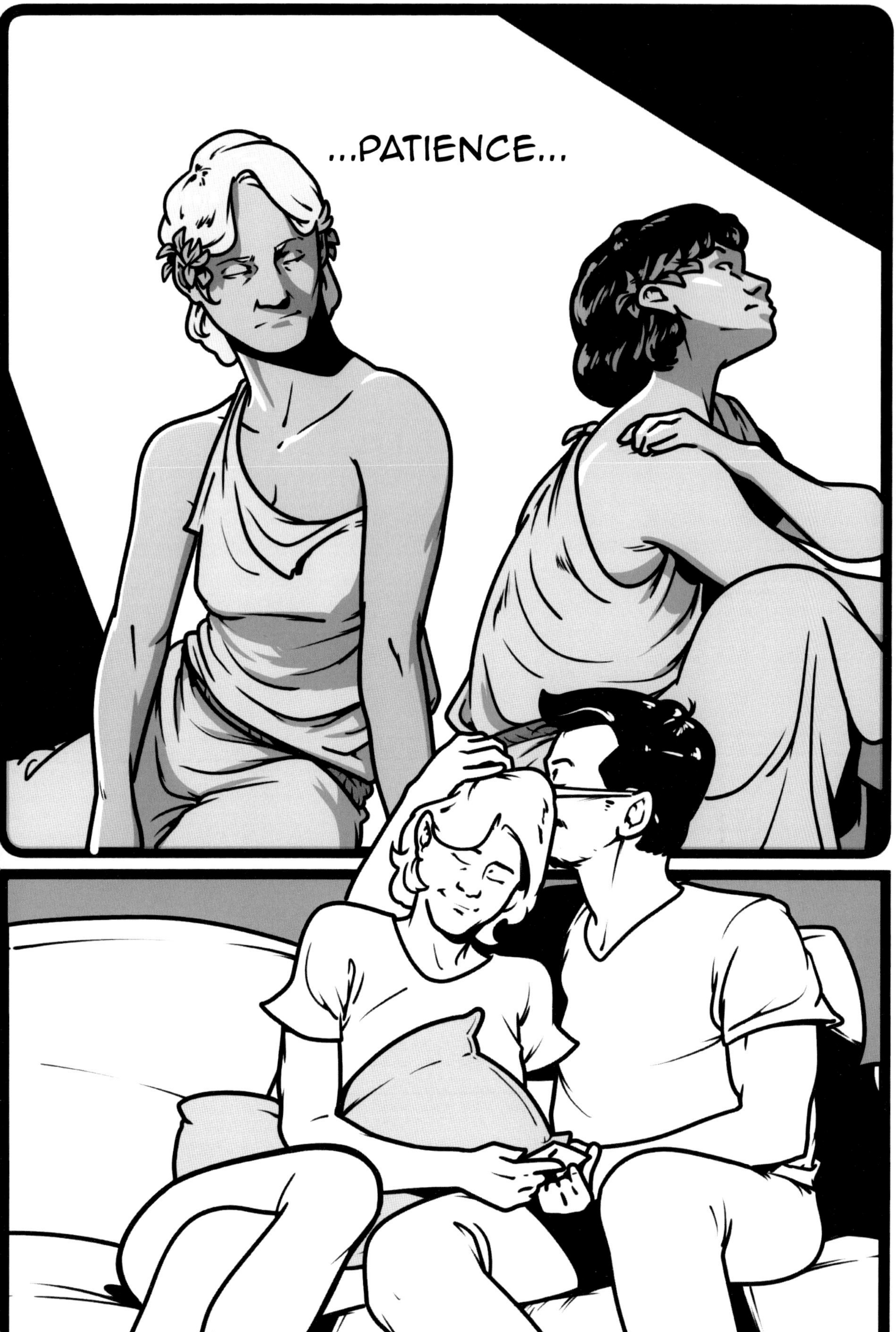
...PATIENCE...

INTERLUDE: PETER AND BEN, IPs FROM AUSTRALIA

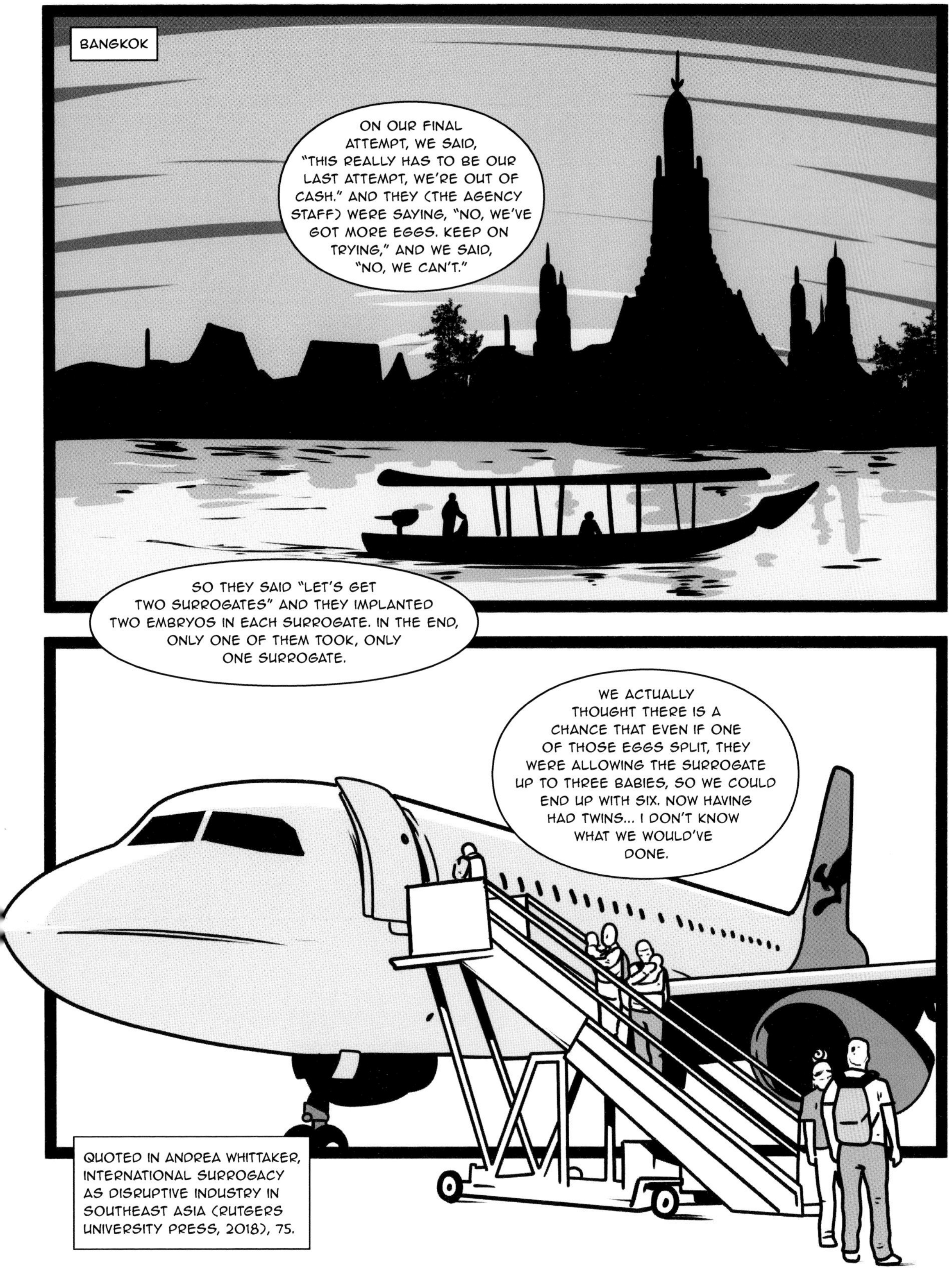
BANGKOK
ON OUR FINAL ATTEMPT, WE SAID, "THIS REALLY HAS TO BE OUR LAST ATTEMPT, WE'RE OUT OF CASH." AND THEY (THE AGENCY STAFF) WERE SAYING, "NO, WE'VE GOT MORE EGGS. KEEP ON TRYING," AND WE SAID, "NO, WE CAN'T."
SO THEY SAID "LET'S GET TWO SURROGATES" AND THEY IMPLANTED TWO EMBRYOS IN EACH SURROGATE. IN THE END, ONLY ONE OF THEM TOOK, ONLY ONE SURROGATE.
WE ACTUALLY THOUGHT THERE IS A CHANCE THAT EVEN IF ONE OF THOSE EGGS SPLIT, THEY WERE ALLOWING THE SURROGATE UP TO THREE BABIES, SO WE COULD END UP WITH SIX. NOW HAVING HAD TWINS... I DON'T KNOW WHAT WE WOULD'VE DONE.

QUOTED IN ANDREA WHITTAKER, INTERNATIONAL SURROGACY AS DISRUPTIVE INDUSTRY IN SOUTHEAST ASIA (RUTGERS UNIVERSITY PRESS, 2018), 75.

-CHAPTER 9-
ROLLER COASTER

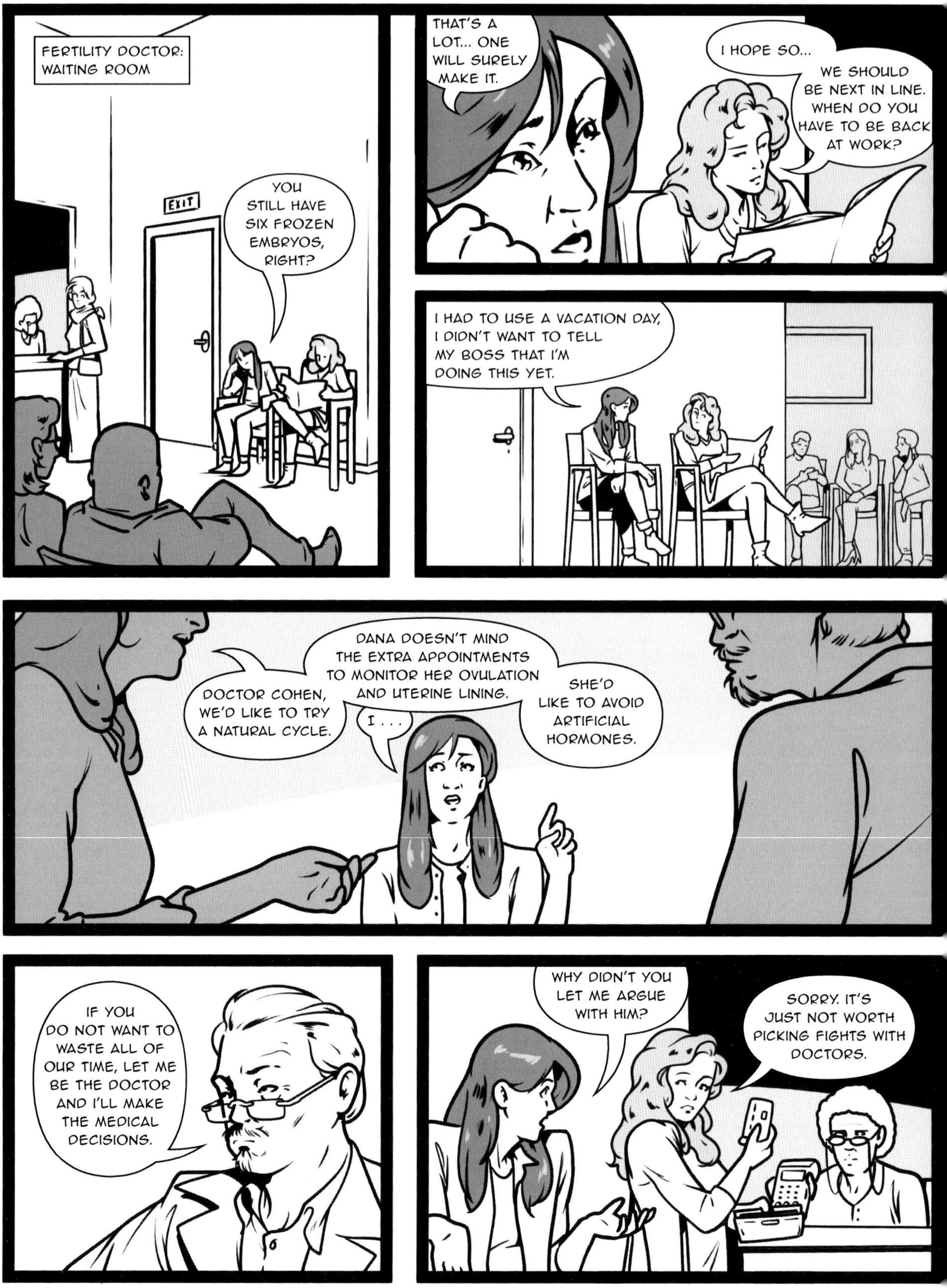
FERTILITY DOCTOR: WAITING ROOM
YOU STILL HAVE SIX FROZEN EMBRYOS, RIGHT?
EXIT
THAT'S A LOT... ONE WILL SURELY MAKE IT.
I HOPE SO...
WE SHOULD BE NEXT IN LINE. WHEN DO YOU HAVE TO BE BACK AT WORK?
I HAD TO USE A VACATION DAY, I DIDN'T WANT TO TELL MY BOSS THAT I'M DOING THIS YET.
DOCTOR COHEN, WE'D LIKE TO TRY A NATURAL CYCLE.
I . . .
DANA DOESN'T MIND THE EXTRA APPOINTMENTS TO MONITOR HER OVULATION AND UTERINE LINING.
SHE'D LIKE TO AVOID ARTIFICIAL HORMONES.
IF YOU DO NOT WANT TO WASTE ALL OF OUR TIME, LET ME BE THE DOCTOR AND I'LL MAKE THE MEDICAL DECISIONS.
WHY DIDN'T YOU LET ME ARGUE WITH HIM?
SORRY. IT'S JUST NOT WORTH PICKING FIGHTS WITH DOCTORS.

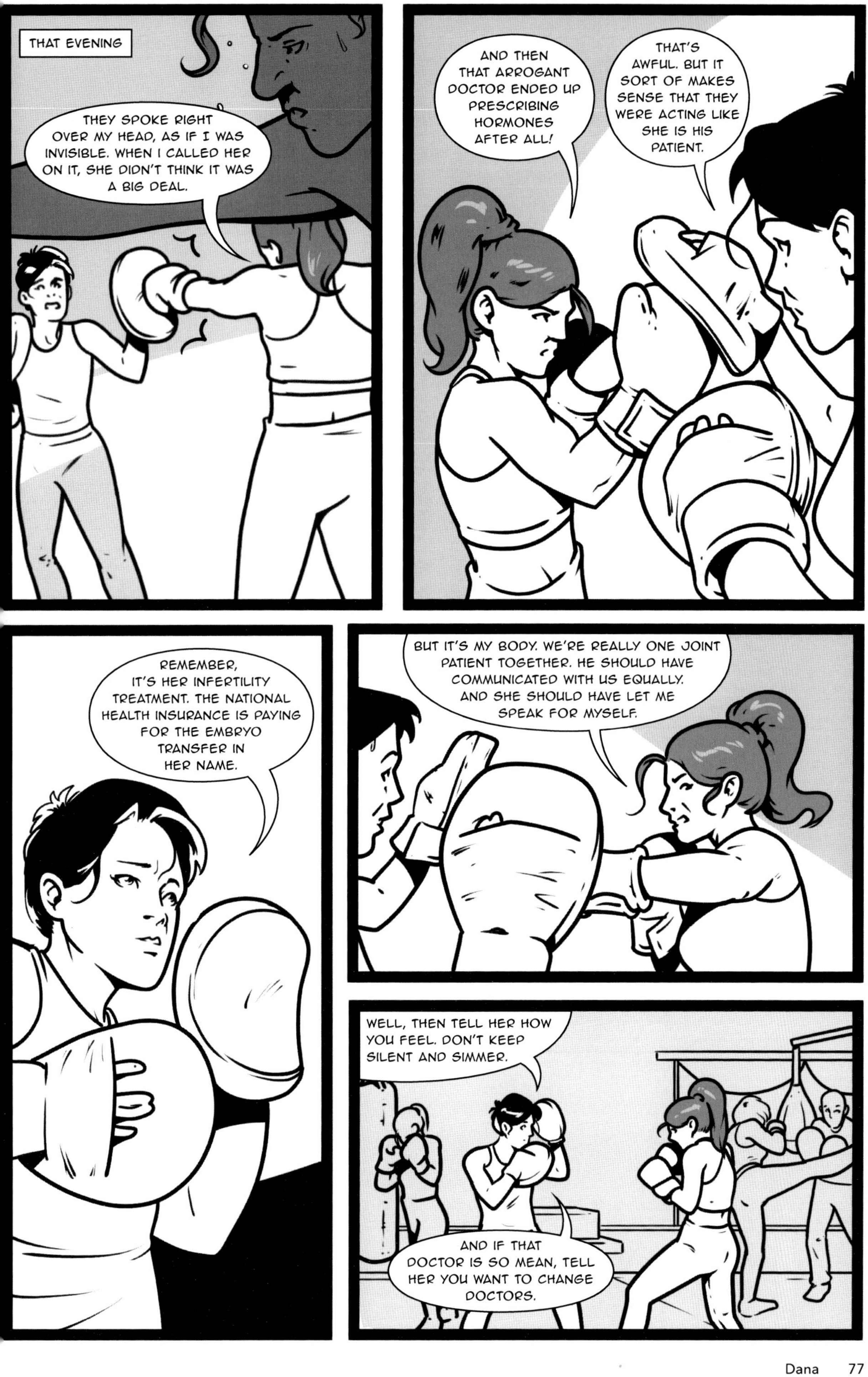
THAT EVENING
THEY SPOKE RIGHT OVER MY HEAD, AS IF I WAS INVISIBLE. WHEN I CALLED HER ON IT, SHE DIDN'T THINK IT WAS A BIG DEAL.
AND THEN THAT ARROGANT DOCTOR ENDED UP PRESCRIBING HORMONES AFTER ALL!
THAT'S AWFUL. BUT IT SORT OF MAKES SENSE THAT THEY WERE ACTING LIKE SHE IS HIS PATIENT.
REMEMBER, IT'S HER INFERTILITY TREATMENT. THE NATIONAL HEALTH INSURANCE IS PAYING FOR THE EMBRYO TRANSFER IN HER NAME.
BUT IT'S MY BODY. WE'RE REALLY ONE JOINT PATIENT TOGETHER. HE SHOULD HAVE COMMUNICATED WITH US EQUALLY. AND SHE SHOULD HAVE LET ME SPEAK FOR MYSELF.
WELL, THEN TELL HER HOW YOU FEEL. DON'T KEEP SILENT AND SIMMER.
AND IF THAT DOCTOR IS SO MEAN, TELL HER YOU WANT TO CHANGE DOCTORS.

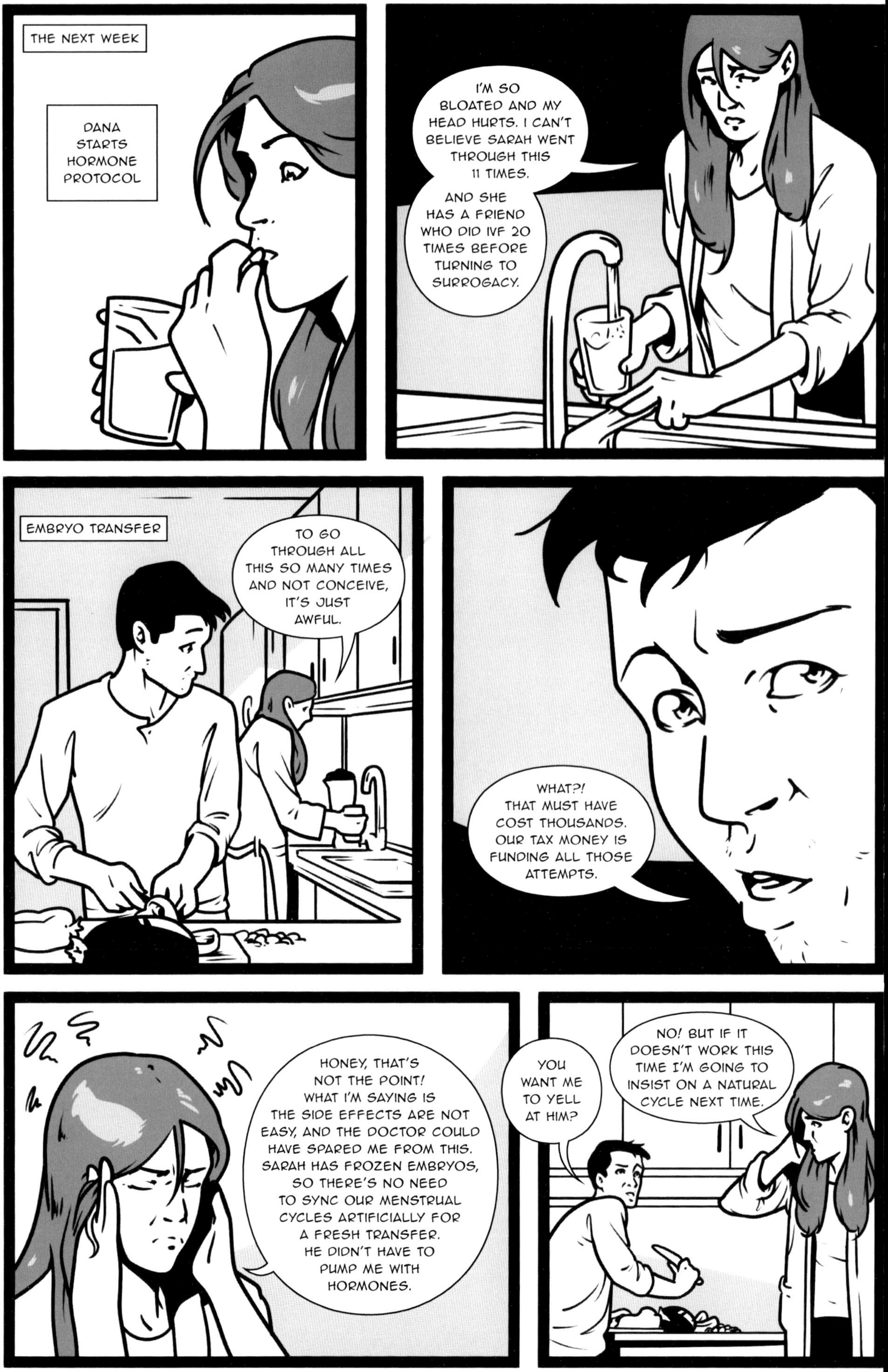
THE NEXT WEEK
DANA STARTS HORMONE PROTOCOL
I'M SO BLOATED AND MY HEAD HURTS. I CAN'T BELIEVE SARAH WENT THROUGH THIS 11 TIMES.
AND SHE HAS A FRIEND WHO DID IVF 20 TIMES BEFORE TURNING TO SURROGACY.
EMBRYO TRANSFER
TO GO THROUGH ALL THIS SO MANY TIMES AND NOT CONCEIVE, IT'S JUST AWFUL.
WHAT?! THAT MUST HAVE COST THOUSANDS. OUR TAX MONEY IS FUNDING ALL THOSE ATTEMPTS.
HONEY, THAT'S NOT THE POINT! WHAT I'M SAYING IS THE SIDE EFFECTS ARE NOT EASY, AND THE DOCTOR COULD HAVE SPARED ME FROM THIS. SARAH HAS FROZEN EMBRYOS, SO THERE'S NO NEED TO SYNC OUR MENSTRUAL CYCLES ARTIFICIALLY FOR A FRESH TRANSFER. HE DIDN'T HAVE TO PUMP ME WITH HORMONES.
YOU WANT ME TO YELL AT HIM?
NO! BUT IF IT DOESN'T WORK THIS TIME I'M GOING TO INSIST ON A NATURAL CYCLE NEXT TIME.

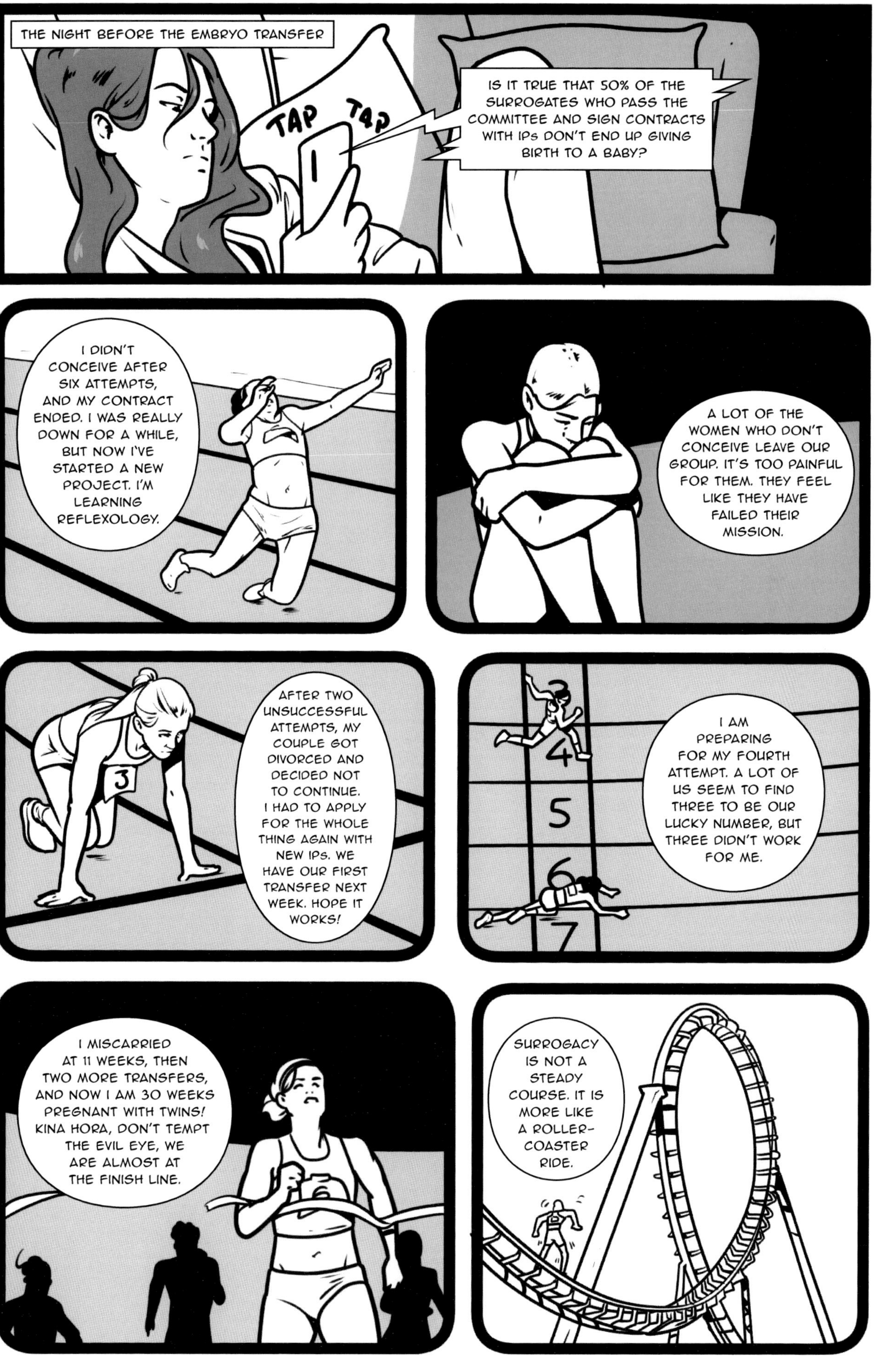
THE NIGHT BEFORE THE EMBRYO TRANSFER
TAP TAP
IS IT TRUE THAT 50% OF THE SURROGATES WHO PASS THE COMMITTEE AND SIGN CONTRACTS WITH IPs DON'T END UP GIVING BIRTH TO A BABY?
I DIDN'T CONCEIVE AFTER SIX ATTEMPTS, AND MY CONTRACT ENDED. I WAS REALLY DOWN FOR A WHILE, BUT NOW I'VE STARTED A NEW PROJECT. I'M LEARNING REFLEXOLOGY.
A LOT OF THE WOMEN WHO DON'T CONCEIVE LEAVE OUR GROUP. IT'S TOO PAINFUL FOR THEM. THEY FEEL LIKE THEY HAVE FAILED THEIR MISSION.
3
AFTER TWO UNSUCCESSFUL ATTEMPTS, MY COUPLE GOT DIVORCED AND DECIDED NOT TO CONTINUE. I HAD TO APPLY FOR THE WHOLE THING AGAIN WITH NEW IPs. WE HAVE OUR FIRST TRANSFER NEXT WEEK. HOPE IT WORKS!
3
4
5
6
7
I AM PREPARING FOR MY FOURTH ATTEMPT. A LOT OF US SEEM TO FIND THREE TO BE OUR LUCKY NUMBER, BUT THREE DIDN'T WORK FOR ME.
I MISCARRIED AT 11 WEEKS, THEN TWO MORE TRANSFERS, AND NOW I AM 30 WEEKS PREGNANT WITH TWINS! KINA HORA, DON'T TEMPT THE EVIL EYE, WE ARE ALMOST AT THE FINISH LINE.
SURROGACY IS NOT A STEADY COURSE. IT IS MORE LIKE A ROLLER-COASTER RIDE.

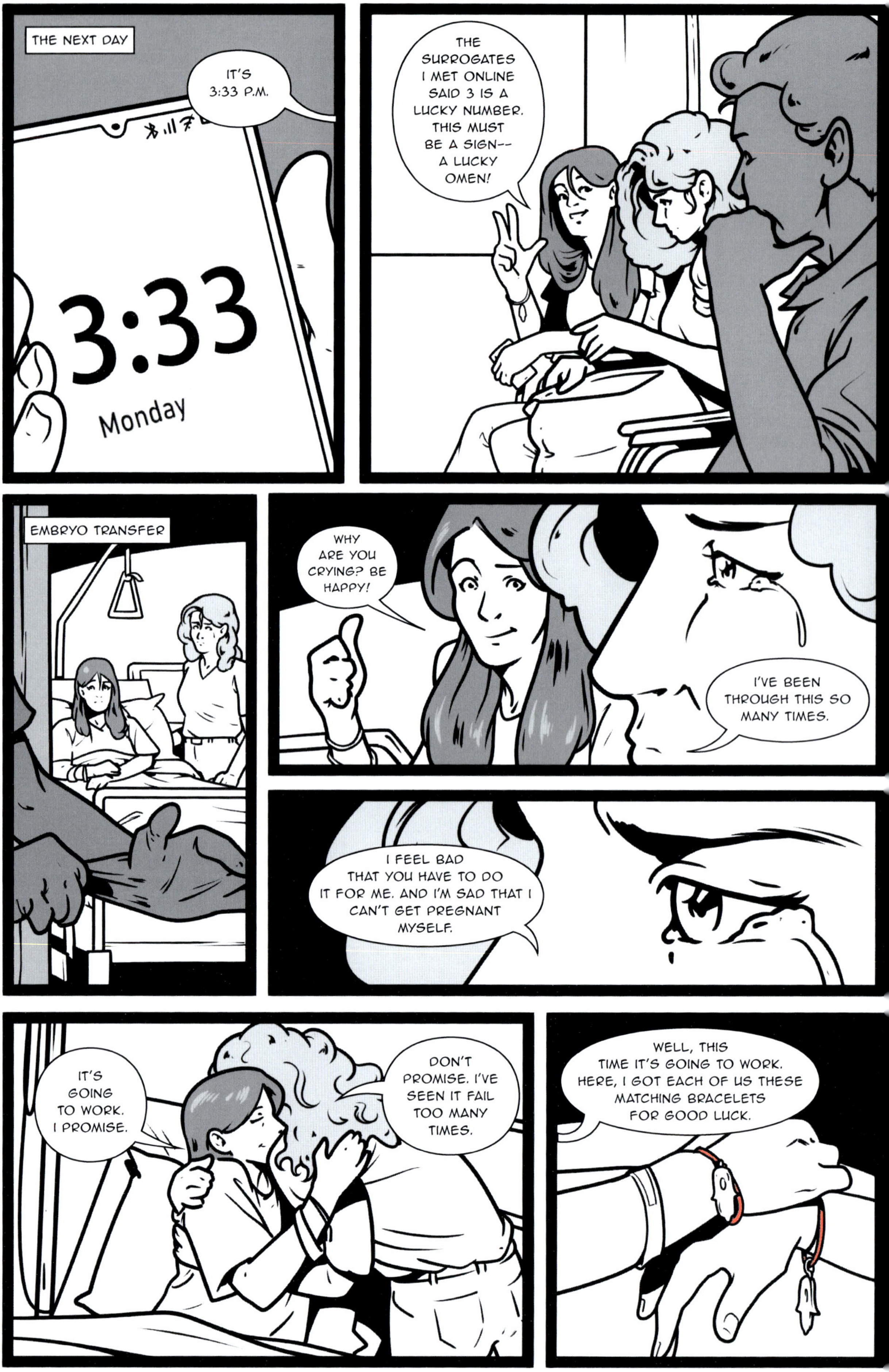
THE NEXT DAY
IT'S 3:33 P.M.
3:33
Monday
THE SURROGATES I MET ONLINE SAID 3 IS A LUCKY NUMBER. THIS MUST BE A SIGN-- A LUCKY OMEN!
EMBRYO TRANSFER
WHY ARE YOU CRYING? BE HAPPY!
I'VE BEEN THROUGH THIS SO MANY TIMES.
I FEEL BAD THAT YOU HAVE TO DO IT FOR ME. AND I'M SAD THAT I CAN'T GET PREGNANT MYSELF.
IT'S GOING TO WORK. I PROMISE.
DON'T PROMISE. I'VE SEEN IT FAIL TOO MANY TIMES.
WELL, THIS TIME IT'S GOING TO WORK. HERE, I GOT EACH OF US THESE MATCHING BRACELETS FOR GOOD LUCK.

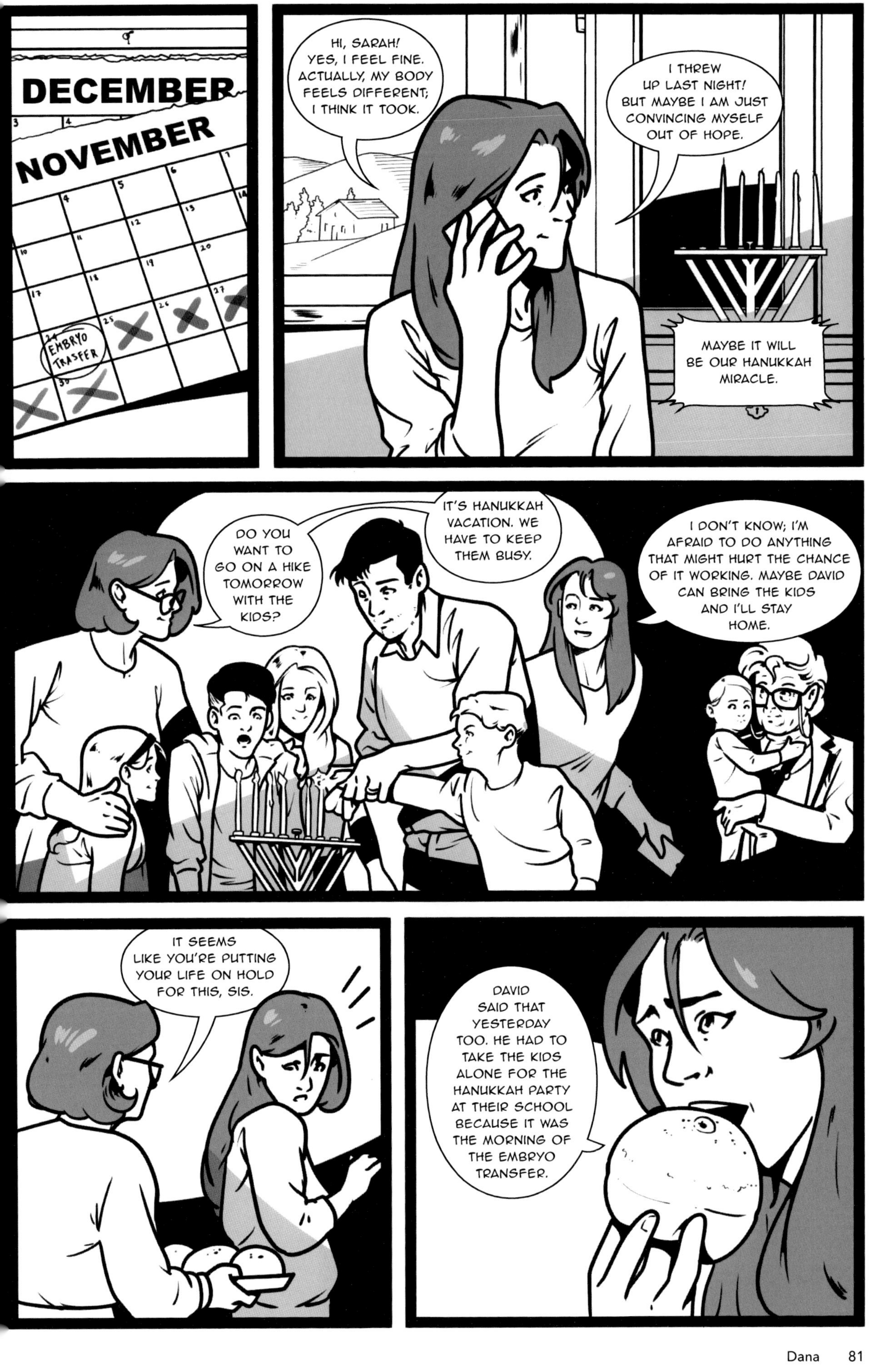
DECEMBER
NOVEMBER
EMBRYO TRASFER
HI, SARAH! YES, I FEEL FINE. ACTUALLY, MY BODY FEELS DIFFERENT; I THINK IT TOOK.
I THREW UP LAST NIGHT! BUT MAYBE I AM JUST CONVINCING MYSELF OUT OF HOPE.
MAYBE IT WILL BE OUR HANUKKAH MIRACLE.
DO YOU WANT TO GO ON A HIKE TOMORROW WITH THE KIDS?
IT'S HANUKKAH VACATION. WE HAVE TO KEEP THEM BUSY.
I DON'T KNOW; I'M AFRAID TO DO ANYTHING THAT MIGHT HURT THE CHANCE OF IT WORKING. MAYBE DAVID CAN BRING THE KIDS AND I'LL STAY HOME.
IT SEEMS LIKE YOU'RE PUTTING YOUR LIFE ON HOLD FOR THIS, SIS.
DAVID SAID THAT YESTERDAY TOO. HE HAD TO TAKE THE KIDS ALONE FOR THE HANUKKAH PARTY AT THEIR SCHOOL BECAUSE IT WAS THE MORNING OF THE EMBRYO TRANSFER.

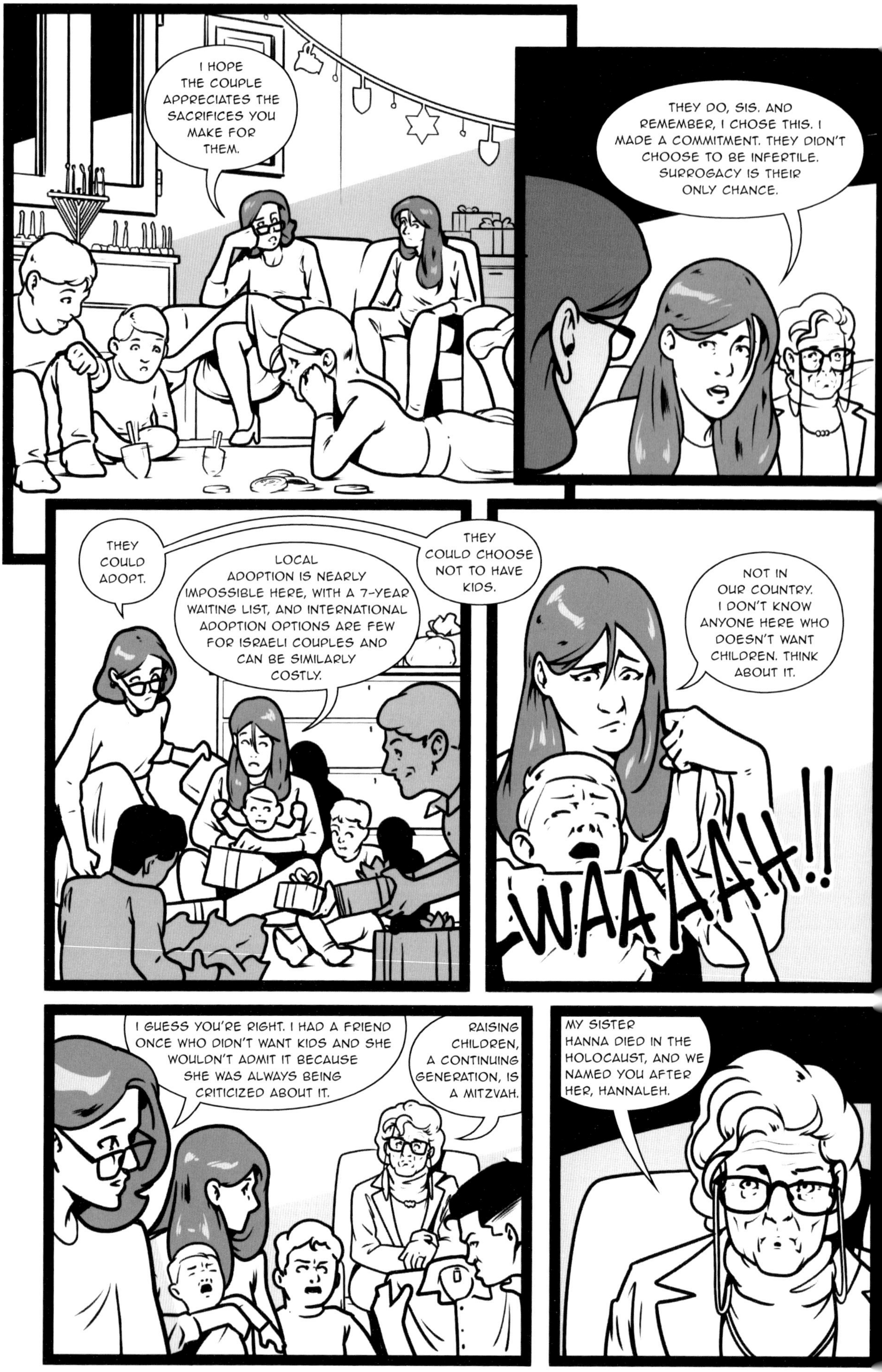
I HOPE THE COUPLE APPRECIATES THE SACRIFICES YOU MAKE FOR THEM.
THEY DO, SIS. AND REMEMBER, I CHOSE THIS. I MADE A COMMITMENT. THEY DIDN'T CHOOSE TO BE INFERTILE. SURROGACY IS THEIR ONLY CHANCE.
THEY COULD ADOPT.
THEY COULD CHOOSE NOT TO HAVE KIDS.
LOCAL ADOPTION IS NEARLY IMPOSSIBLE HERE, WITH A 7-YEAR WAITING LIST, AND INTERNATIONAL ADOPTION OPTIONS ARE FEW FOR ISRAELI COUPLES AND CAN BE SIMILARLY COSTLY.
NOT IN OUR COUNTRY. I DON'T KNOW ANYONE HERE WHO DOESN'T WANT CHILDREN. THINK ABOUT IT.
WAAAAH!!
I GUESS YOU'RE RIGHT. I HAD A FRIEND ONCE WHO DIDN'T WANT KIDS AND SHE WOULDN'T ADMIT IT BECAUSE SHE WAS ALWAYS BEING CRITICIZED ABOUT IT.
RAISING CHILDREN, A CONTINUING GENERATION, IS A MITZVAH.
MY SISTER HANNA DIED IN THE HOLOCAUST, AND WE NAMED YOU AFTER HER, HANNALEH.

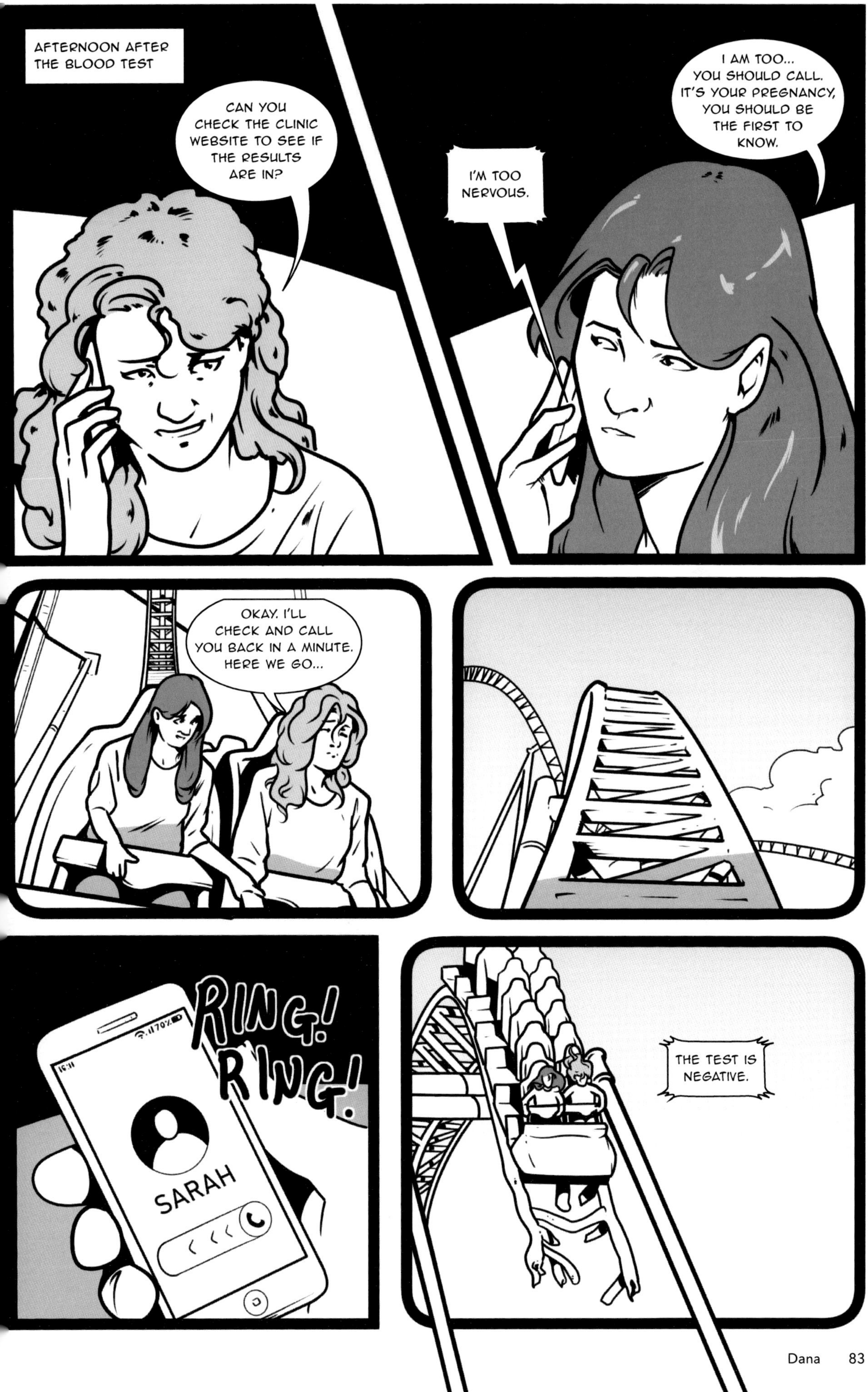
AFTERNOON AFTER THE BLOOD TEST
CAN YOU CHECK THE CLINIC WEBSITE TO SEE IF THE RESULTS ARE IN?
I'M TOO NERVOUS.
I AM TOO... YOU SHOULD CALL. IT'S YOUR PREGNANCY, YOU SHOULD BE THE FIRST TO KNOW.
OKAY. I'LL CHECK AND CALL YOU BACK IN A MINUTE. HERE WE GO...
RING! RING!
SARAH
THE TEST IS NEGATIVE.

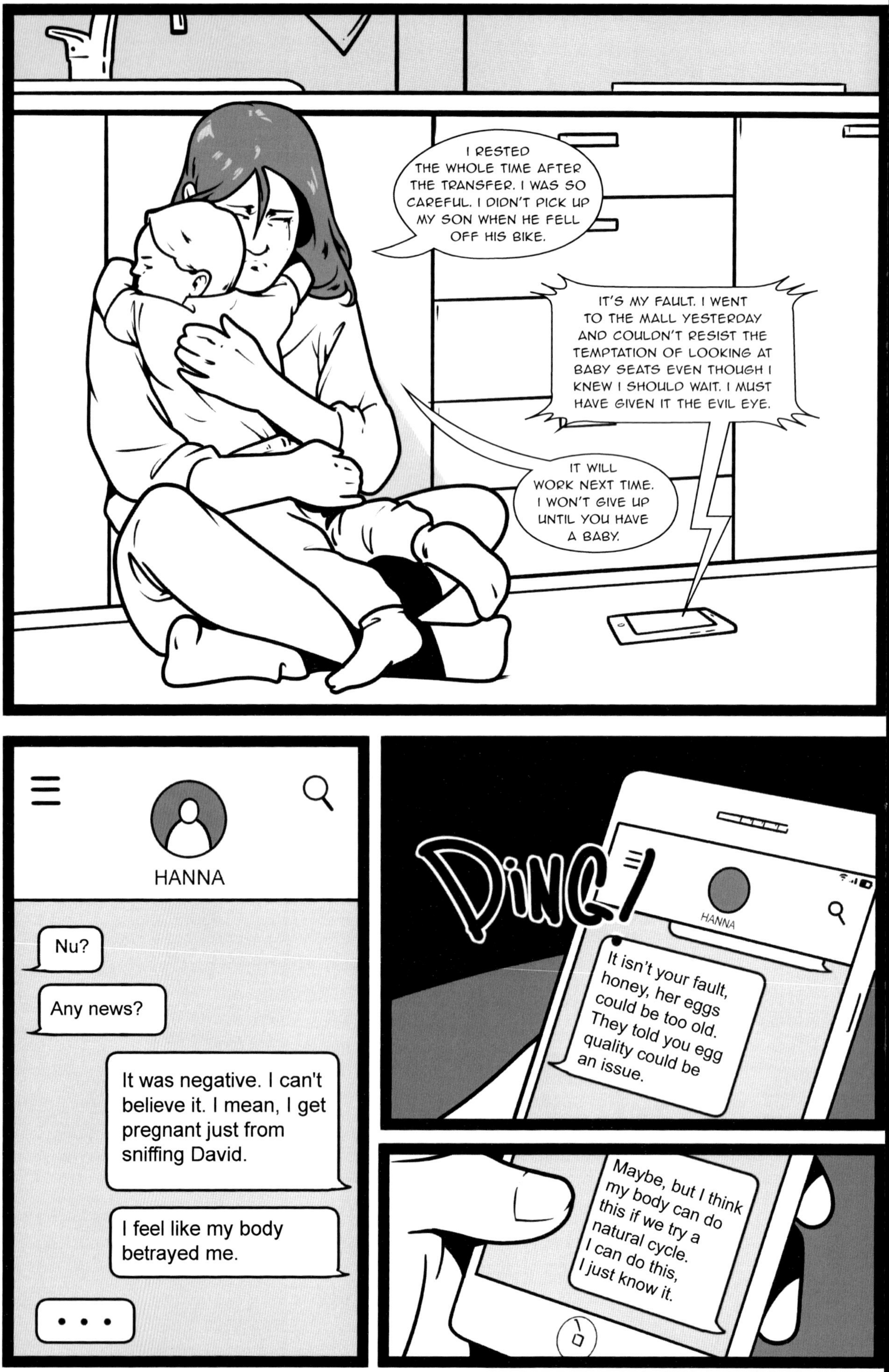
I RESTED THE WHOLE TIME AFTER THE TRANSFER. I WAS SO CAREFUL. I DIDN'T PICK UP MY SON WHEN HE FELL OFF HIS BIKE.
IT'S MY FAULT. I WENT TO THE MALL YESTERDAY AND COULDN'T RESIST THE TEMPTATION OF LOOKING AT BABY SEATS EVEN THOUGH I KNEW I SHOULD WAIT. I MUST HAVE GIVEN IT THE EVIL EYE.
IT WILL WORK NEXT TIME. I WON'T GIVE UP UNTIL YOU HAVE A BABY.
HANNA
Nu?
Any news?
It was negative. I can't believe it. I mean, I get pregnant just from sniffing David.
I feel like my body betrayed me.
DING!
HANNA
It isn't your fault, honey, her eggs could be too old. They told you egg quality could be an issue.
Maybe, but I think my body can do this if we try a natural cycle. I can do this, I just know it.

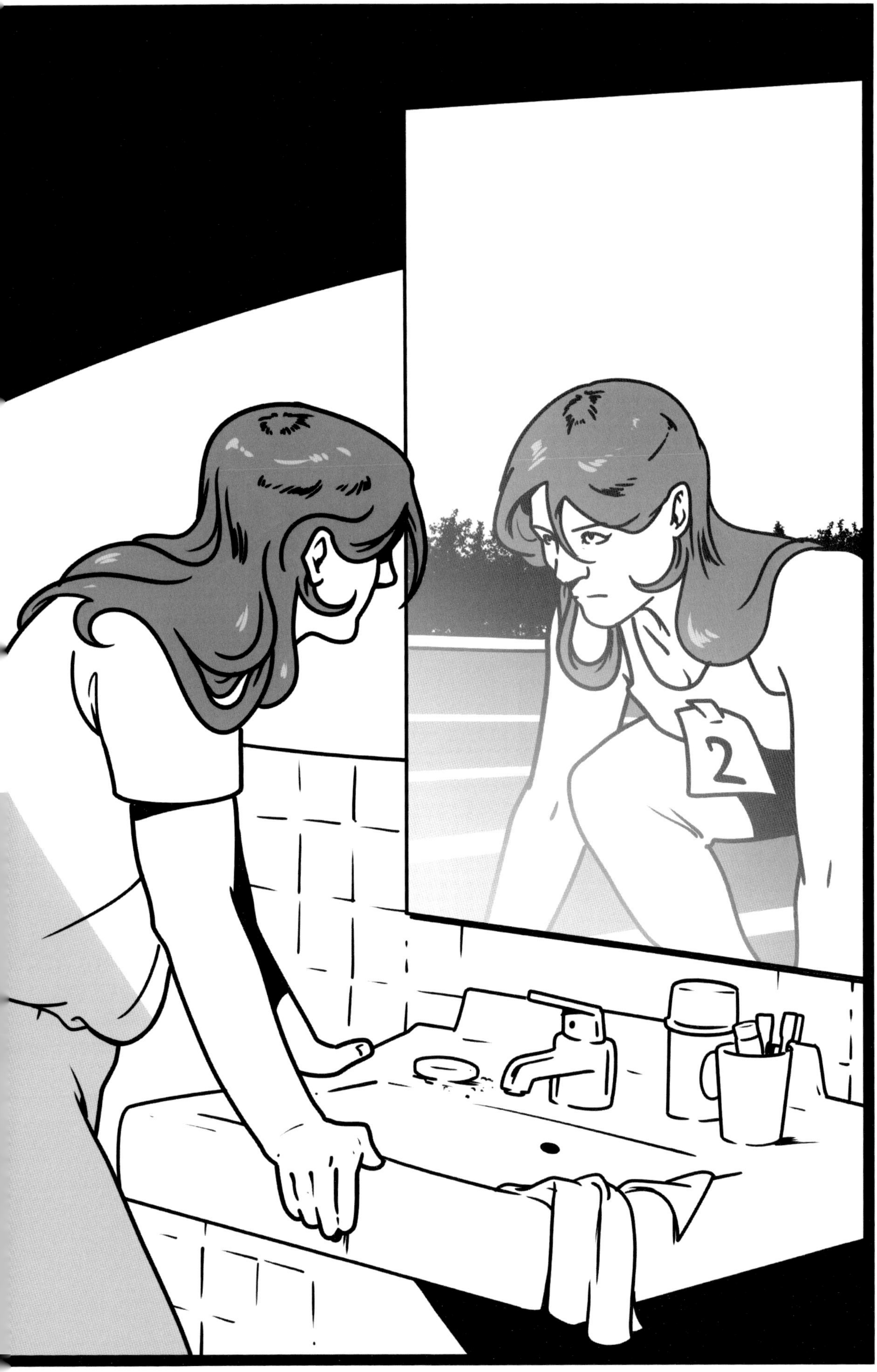
2

-CHAPTER 10-
THE FERRIS WHEEL

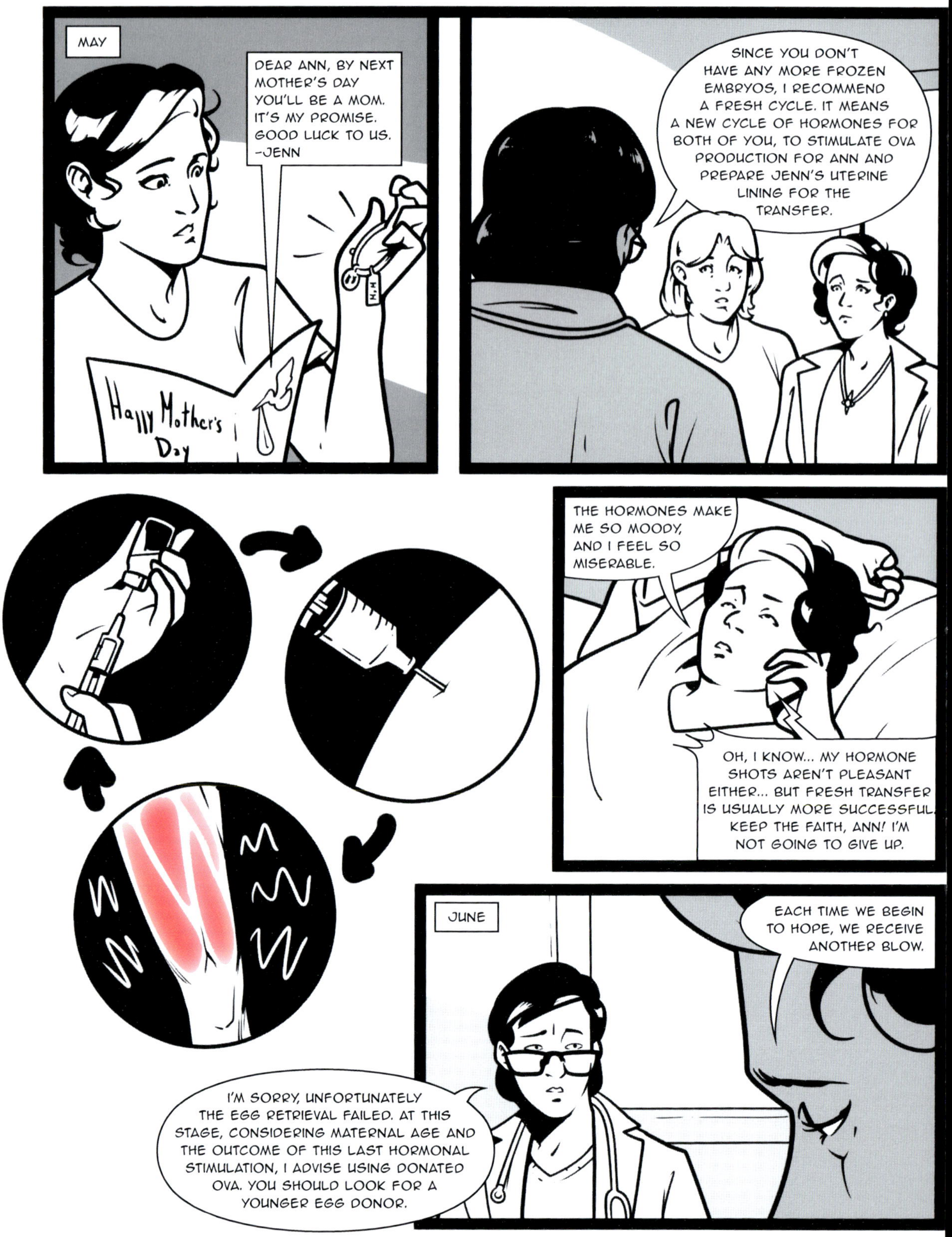

MAY
DEAR ANN, BY NEXT MOTHER'S DAY YOU'LL BE A MOM. IT'S MY PROMISE. GOOD LUCK TO US. -JENN
Happy Mother's Day
SINCE YOU DON'T HAVE ANY MORE FROZEN EMBRYOS, I RECOMMEND A FRESH CYCLE. IT MEANS A NEW CYCLE OF HORMONES FOR BOTH OF YOU, TO STIMULATE OVA PRODUCTION FOR ANN AND PREPARE JENN'S UTERINE LINING FOR THE TRANSFER.
THE HORMONES MAKE ME SO MOODY, AND I FEEL SO MISERABLE.
OH, I KNOW... MY HORMONE SHOTS AREN'T PLEASANT EITHER... BUT FRESH TRANSFER IS USUALLY MORE SUCCESSFUL. KEEP THE FAITH, ANN! I'M NOT GOING TO GIVE UP.
JUNE
EACH TIME WE BEGIN TO HOPE, WE RECEIVE ANOTHER BLOW.
I'M SORRY, UNFORTUNATELY THE EGG RETRIEVAL FAILED. AT THIS STAGE, CONSIDERING MATERNAL AGE AND THE OUTCOME OF THIS LAST HORMONAL STIMULATION, I ADVISE USING DONATED OVA. YOU SHOULD LOOK FOR A YOUNGER EGG DONOR.

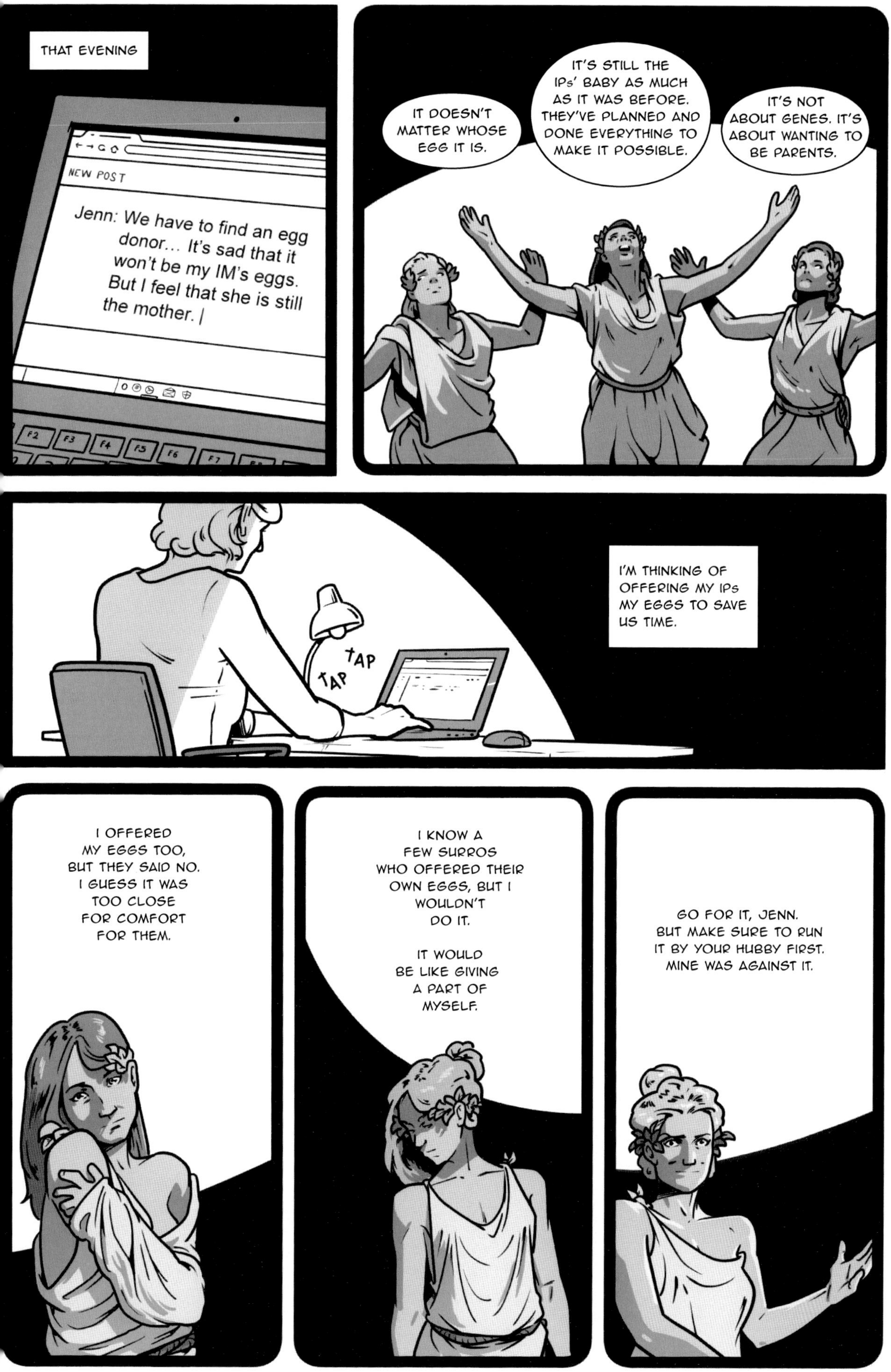
THAT EVENING
NEW POST
Jenn: We have to find an egg donor... It's sad that it won't be my IM's eggs. But I feel that she is still the mother. |
IT DOESN'T MATTER WHOSE EGG IT IS.
IT'S STILL THE IPs' BABY AS MUCH AS IT WAS BEFORE. THEY'VE PLANNED AND DONE EVERYTHING TO MAKE IT POSSIBLE.
IT'S NOT ABOUT GENES. IT'S ABOUT WANTING TO BE PARENTS.
I'M THINKING OF OFFERING MY IPs MY EGGS TO SAVE US TIME.
TAP
TAP
I OFFERED MY EGGS TOO, BUT THEY SAID NO. I GUESS IT WAS TOO CLOSE FOR COMFORT FOR THEM.
I KNOW A FEW SURROS WHO OFFERED THEIR OWN EGGS, BUT I WOULDN'T DO IT.
IT WOULD BE LIKE GIVING A PART OF MYSELF.
GO FOR IT, JENN. BUT MAKE SURE TO RUN IT BY YOUR HUBBY FIRST. MINE WAS AGAINST IT.

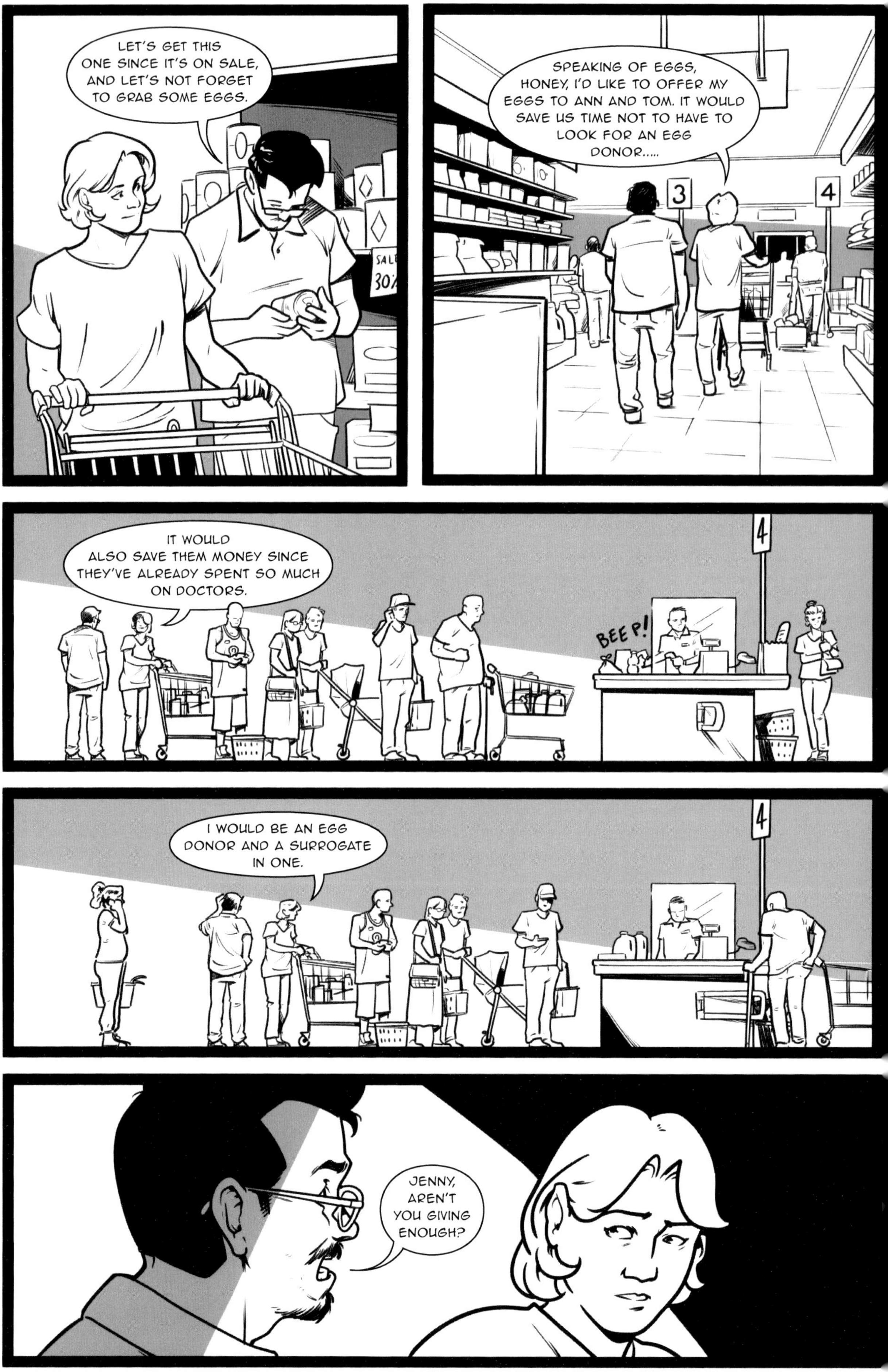
LET'S GET THIS ONE SINCE IT'S ON SALE, AND LET'S NOT FORGET TO GRAB SOME EGGS.
SALE 30%
SPEAKING OF EGGS, HONEY, I'D LIKE TO OFFER MY EGGS TO ANN AND TOM. IT WOULD SAVE US TIME NOT TO HAVE TO LOOK FOR AN EGG DONOR.....
3
4
IT WOULD ALSO SAVE THEM MONEY SINCE THEY'VE ALREADY SPENT SO MUCH ON DOCTORS.
BEEP!
4
I WOULD BE AN EGG DONOR AND A SURROGATE IN ONE.
4
JENNY, AREN'T YOU GIVING ENOUGH?

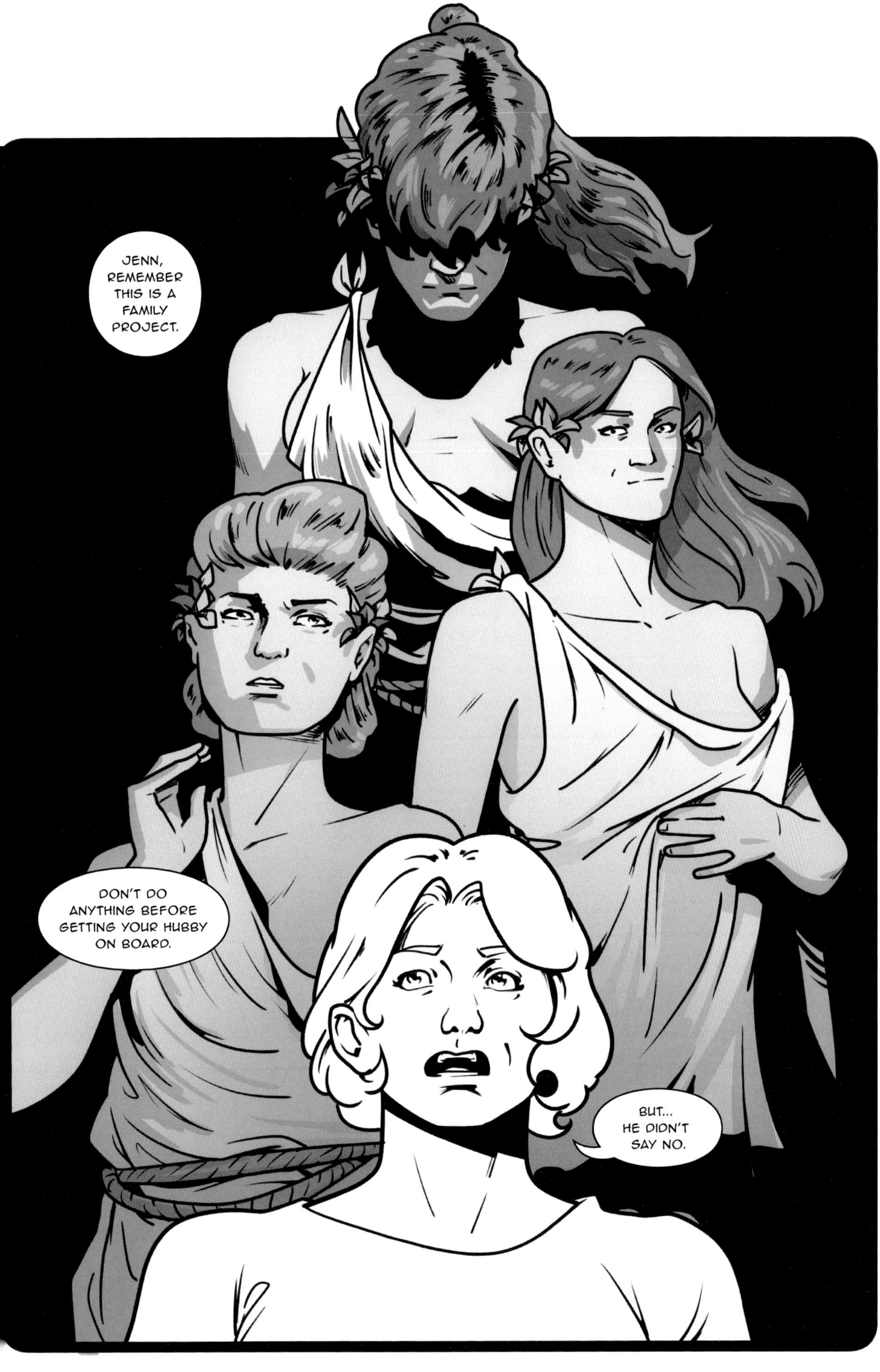
JENN, REMEMBER THIS IS A FAMILY PROJECT.
DON'T DO ANYTHING BEFORE GETTING YOUR HUBBY ON BOARD.
BUT... HE DIDN'T SAY NO.

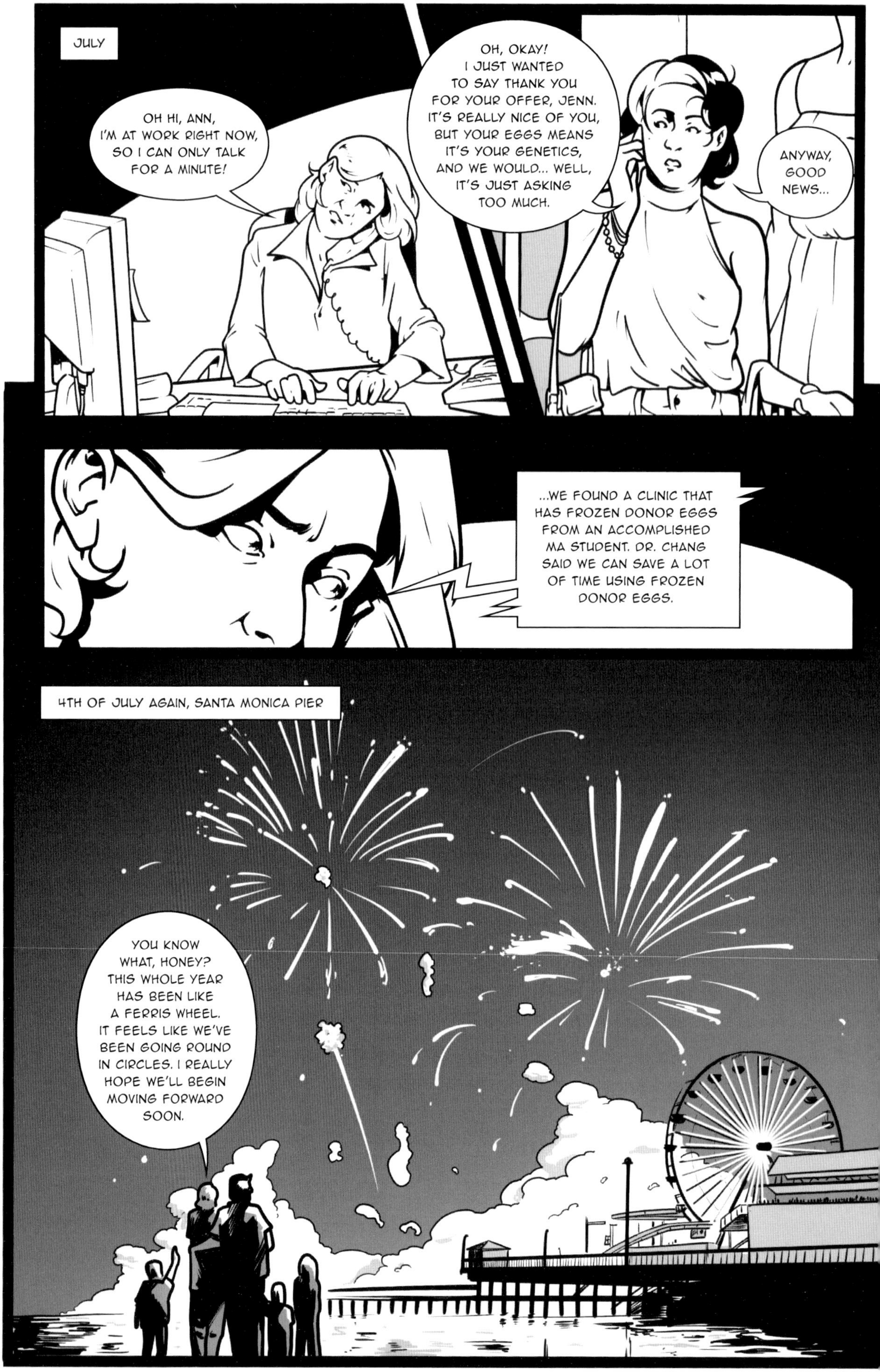
JULY
OH HI, ANN, I'M AT WORK RIGHT NOW, SO I CAN ONLY TALK FOR A MINUTE!
OH, OKAY! I JUST WANTED TO SAY THANK YOU FOR YOUR OFFER, JENN. IT'S REALLY NICE OF YOU, BUT YOUR EGGS MEANS IT'S YOUR GENETICS, AND WE WOULD... WELL, IT'S JUST ASKING TOO MUCH.
ANYWAY, GOOD NEWS...
...WE FOUND A CLINIC THAT HAS FROZEN DONOR EGGS FROM AN ACCOMPLISHED MA STUDENT. DR. CHANG SAID WE CAN SAVE A LOT OF TIME USING FROZEN DONOR EGGS.
4TH OF JULY AGAIN, SANTA MONICA PIER
YOU KNOW WHAT, HONEY? THIS WHOLE YEAR HAS BEEN LIKE A FERRIS WHEEL. IT FEELS LIKE WE'VE BEEN GOING ROUND IN CIRCLES. I REALLY HOPE WE'LL BEGIN MOVING FORWARD SOON.

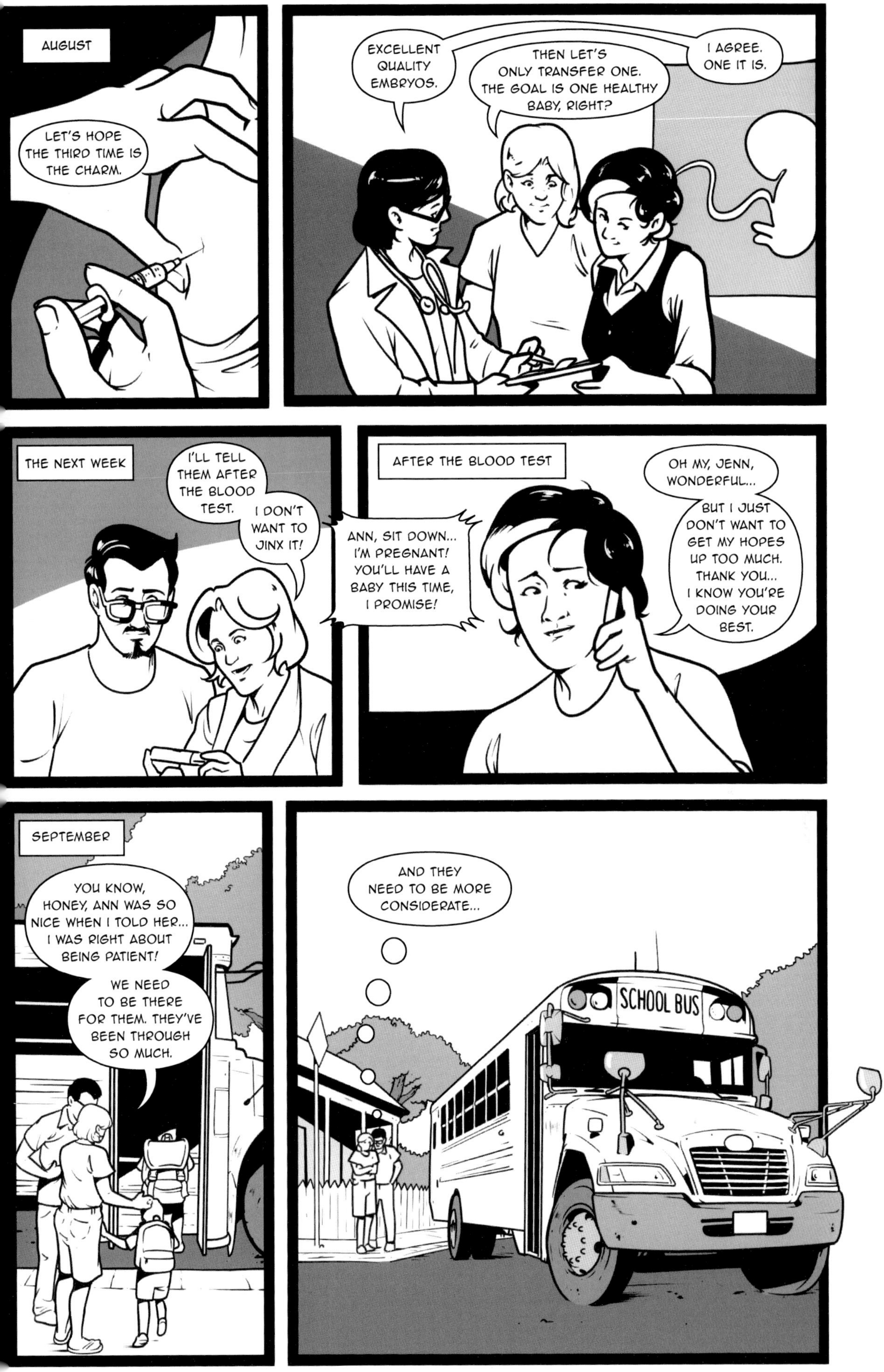
AUGUST
LET'S HOPE THE THIRD TIME IS THE CHARM.
EXCELLENT QUALITY EMBRYOS.
THEN LET'S ONLY TRANSFER ONE. THE GOAL IS ONE HEALTHY BABY, RIGHT?
I AGREE. ONE IT IS.
THE NEXT WEEK
I'LL TELL THEM AFTER THE BLOOD TEST.
I DON'T WANT TO JINX IT!
AFTER THE BLOOD TEST
ANN, SIT DOWN... I'M PREGNANT! YOU'LL HAVE A BABY THIS TIME, I PROMISE!
OH MY, JENN, WONDERFUL...
BUT I JUST DON'T WANT TO GET MY HOPES UP TOO MUCH. THANK YOU... I KNOW YOU'RE DOING YOUR BEST.
SEPTEMBER
YOU KNOW, HONEY, ANN WAS SO NICE WHEN I TOLD HER... I WAS RIGHT ABOUT BEING PATIENT!
WE NEED TO BE THERE FOR THEM. THEY'VE BEEN THROUGH SO MUCH.
AND THEY NEED TO BE MORE CONSIDERATE...
SCHOOL BUS

INTERLUDE: HASOMATI, SURROGATE IN STATE OF GUJARAT, INDIA

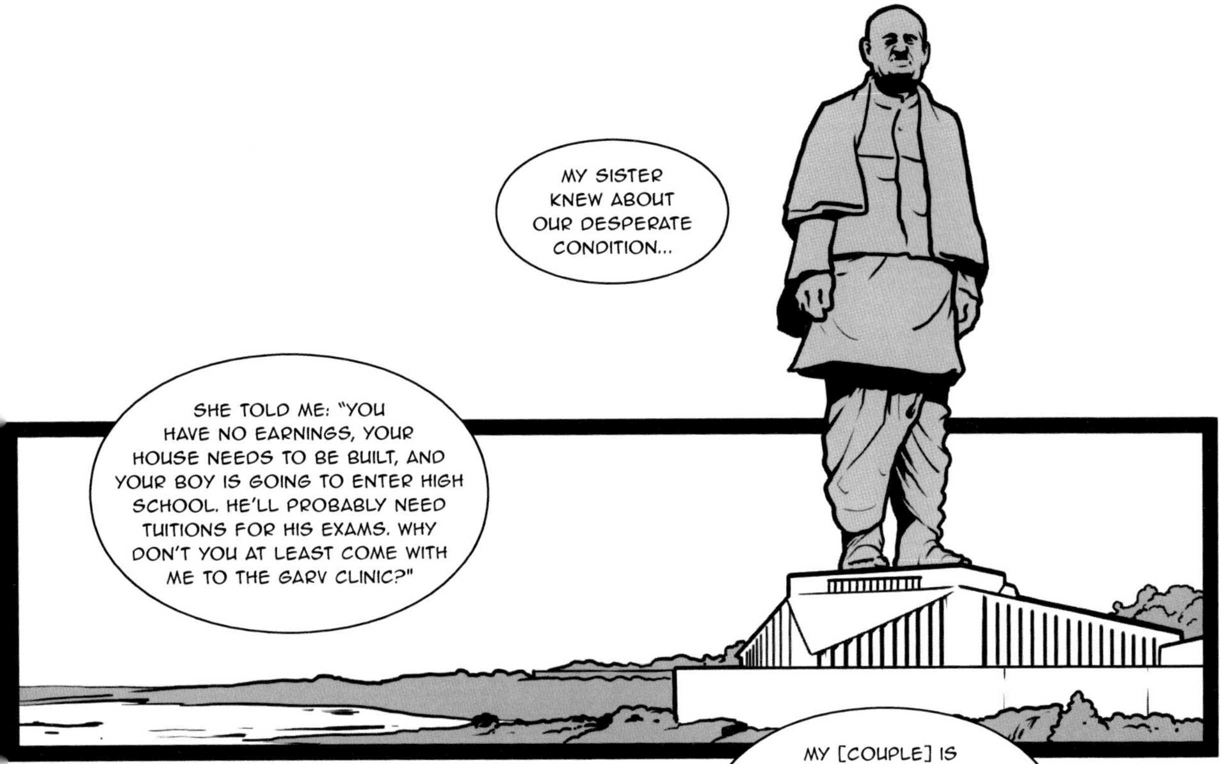
MY SISTER KNEW ABOUT OUR DESPERATE CONDITION...
SHE TOLD ME: "YOU HAVE NO EARNINGS, YOUR HOUSE NEEDS TO BE BUILT, AND YOUR BOY IS GOING TO ENTER HIGH SCHOOL. HE'LL PROBABLY NEED TUITIONS FOR HIS EXAMS. WHY DON'T YOU AT LEAST COME WITH ME TO THE GARV CLINIC?"

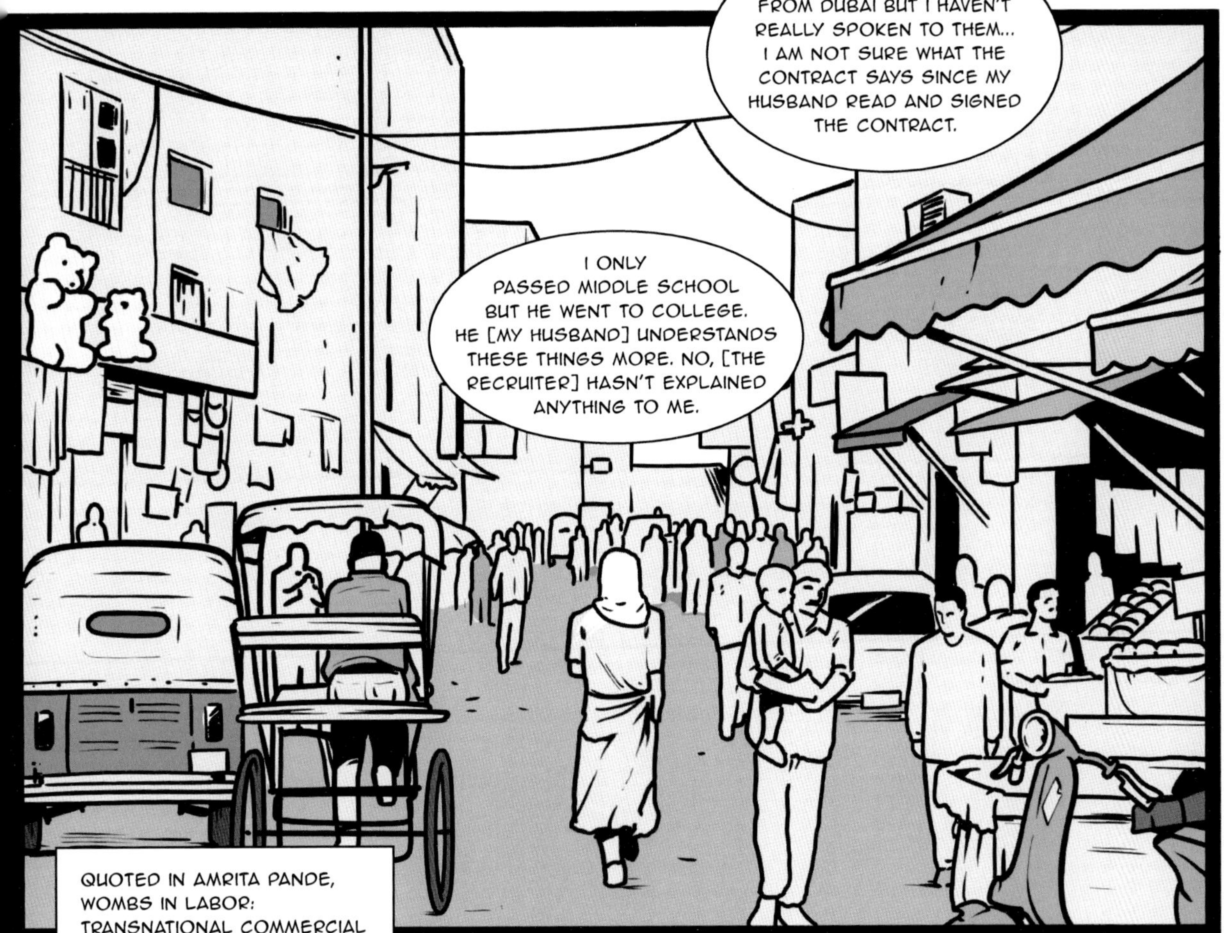
MY [COUPLE] IS FROM DUBAI BUT I HAVEN'T REALLY SPOKEN TO THEM... I AM NOT SURE WHAT THE CONTRACT SAYS SINCE MY HUSBAND READ AND SIGNED THE CONTRACT.
I ONLY PASSED MIDDLE SCHOOL BUT HE WENT TO COLLEGE. HE [MY HUSBAND] UNDERSTANDS THESE THINGS MORE. NO, [THE RECRUITER] HASN'T EXPLAINED ANYTHING TO ME.

QUOTED IN AMRITA PANDE, WOMBS IN LABOR: TRANSNATIONAL COMMERCIAL SURROGACY IN INDIA (COLUMBIA UNIVERSITY PRESS, 2014), 109.

-CHAPTER 11-
HEARTBEAT

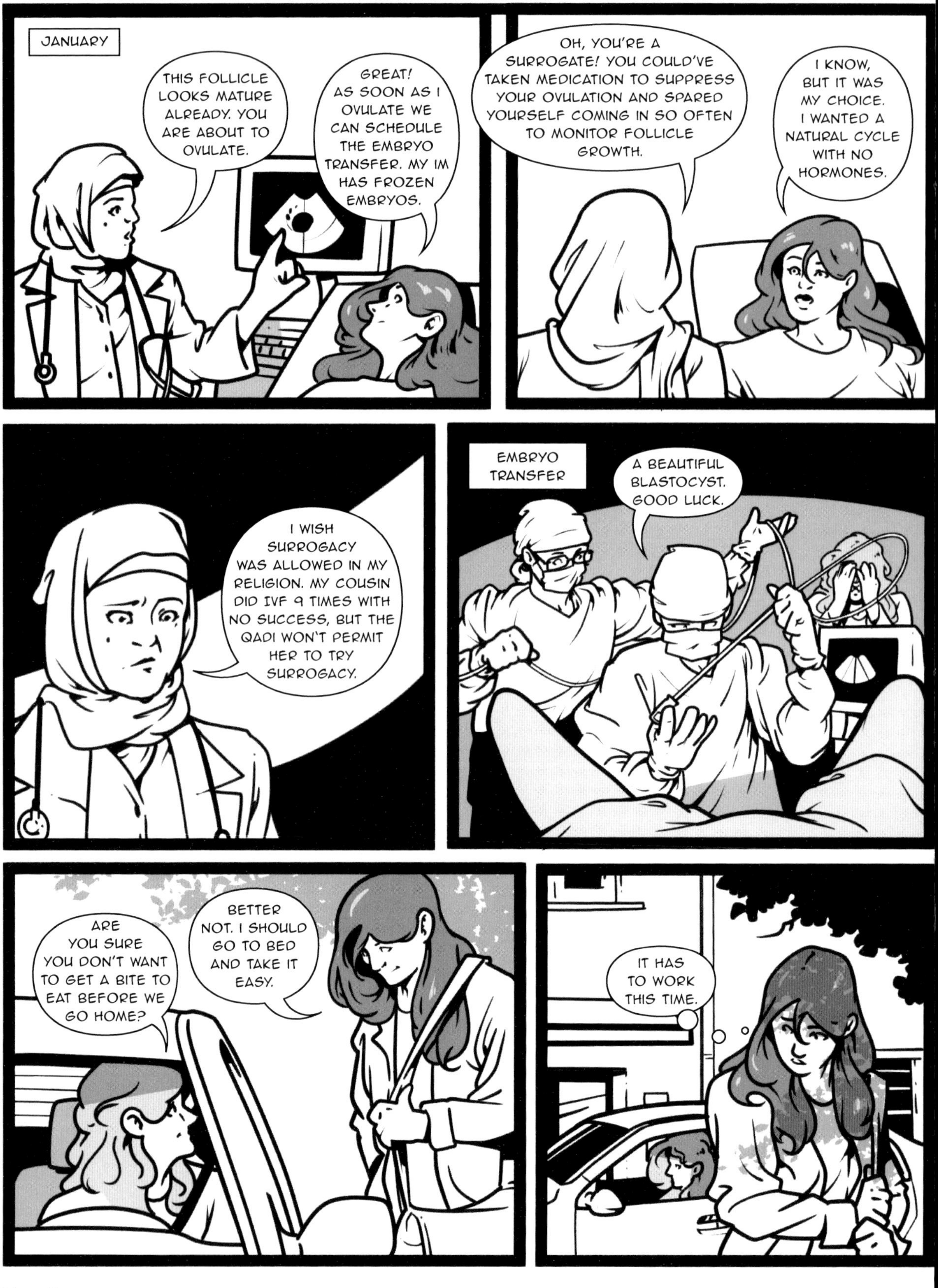

JANUARY
THIS FOLLICLE LOOKS MATURE ALREADY. YOU ARE ABOUT TO OVULATE.
GREAT! AS SOON AS I OVULATE WE CAN SCHEDULE THE EMBRYO TRANSFER. MY IM HAS FROZEN EMBRYOS.
OH, YOU'RE A SURROGATE! YOU COULD'VE TAKEN MEDICATION TO SUPPRESS YOUR OVULATION AND SPARED YOURSELF COMING IN SO OFTEN TO MONITOR FOLLICLE GROWTH.
I KNOW, BUT IT WAS MY CHOICE. I WANTED A NATURAL CYCLE WITH NO HORMONES.
I WISH SURROGACY WAS ALLOWED IN MY RELIGION. MY COUSIN DID IVF 9 TIMES WITH NO SUCCESS, BUT THE QADI WON'T PERMIT HER TO TRY SURROGACY.
EMBRYO TRANSFER
A BEAUTIFUL BLASTOCYST. GOOD LUCK.
ARE YOU SURE YOU DON'T WANT TO GET A BITE TO EAT BEFORE WE GO HOME?
BETTER NOT. I SHOULD GO TO BED AND TAKE IT EASY.
IT HAS TO WORK THIS TIME.

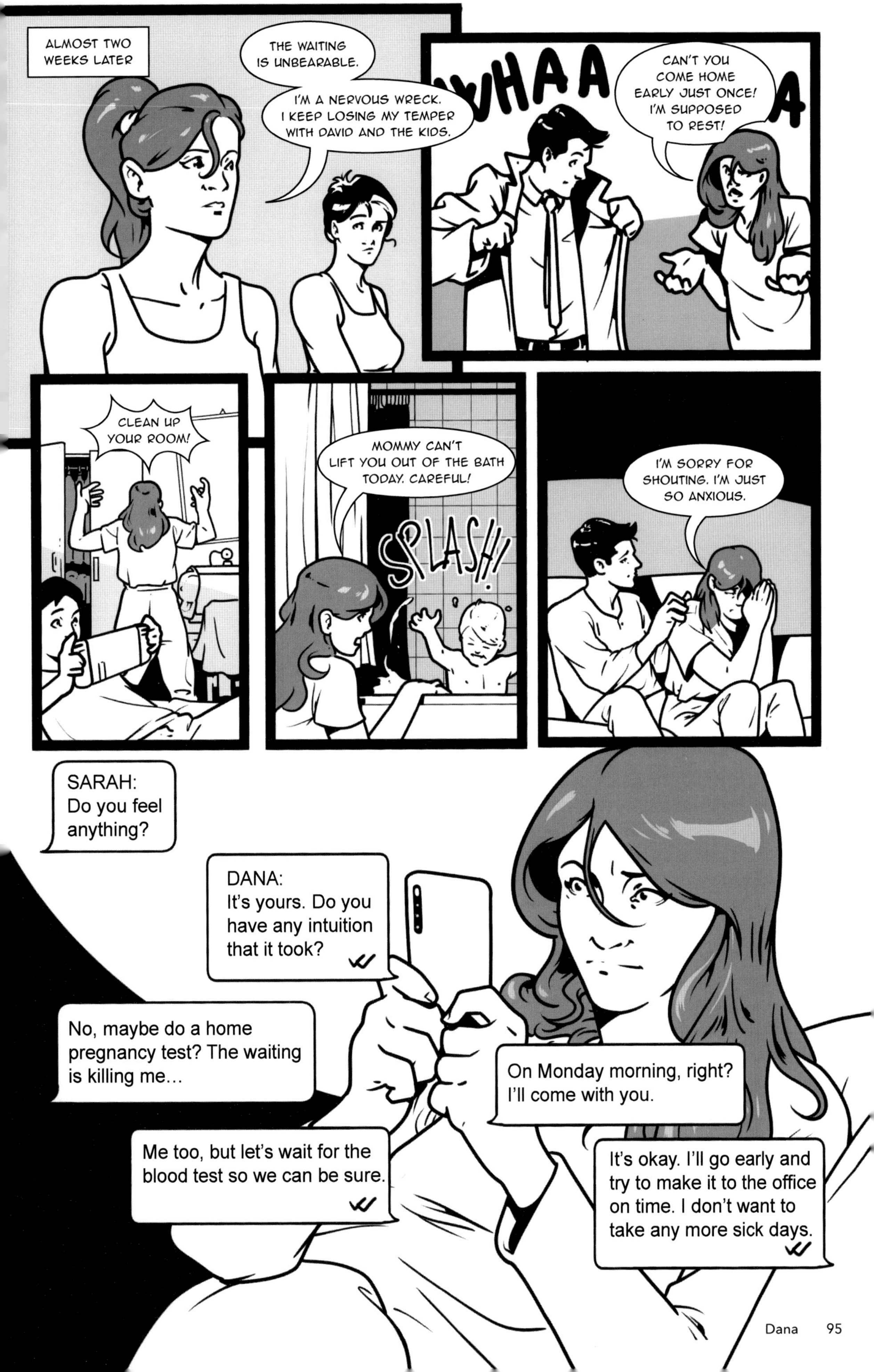
ALMOST TWO WEEKS LATER
THE WAITING IS UNBEARABLE.
I'M A NERVOUS WRECK. I KEEP LOSING MY TEMPER WITH DAVID AND THE KIDS.
WHAA A A
CAN'T YOU COME HOME EARLY JUST ONCE! I'M SUPPOSED TO REST!
CLEAN UP YOUR ROOM!
MOMMY CAN'T LIFT YOU OUT OF THE BATH TODAY. CAREFUL!
SPLASH!
I'M SORRY FOR SHOUTING. I'M JUST SO ANXIOUS.
SARAH: Do you feel anything?
DANA: It's yours. Do you have any intuition that it took?
No, maybe do a home pregnancy test? The waiting is killing me…
Me too, but let's wait for the blood test so we can be sure.
On Monday morning, right? I'll come with you.
It's okay. I'll go early and try to make it to the office on time. I don't want to take any more sick days.

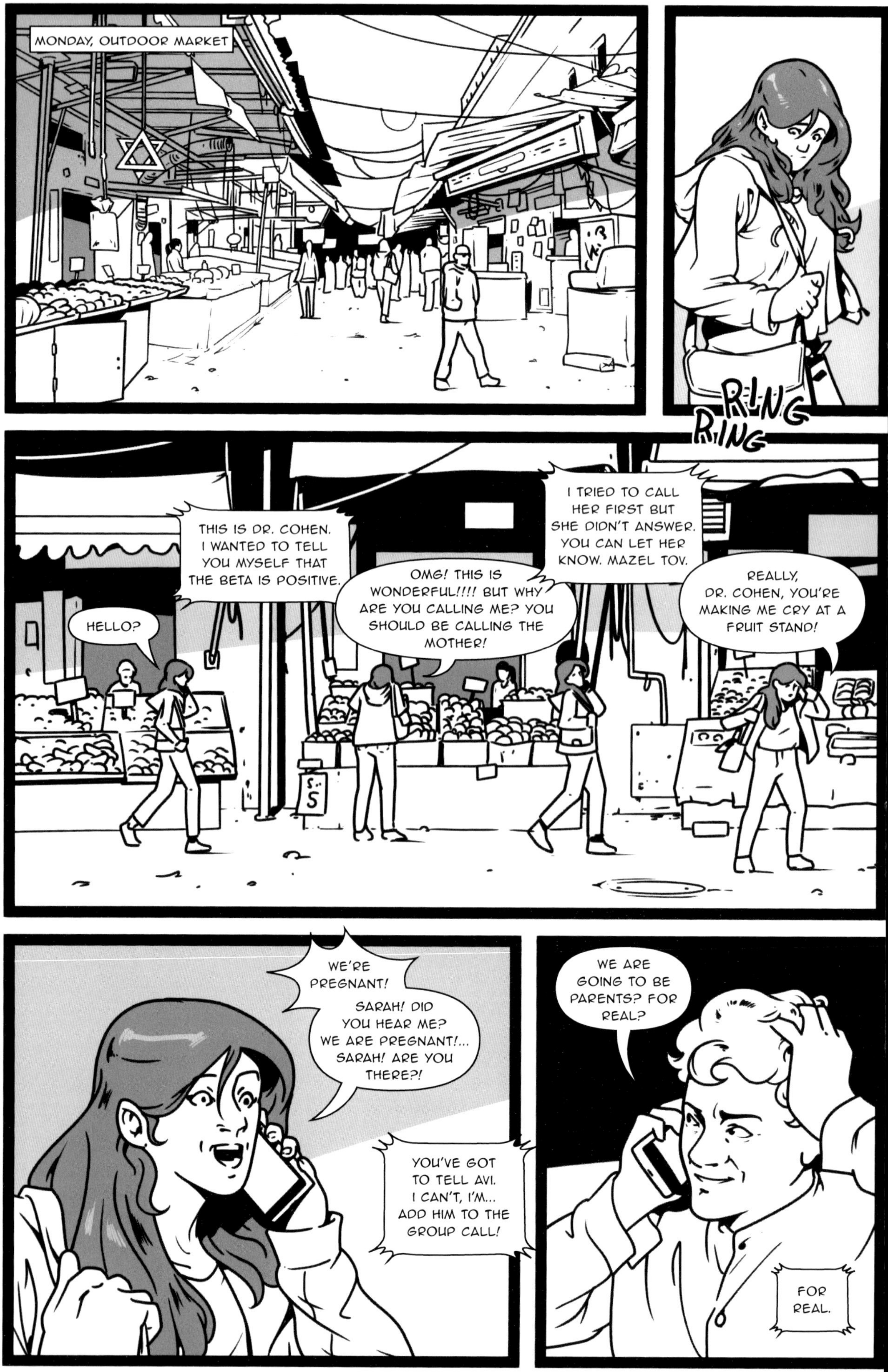
MONDAY, OUTDOOR MARKET
RING
RING
HELLO?
THIS IS DR. COHEN. I WANTED TO TELL YOU MYSELF THAT THE BETA IS POSITIVE.
OMG! THIS IS WONDERFUL!!!! BUT WHY ARE YOU CALLING ME? YOU SHOULD BE CALLING THE MOTHER!
I TRIED TO CALL HER FIRST BUT SHE DIDN'T ANSWER. YOU CAN LET HER KNOW. MAZEL TOV.
REALLY, DR. COHEN, YOU'RE MAKING ME CRY AT A FRUIT STAND!
WE'RE PREGNANT!
SARAH! DID YOU HEAR ME? WE ARE PREGNANT!... SARAH! ARE YOU THERE?!
YOU'VE GOT TO TELL AVI. I CAN'T, I'M... ADD HIM TO THE GROUP CALL!
WE ARE GOING TO BE PARENTS? FOR REAL?
FOR REAL.

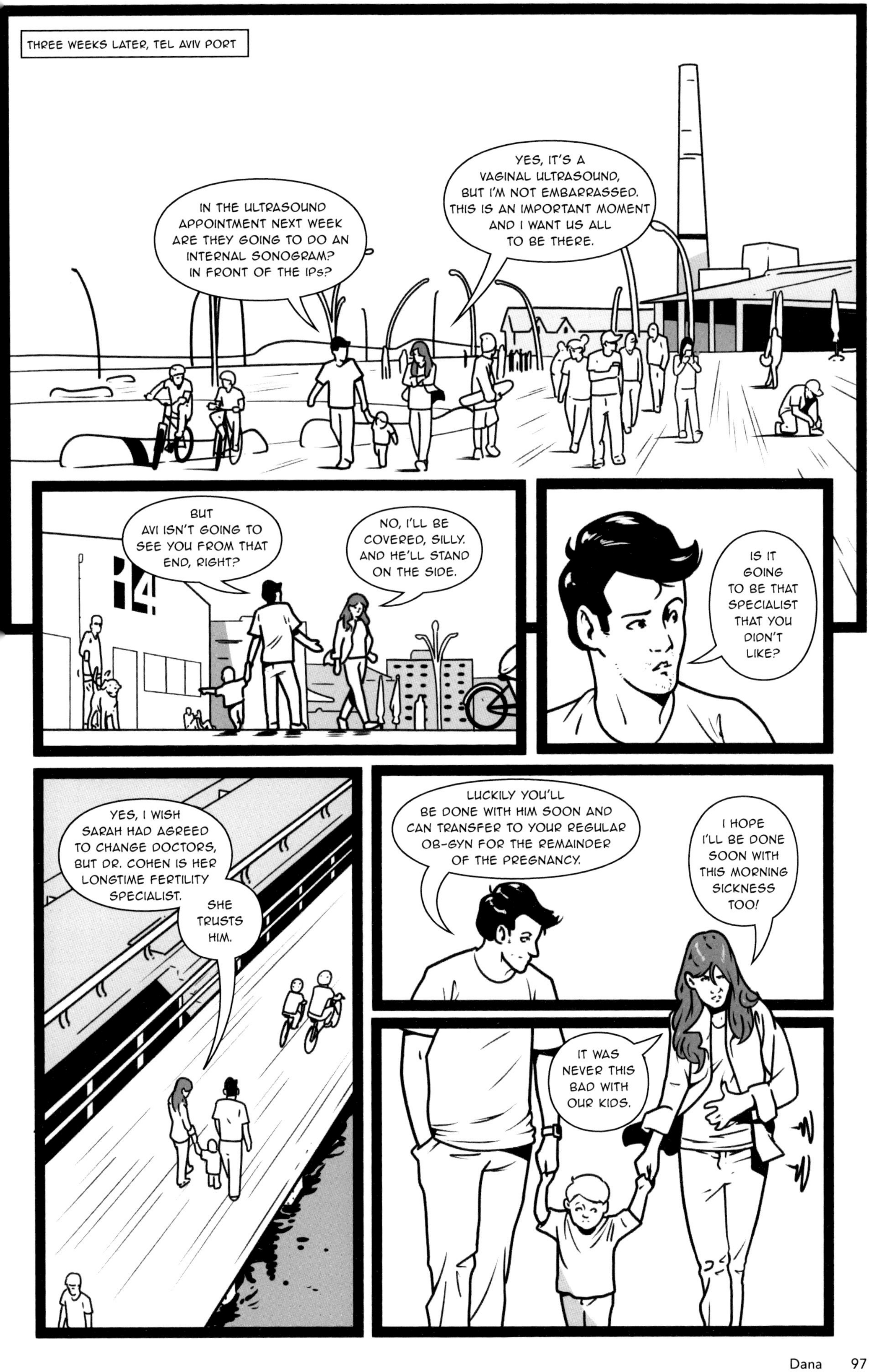
THREE WEEKS LATER, TEL AVIV PORT
IN THE ULTRASOUND APPOINTMENT NEXT WEEK ARE THEY GOING TO DO AN INTERNAL SONOGRAM? IN FRONT OF THE IPs?
YES, IT'S A VAGINAL ULTRASOUND, BUT I'M NOT EMBARRASSED. THIS IS AN IMPORTANT MOMENT AND I WANT US ALL TO BE THERE.
BUT AVI ISN'T GOING TO SEE YOU FROM THAT END, RIGHT?
NO, I'LL BE COVERED, SILLY. AND HE'LL STAND ON THE SIDE.
IS IT GOING TO BE THAT SPECIALIST THAT YOU DIDN'T LIKE?
YES, I WISH SARAH HAD AGREED TO CHANGE DOCTORS, BUT DR. COHEN IS HER LONGTIME FERTILITY SPECIALIST.
SHE TRUSTS HIM.
LUCKILY YOU'LL BE DONE WITH HIM SOON AND CAN TRANSFER TO YOUR REGULAR OB-GYN FOR THE REMAINDER OF THE PREGNANCY.
I HOPE I'LL BE DONE SOON WITH THIS MORNING SICKNESS TOO!
IT WAS NEVER THIS BAD WITH OUR KIDS.

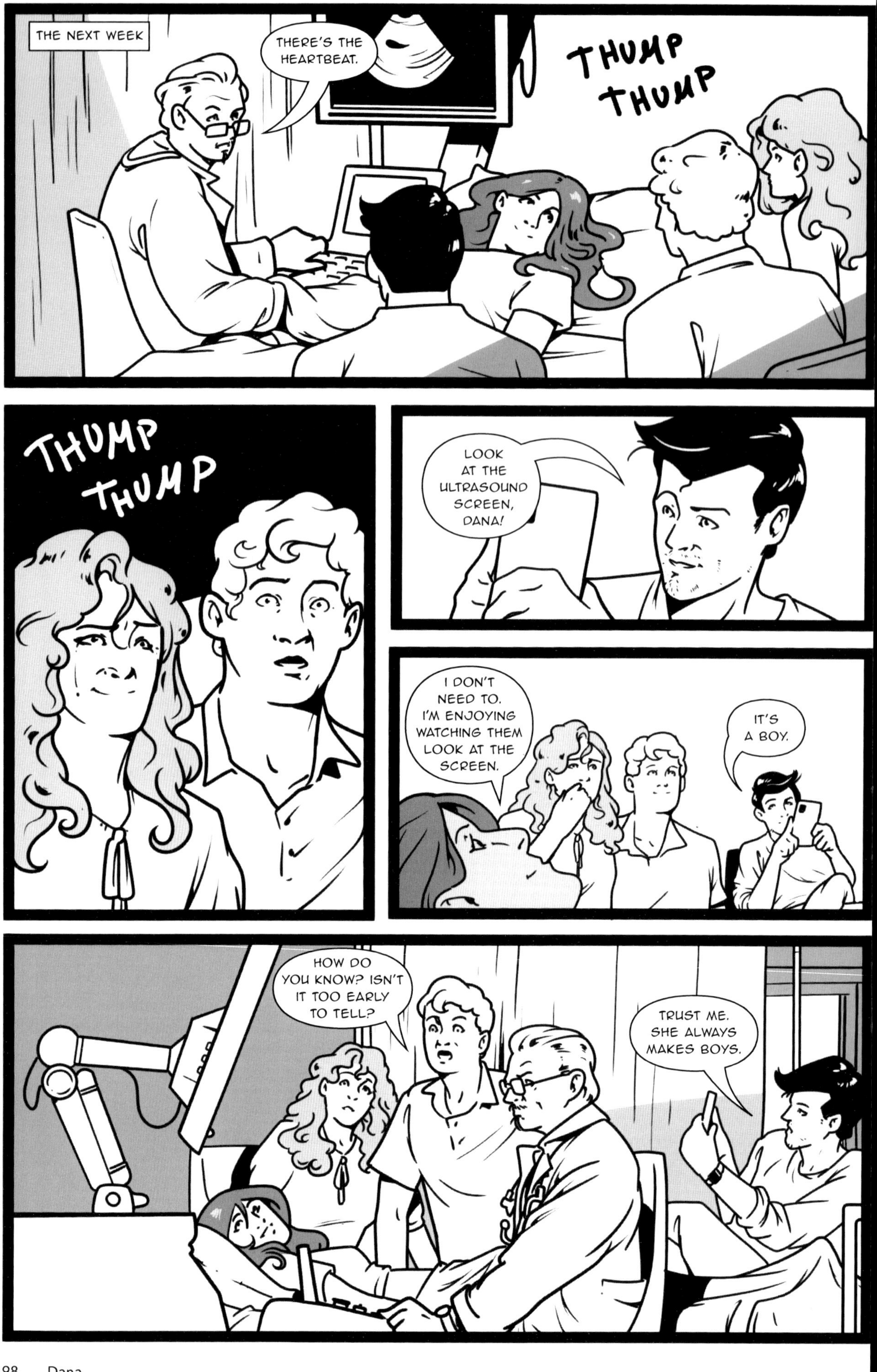
THE NEXT WEEK
THERE'S THE HEARTBEAT.
THUMP THUMP
THUMP THUMP
LOOK AT THE ULTRASOUND SCREEN, DANA!
I DON'T NEED TO. I'M ENJOYING WATCHING THEM LOOK AT THE SCREEN.
IT'S A BOY.
HOW DO YOU KNOW? ISN'T IT TOO EARLY TO TELL?
TRUST ME. SHE ALWAYS MAKES BOYS.

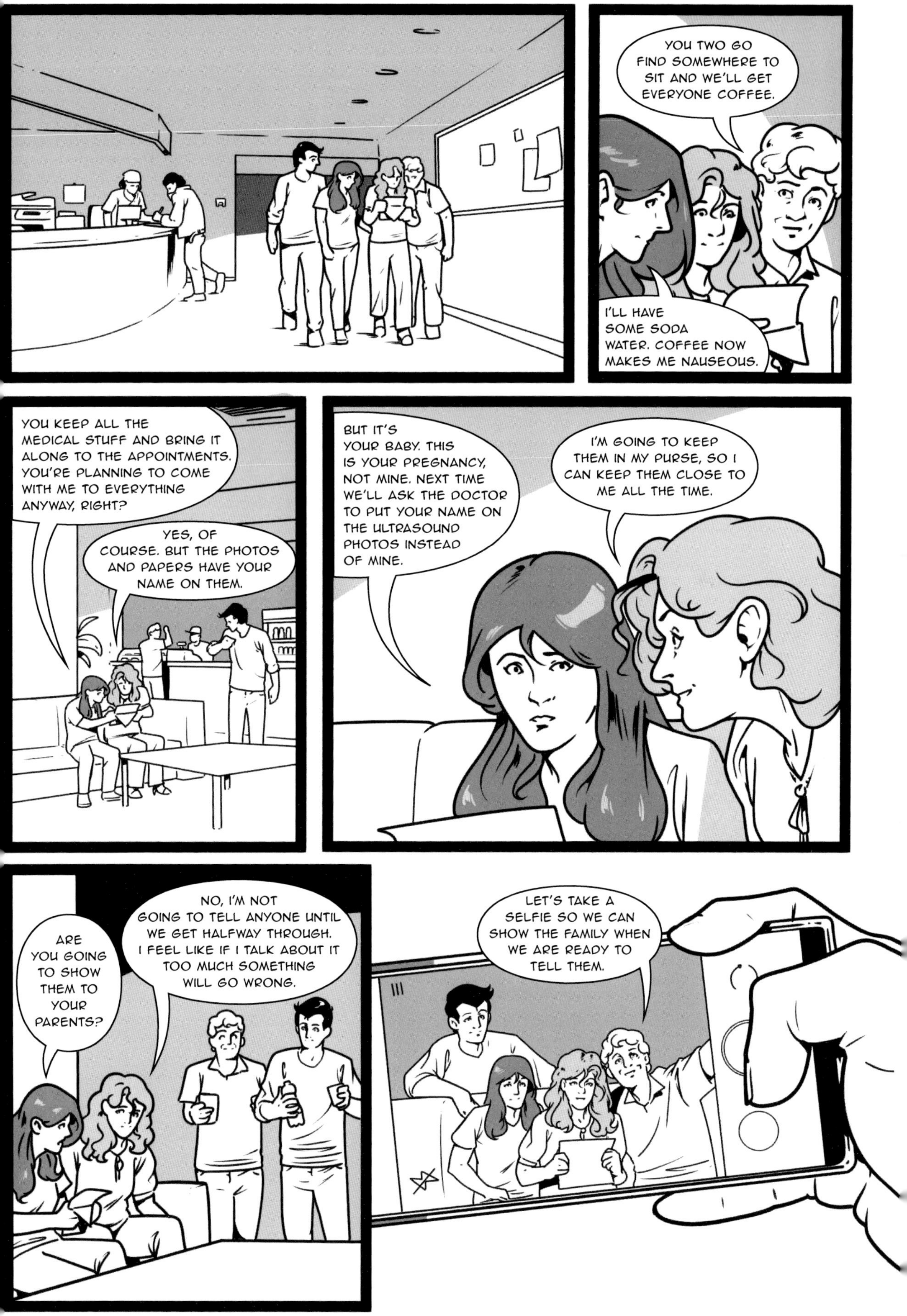
YOU TWO GO FIND SOMEWHERE TO SIT AND WE'LL GET EVERYONE COFFEE.
I'LL HAVE SOME SODA WATER. COFFEE NOW MAKES ME NAUSEOUS.
YOU KEEP ALL THE MEDICAL STUFF AND BRING IT ALONG TO THE APPOINTMENTS. YOU'RE PLANNING TO COME WITH ME TO EVERYTHING ANYWAY, RIGHT?
YES, OF COURSE. BUT THE PHOTOS AND PAPERS HAVE YOUR NAME ON THEM.
BUT IT'S YOUR BABY. THIS IS YOUR PREGNANCY, NOT MINE. NEXT TIME WE'LL ASK THE DOCTOR TO PUT YOUR NAME ON THE ULTRASOUND PHOTOS INSTEAD OF MINE.
I'M GOING TO KEEP THEM IN MY PURSE, SO I CAN KEEP THEM CLOSE TO ME ALL THE TIME.
ARE YOU GOING TO SHOW THEM TO YOUR PARENTS?
NO, I'M NOT GOING TO TELL ANYONE UNTIL WE GET HALFWAY THROUGH. I FEEL LIKE IF I TALK ABOUT IT TOO MUCH SOMETHING WILL GO WRONG.
LET'S TAKE A SELFIE SO WE CAN SHOW THE FAMILY WHEN WE ARE READY TO TELL THEM.

-CHAPTER 12-
TELLING THE KIDS

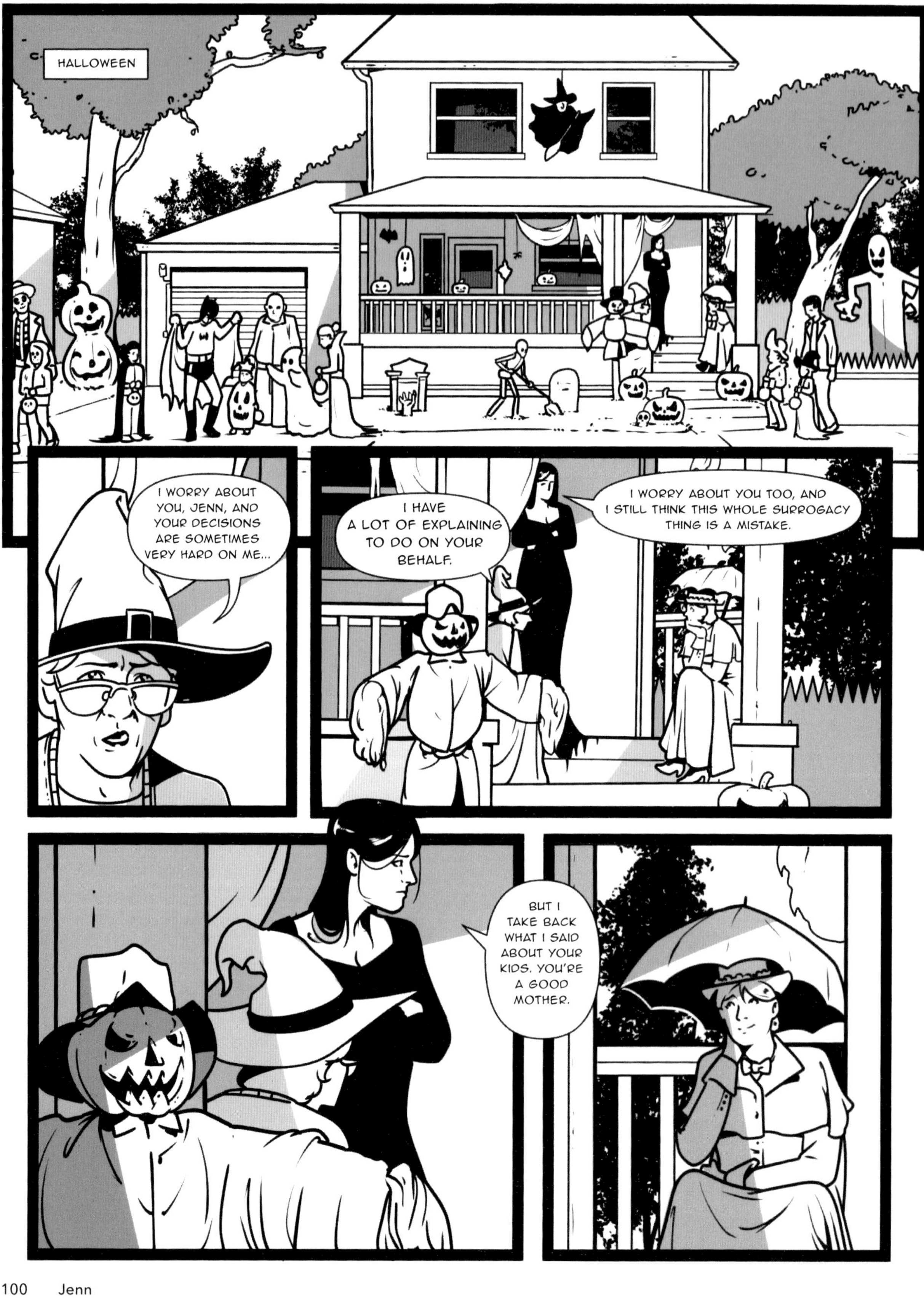

HALLOWEEN
I WORRY ABOUT YOU, JENN, AND YOUR DECISIONS ARE SOMETIMES VERY HARD ON ME...
I HAVE A LOT OF EXPLAINING TO DO ON YOUR BEHALF.
I WORRY ABOUT YOU TOO, AND I STILL THINK THIS WHOLE SURROGACY THING IS A MISTAKE.
BUT I TAKE BACK WHAT I SAID ABOUT YOUR KIDS. YOU'RE A GOOD MOTHER.

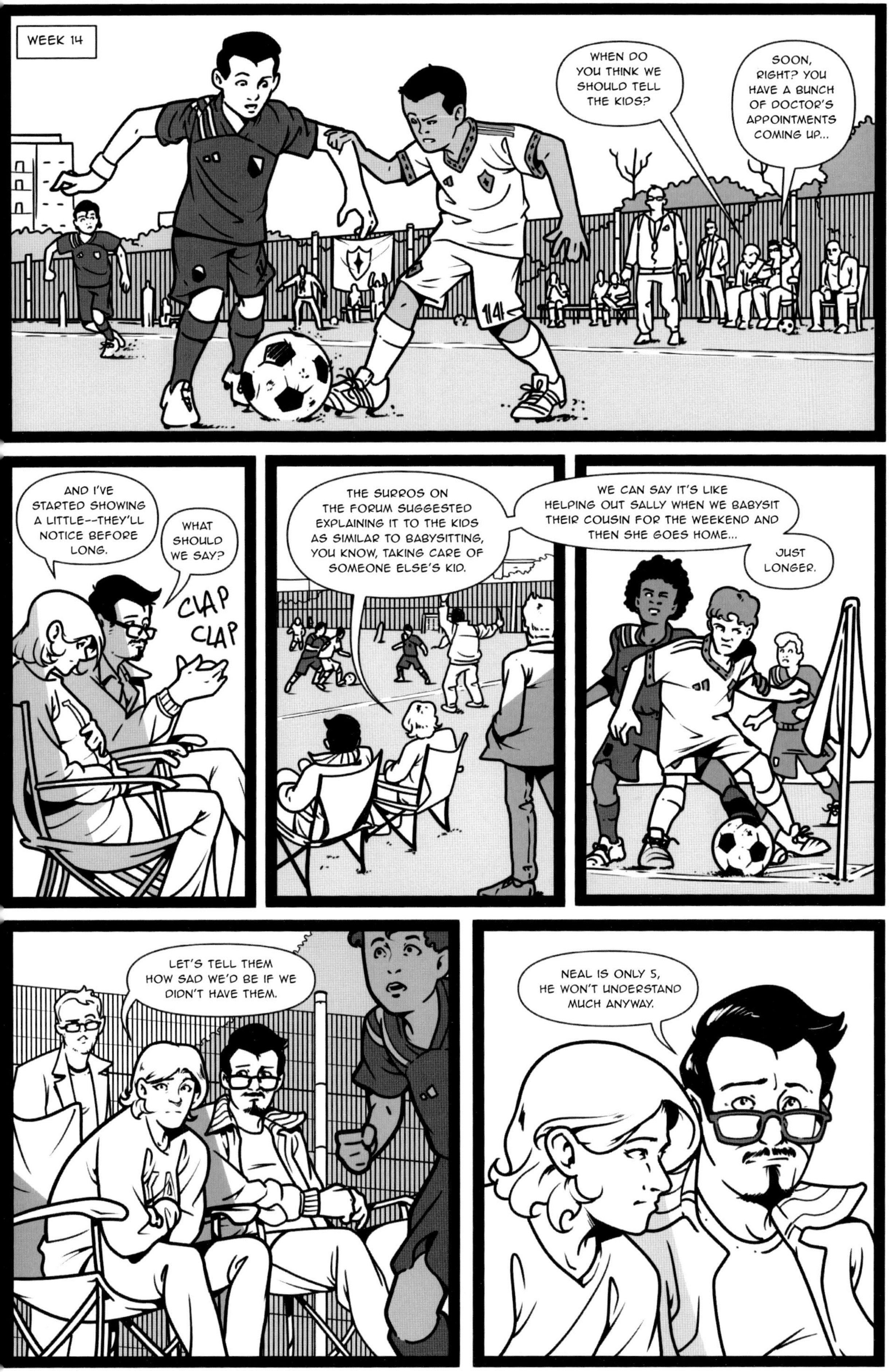
WEEK 14
WHEN DO YOU THINK WE SHOULD TELL THE KIDS?
SOON, RIGHT? YOU HAVE A BUNCH OF DOCTOR'S APPOINTMENTS COMING UP...
AND I'VE STARTED SHOWING A LITTLE--THEY'LL NOTICE BEFORE LONG.
WHAT SHOULD WE SAY?
CLAP CLAP
THE SURROS ON THE FORUM SUGGESTED EXPLAINING IT TO THE KIDS AS SIMILAR TO BABYSITTING, YOU KNOW, TAKING CARE OF SOMEONE ELSE'S KID.
WE CAN SAY IT'S LIKE HELPING OUT SALLY WHEN WE BABYSIT THEIR COUSIN FOR THE WEEKEND AND THEN SHE GOES HOME...
JUST LONGER.
LET'S TELL THEM HOW SAD WE'D BE IF WE DIDN'T HAVE THEM.
NEAL IS ONLY 5, HE WON'T UNDERSTAND MUCH ANYWAY.

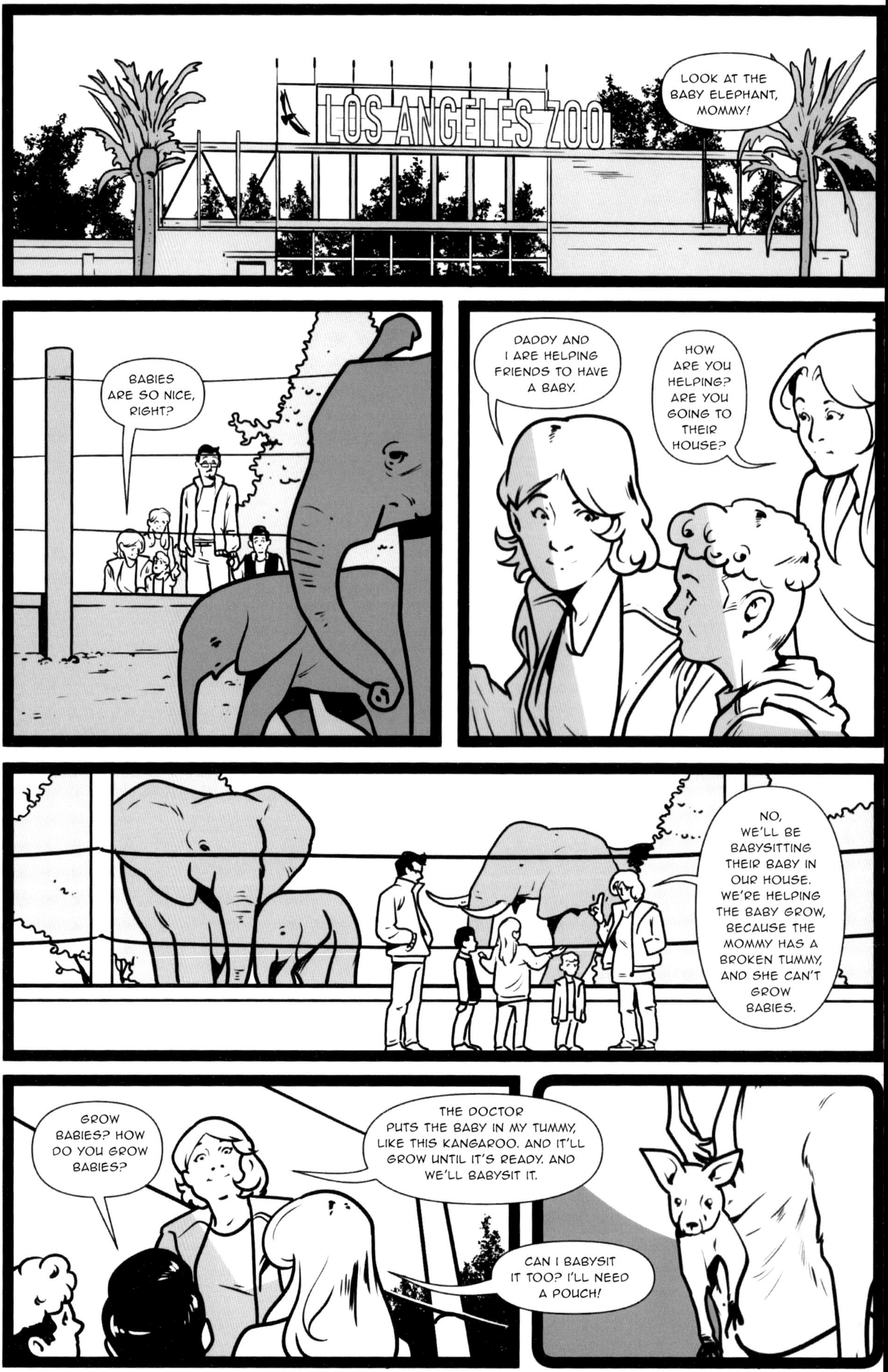
LOS ANGELES ZOO
LOOK AT THE BABY ELEPHANT, MOMMY!
BABIES ARE SO NICE, RIGHT?
DADDY AND I ARE HELPING FRIENDS TO HAVE A BABY.
HOW ARE YOU HELPING? ARE YOU GOING TO THEIR HOUSE?
NO, WE'LL BE BABYSITTING THEIR BABY IN OUR HOUSE. WE'RE HELPING THE BABY GROW, BECAUSE THE MOMMY HAS A BROKEN TUMMY, AND SHE CAN'T GROW BABIES.
GROW BABIES? HOW DO YOU GROW BABIES?
THE DOCTOR PUTS THE BABY IN MY TUMMY, LIKE THIS KANGAROO. AND IT'LL GROW UNTIL IT'S READY. AND WE'LL BABYSIT IT.
CAN I BABYSIT IT TOO? I'LL NEED A POUCH!

WE NEED TO TAKE VERY GOOD CARE OF THE BABY WHILE IT'S GROWING INSIDE ME, BECAUSE IT NEEDS WARMTH AND CARE.
THE PARENTS TRUST US TO HELP IT GROW UNTIL IT GOES HOME.
JUST LIKE HOW AUNT SALLY TRUSTS US TO TAKE GOOD CARE OF TIFFANY WHEN WE BABYSIT HER. IT'S THE SAME WITH THIS BABY.
WHEN WILL IT BE READY TO LEAVE?
IN A FEW MONTHS, BUT DURING THAT TIME WE NEED YOUR HELP, GUYS!
HELP HOW? I HATE TO MAKE MY BED...
CHRISTY, YOU CAN HELP BY PUTTING YOUR TOYS AWAY, SO THAT WE DON'T TRIP ON THEM! THAT WOULD BE SUCH A GREAT HELP.
WHO ARE THESE FRIENDS YOU'RE HELPING?
YOU SEE, THE BABY HAS ITS OWN HOME, AND THE PARENTS ARE WAITING AND SO EXCITED TO MEET THEIR BABY... LIKE WE WERE WHEN YOU ARRIVED.
CAN YOU IMAGINE US NOT HAVING YOU?
I CAN IMAGINE NOT HAVING NEAL... HE TAKES MY STUFF AND HIDES IT.
HE'S ANNOYING.
I DON'T WANT ANOTHER BROTHER ANYWAY. BUT CAN WE HAVE A BABY ELEPHANT?

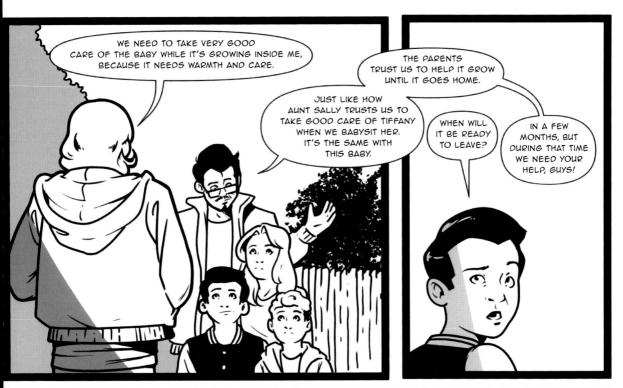

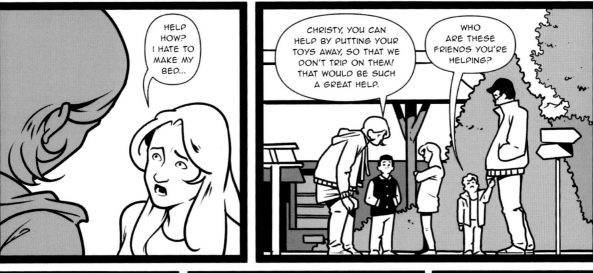

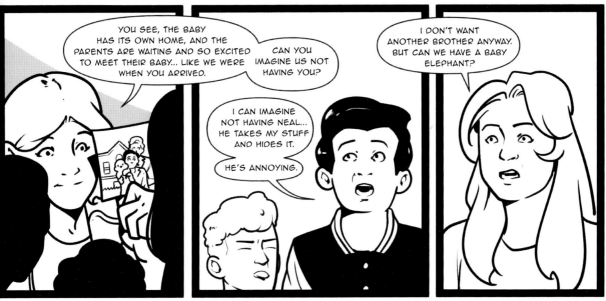

INTERLUDE: INDIRANI, SURROGATE IN BANGALORE, INDIA

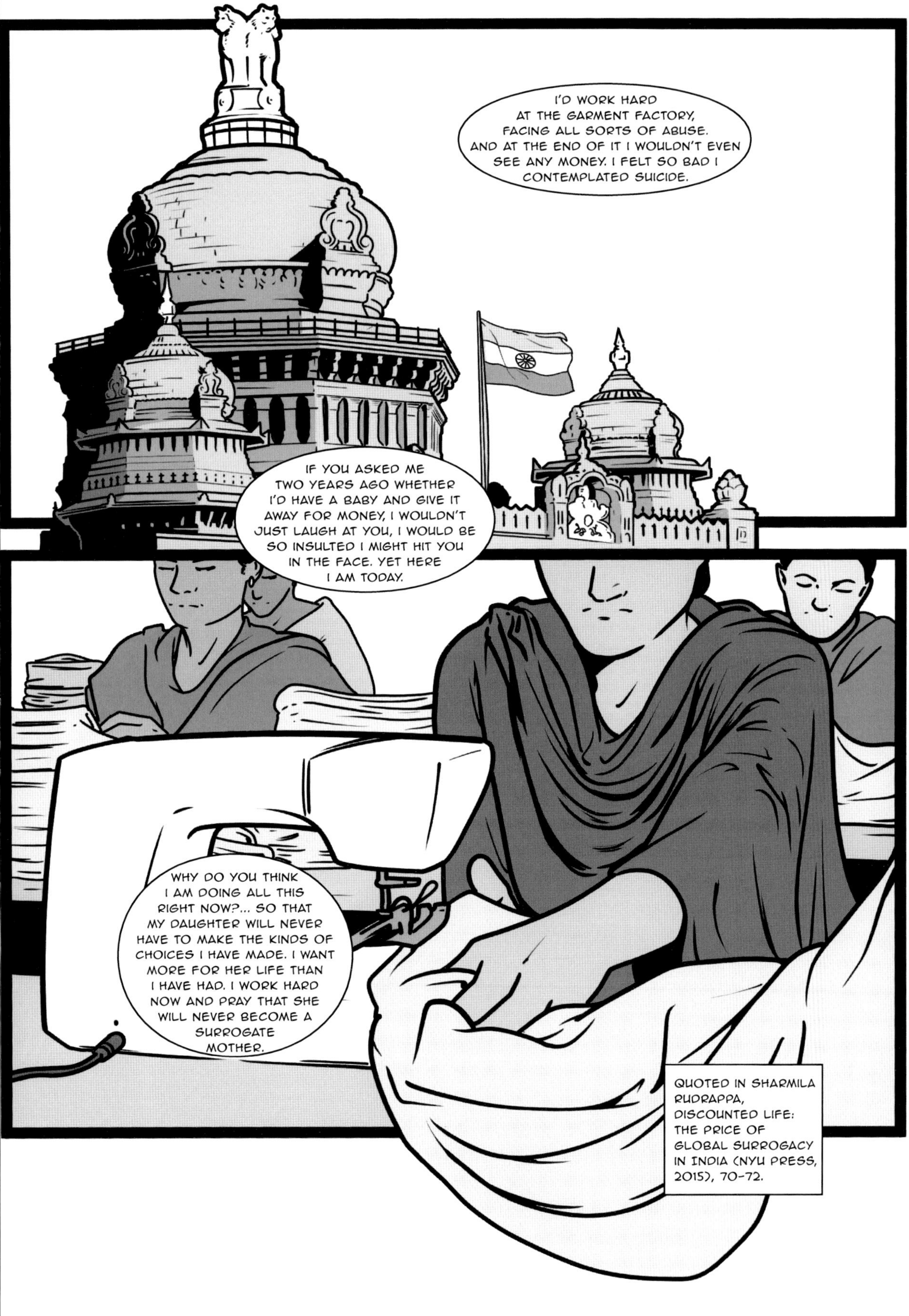
I'D WORK HARD AT THE GARMENT FACTORY, FACING ALL SORTS OF ABUSE. AND AT THE END OF IT I WOULDN'T EVEN SEE ANY MONEY. I FELT SO BAD I CONTEMPLATED SUICIDE.
IF YOU ASKED ME TWO YEARS AGO WHETHER I'D HAVE A BABY AND GIVE IT AWAY FOR MONEY, I WOULDN'T JUST LAUGH AT YOU, I WOULD BE SO INSULTED I MIGHT HIT YOU IN THE FACE. YET HERE I AM TODAY.
WHY DO YOU THINK I AM DOING ALL THIS RIGHT NOW?... SO THAT MY DAUGHTER WILL NEVER HAVE TO MAKE THE KINDS OF CHOICES I HAVE MADE. I WANT MORE FOR HER LIFE THAN I HAVE HAD. I WORK HARD NOW AND PRAY THAT SHE WILL NEVER BECOME A SURROGATE MOTHER.
QUOTED IN SHARMILA RUDRAPPA, DISCOUNTED LIFE: THE PRICE OF GLOBAL SURROGACY IN INDIA (NYU PRESS, 2015), 70–72.

-CHAPTER 13-
TESTING BOUNDARIES

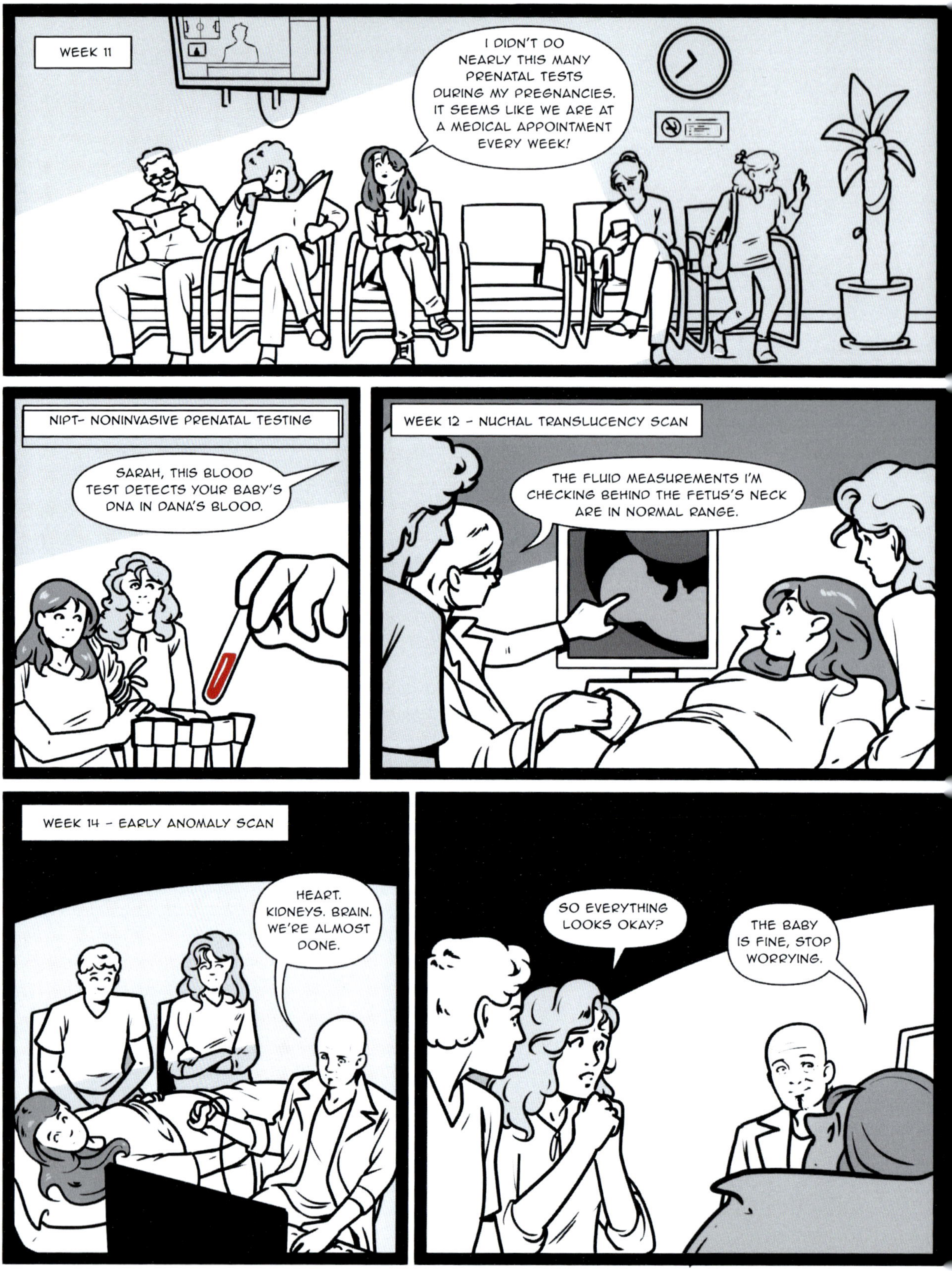

WEEK 11
I DIDN'T DO NEARLY THIS MANY PRENATAL TESTS DURING MY PREGNANCIES. IT SEEMS LIKE WE ARE AT A MEDICAL APPOINTMENT EVERY WEEK!
NIPT- NONINVASIVE PRENATAL TESTING
SARAH, THIS BLOOD TEST DETECTS YOUR BABY'S DNA IN DANA'S BLOOD.
WEEK 12 - NUCHAL TRANSLUCENCY SCAN
THE FLUID MEASUREMENTS I'M CHECKING BEHIND THE FETUS'S NECK ARE IN NORMAL RANGE.
WEEK 14 - EARLY ANOMALY SCAN
HEART. KIDNEYS. BRAIN. WE'RE ALMOST DONE.
SO EVERYTHING LOOKS OKAY?
THE BABY IS FINE, STOP WORRYING.

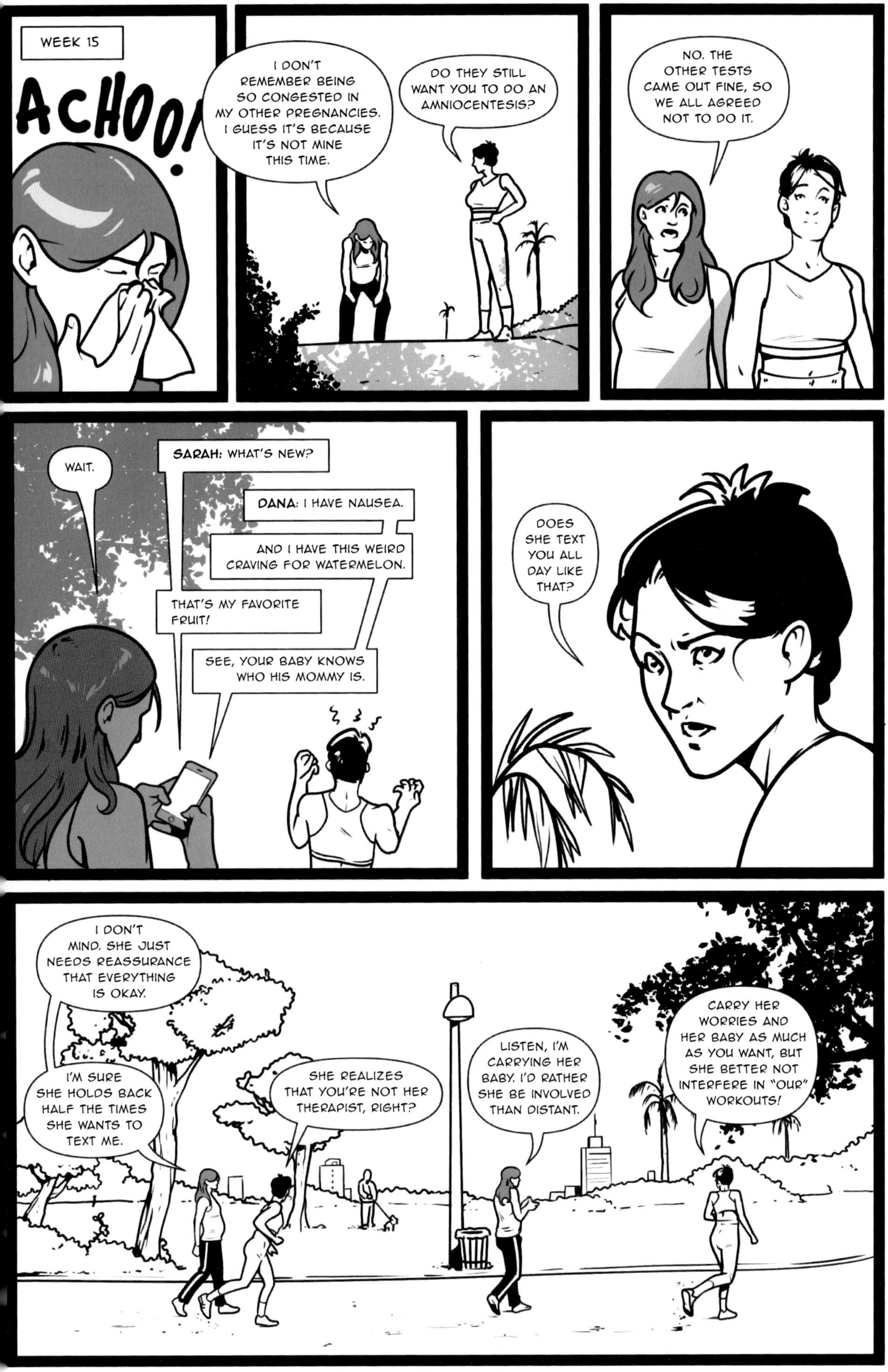
WEEK 15
ACHOO!
I DON'T REMEMBER BEING SO CONGESTED IN MY OTHER PREGNANCIES. I GUESS IT'S BECAUSE IT'S NOT MINE THIS TIME.
DO THEY STILL WANT YOU TO DO AN AMNIOCENTESIS?
NO. THE OTHER TESTS CAME OUT FINE, SO WE ALL AGREED NOT TO DO IT.
WAIT.
SARAH: WHAT'S NEW?
DANA: I HAVE NAUSEA.
AND I HAVE THIS WEIRD CRAVING FOR WATERMELON.
THAT'S MY FAVORITE FRUIT!
SEE, YOUR BABY KNOWS WHO HIS MOMMY IS.
DOES SHE TEXT YOU ALL DAY LIKE THAT?
I DON'T MIND. SHE JUST NEEDS REASSURANCE THAT EVERYTHING IS OKAY.
I'M SURE SHE HOLDS BACK HALF THE TIMES SHE WANTS TO TEXT ME.
SHE REALIZES THAT YOU'RE NOT HER THERAPIST, RIGHT?
LISTEN, I'M CARRYING HER BABY. I'D RATHER SHE BE INVOLVED THAN DISTANT.
CARRY HER WORRIES AND HER BABY AS MUCH AS YOU WANT, BUT SHE BETTER NOT INTERFERE IN "OUR" WORKOUTS!

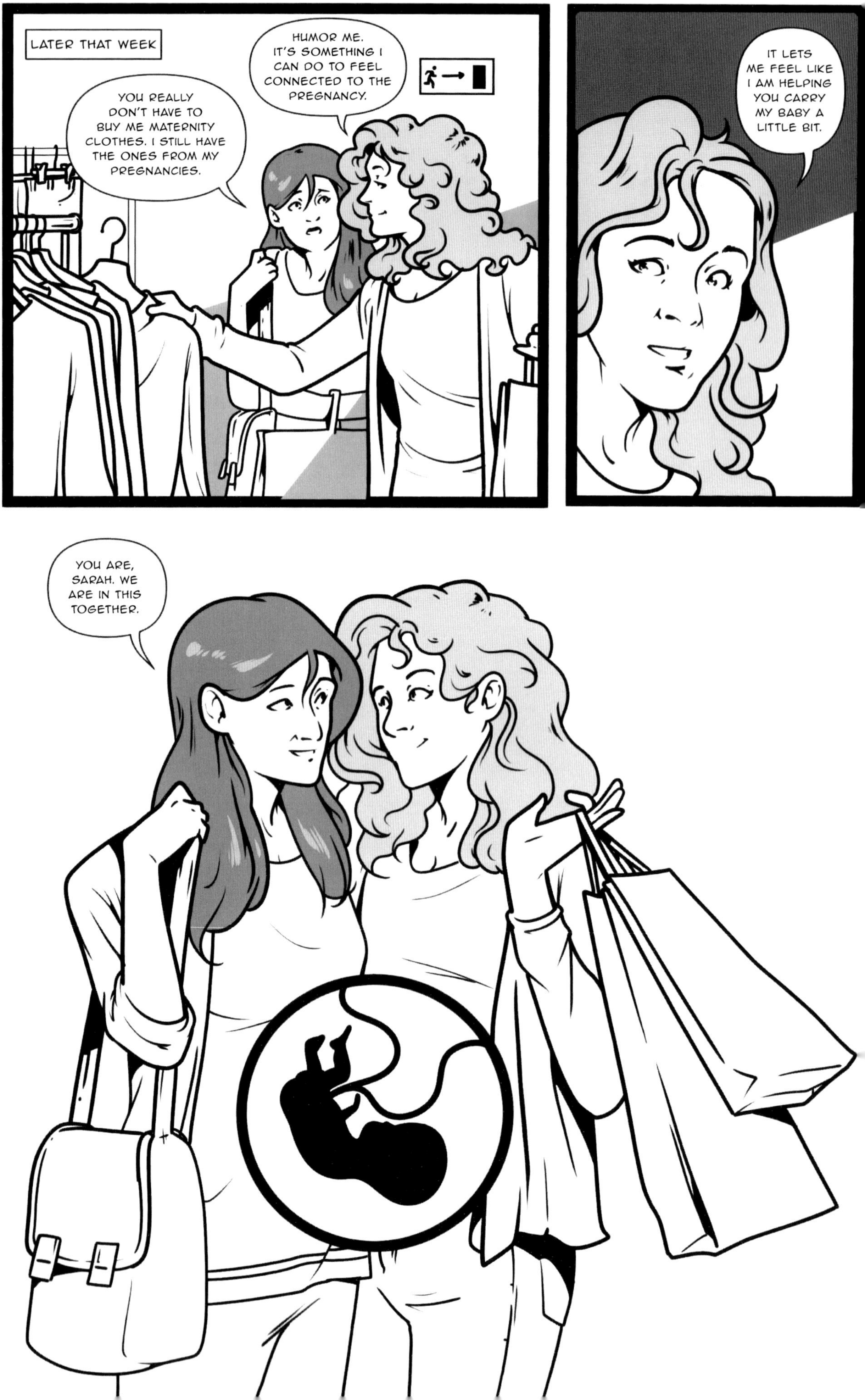
LATER THAT WEEK
YOU REALLY DON'T HAVE TO BUY ME MATERNITY CLOTHES. I STILL HAVE THE ONES FROM MY PREGNANCIES.
HUMOR ME. IT'S SOMETHING I CAN DO TO FEEL CONNECTED TO THE PREGNANCY.
IT LETS ME FEEL LIKE I AM HELPING YOU CARRY MY BABY A LITTLE BIT.
YOU ARE, SARAH. WE ARE IN THIS TOGETHER.

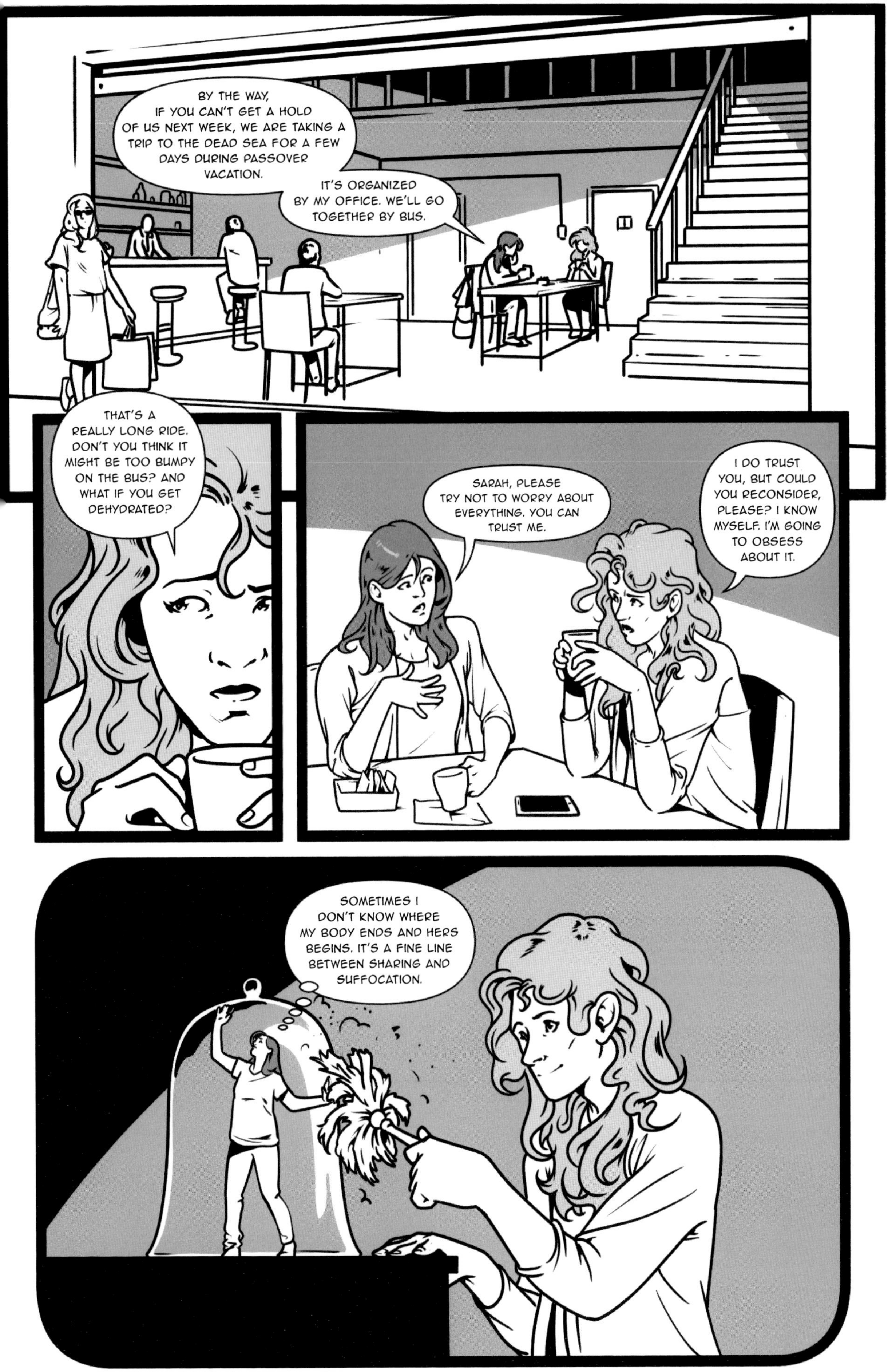
BY THE WAY, IF YOU CAN'T GET A HOLD OF US NEXT WEEK, WE ARE TAKING A TRIP TO THE DEAD SEA FOR A FEW DAYS DURING PASSOVER VACATION.
IT'S ORGANIZED BY MY OFFICE. WE'LL GO TOGETHER BY BUS.
THAT'S A REALLY LONG RIDE. DON'T YOU THINK IT MIGHT BE TOO BUMPY ON THE BUS? AND WHAT IF YOU GET DEHYDRATED?
SARAH, PLEASE TRY NOT TO WORRY ABOUT EVERYTHING. YOU CAN TRUST ME.
I DO TRUST YOU, BUT COULD YOU RECONSIDER, PLEASE? I KNOW MYSELF. I'M GOING TO OBSESS ABOUT IT.
SOMETIMES I DON'T KNOW WHERE MY BODY ENDS AND HERS BEGINS. IT'S A FINE LINE BETWEEN SHARING AND SUFFOCATION.

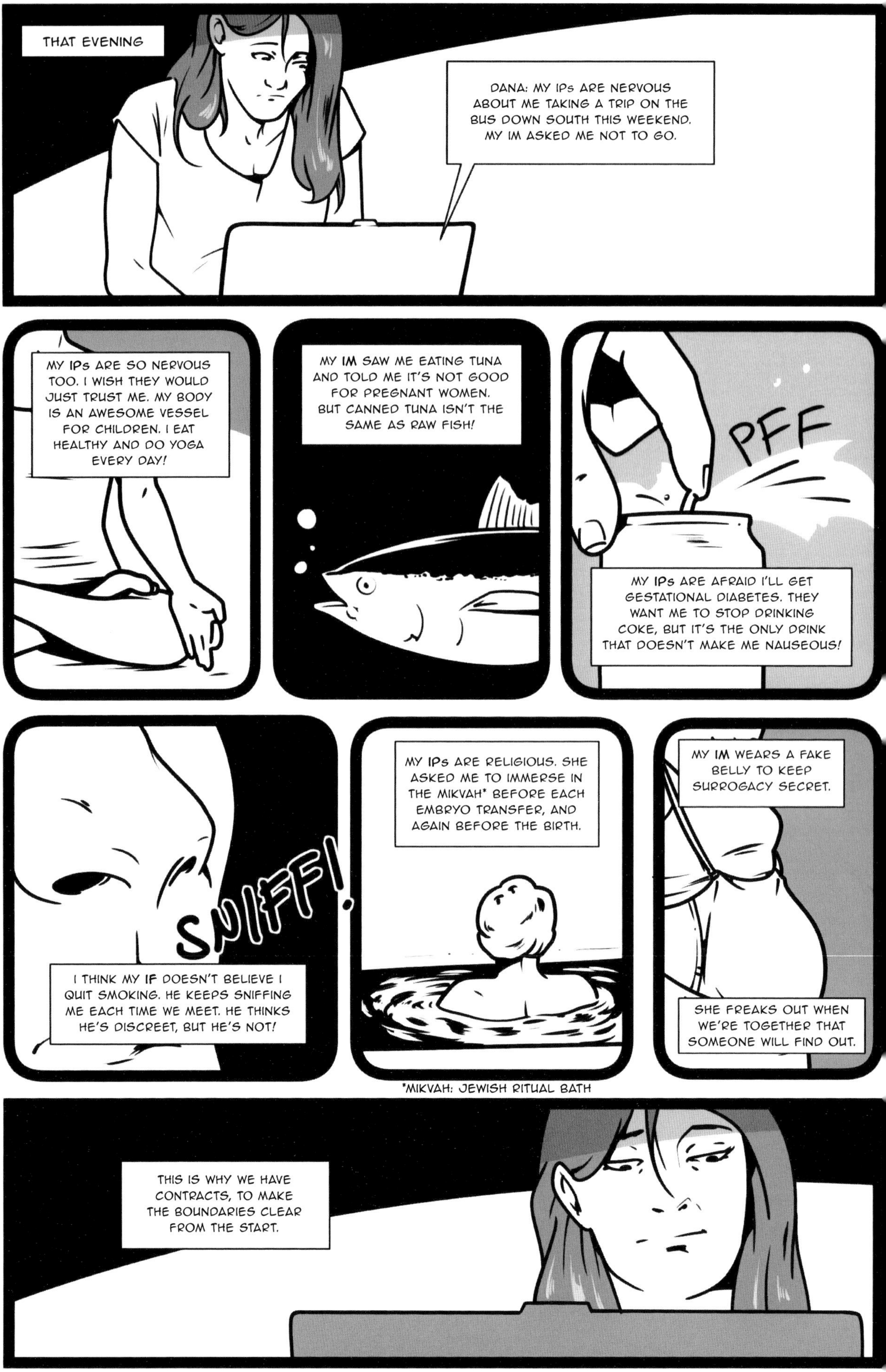
THAT EVENING
DANA: MY IPs ARE NERVOUS ABOUT ME TAKING A TRIP ON THE BUS DOWN SOUTH THIS WEEKEND. MY IM ASKED ME NOT TO GO.
MY IPs ARE SO NERVOUS TOO. I WISH THEY WOULD JUST TRUST ME. MY BODY IS AN AWESOME VESSEL FOR CHILDREN. I EAT HEALTHY AND DO YOGA EVERY DAY!
MY IM SAW ME EATING TUNA AND TOLD ME IT'S NOT GOOD FOR PREGNANT WOMEN. BUT CANNED TUNA ISN'T THE SAME AS RAW FISH!
PFF
MY IPs ARE AFRAID I'LL GET GESTATIONAL DIABETES. THEY WANT ME TO STOP DRINKING COKE, BUT IT'S THE ONLY DRINK THAT DOESN'T MAKE ME NAUSEOUS!
SNIFF!
I THINK MY IF DOESN'T BELIEVE I QUIT SMOKING. HE KEEPS SNIFFING ME EACH TIME WE MEET. HE THINKS HE'S DISCREET, BUT HE'S NOT!
MY IPs ARE RELIGIOUS. SHE ASKED ME TO IMMERSE IN THE MIKVAH* BEFORE EACH EMBRYO TRANSFER, AND AGAIN BEFORE THE BIRTH.
MY IM WEARS A FAKE BELLY TO KEEP SURROGACY SECRET.
SHE FREAKS OUT WHEN WE'RE TOGETHER THAT SOMEONE WILL FIND OUT.
*MIKVAH: JEWISH RITUAL BATH
THIS IS WHY WE HAVE CONTRACTS, TO MAKE THE BOUNDARIES CLEAR FROM THE START.

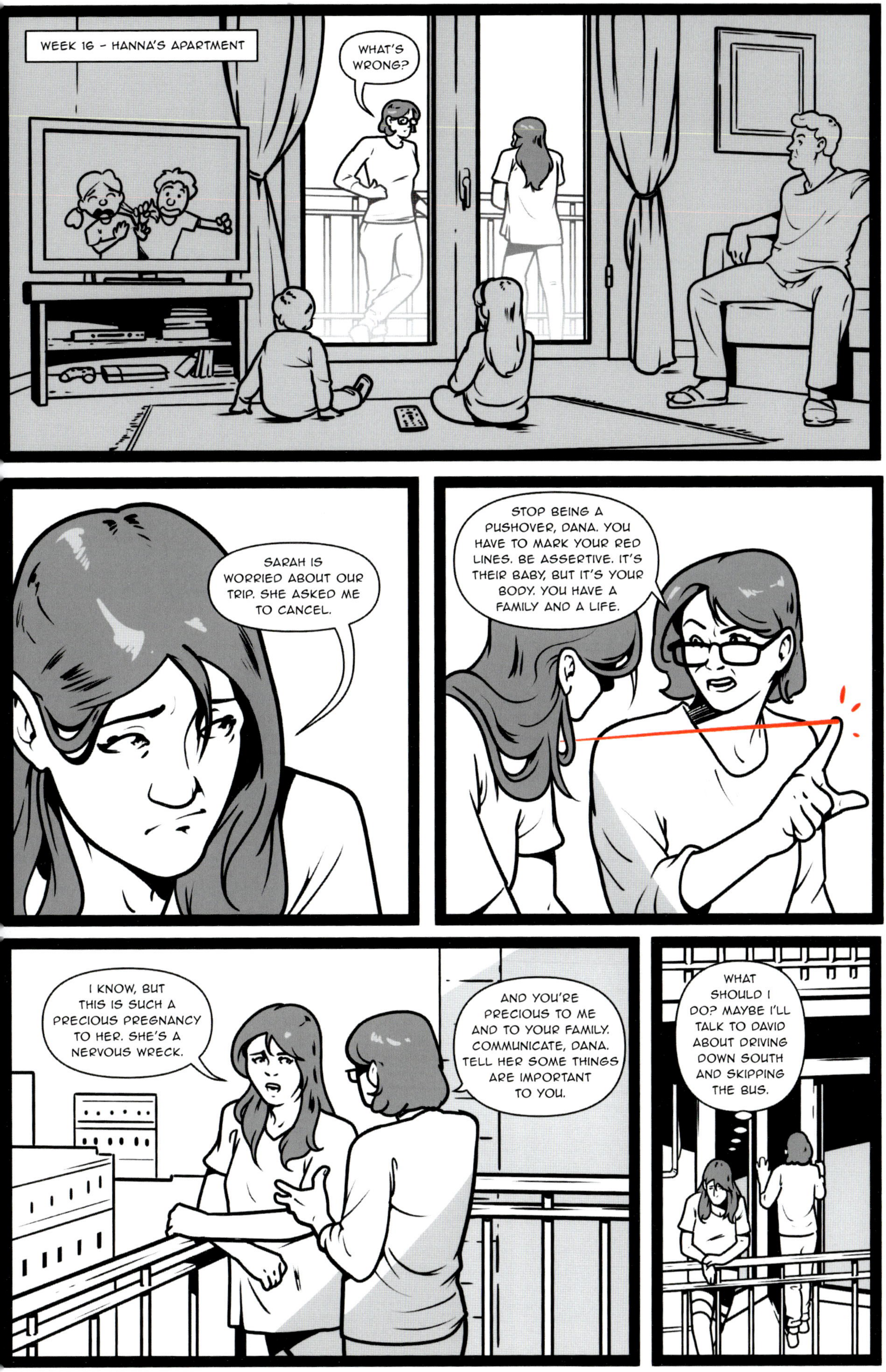
WEEK 16 – HANNA'S APARTMENT
WHAT'S WRONG?
SARAH IS WORRIED ABOUT OUR TRIP. SHE ASKED ME TO CANCEL.
STOP BEING A PUSHOVER, DANA. YOU HAVE TO MARK YOUR RED LINES. BE ASSERTIVE. IT'S THEIR BABY, BUT IT'S YOUR BODY. YOU HAVE A FAMILY AND A LIFE.
I KNOW, BUT THIS IS SUCH A PRECIOUS PREGNANCY TO HER. SHE'S A NERVOUS WRECK.
AND YOU'RE PRECIOUS TO ME AND TO YOUR FAMILY. COMMUNICATE, DANA. TELL HER SOME THINGS ARE IMPORTANT TO YOU.
WHAT SHOULD I DO? MAYBE I'LL TALK TO DAVID ABOUT DRIVING DOWN SOUTH AND SKIPPING THE BUS.

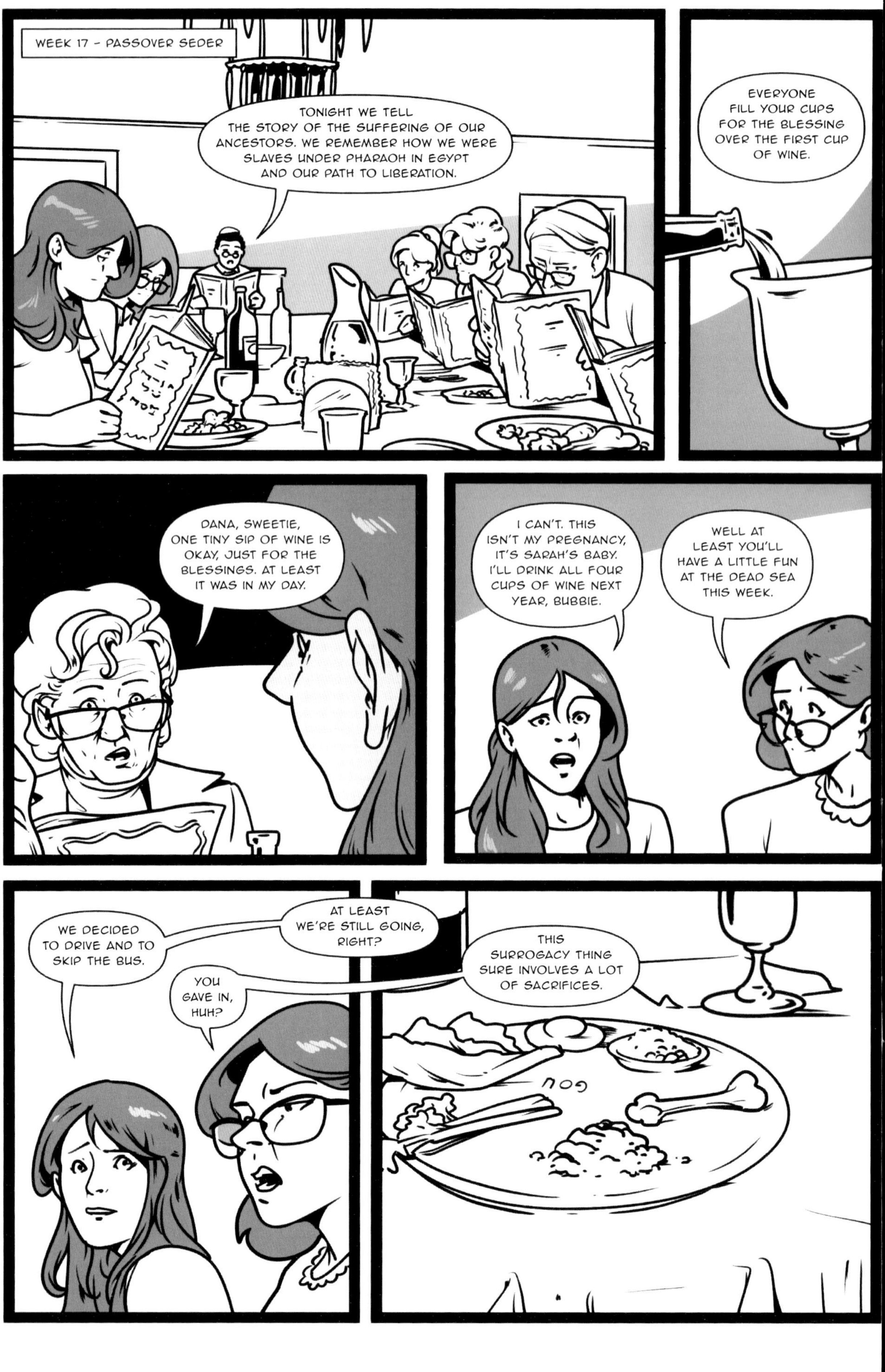
WEEK 17 - PASSOVER SEDER
TONIGHT WE TELL THE STORY OF THE SUFFERING OF OUR ANCESTORS. WE REMEMBER HOW WE WERE SLAVES UNDER PHARAOH IN EGYPT AND OUR PATH TO LIBERATION.
EVERYONE FILL YOUR CUPS FOR THE BLESSING OVER THE FIRST CUP OF WINE.
DANA, SWEETIE, ONE TINY SIP OF WINE IS OKAY, JUST FOR THE BLESSINGS. AT LEAST IT WAS IN MY DAY.
I CAN'T. THIS ISN'T MY PREGNANCY, IT'S SARAH'S BABY. I'LL DRINK ALL FOUR CUPS OF WINE NEXT YEAR, BUBBIE.
WELL AT LEAST YOU'LL HAVE A LITTLE FUN AT THE DEAD SEA THIS WEEK.
WE DECIDED TO DRIVE AND TO SKIP THE BUS.
AT LEAST WE'RE STILL GOING, RIGHT?
YOU GAVE IN, HUH?
THIS SURROGACY THING SURE INVOLVES A LOT OF SACRIFICES.

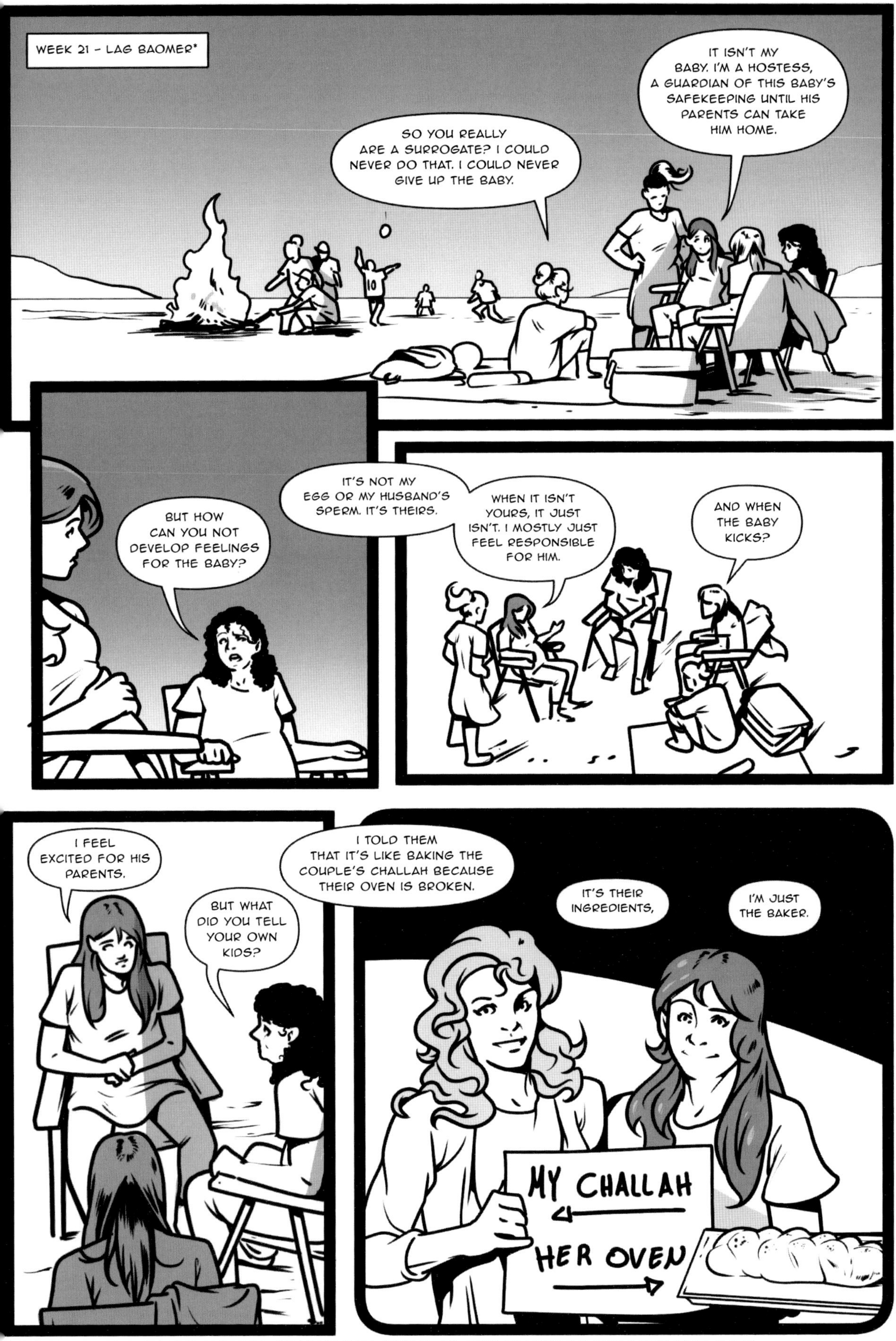
WEEK 21 – LAG BAOMER*
SO YOU REALLY ARE A SURROGATE? I COULD NEVER DO THAT. I COULD NEVER GIVE UP THE BABY.
IT ISN'T MY BABY. I'M A HOSTESS, A GUARDIAN OF THIS BABY'S SAFEKEEPING UNTIL HIS PARENTS CAN TAKE HIM HOME.
10
BUT HOW CAN YOU NOT DEVELOP FEELINGS FOR THE BABY?
IT'S NOT MY EGG OR MY HUSBAND'S SPERM. IT'S THEIRS.
WHEN IT ISN'T YOURS, IT JUST ISN'T. I MOSTLY JUST FEEL RESPONSIBLE FOR HIM.
AND WHEN THE BABY KICKS?
I FEEL EXCITED FOR HIS PARENTS.
BUT WHAT DID YOU TELL YOUR OWN KIDS?
I TOLD THEM THAT IT'S LIKE BAKING THE COUPLE'S CHALLAH BECAUSE THEIR OVEN IS BROKEN.
IT'S THEIR INGREDIENTS,
I'M JUST THE BAKER.
MY CHALLAH
HER OVEN

*A HOLIDAY WHEN IT IS CUSTOMARY FOR JEWISH ISRAELI SCHOOLCHILDREN TO LIGHT BONFIRES WITH THEIR CLASS

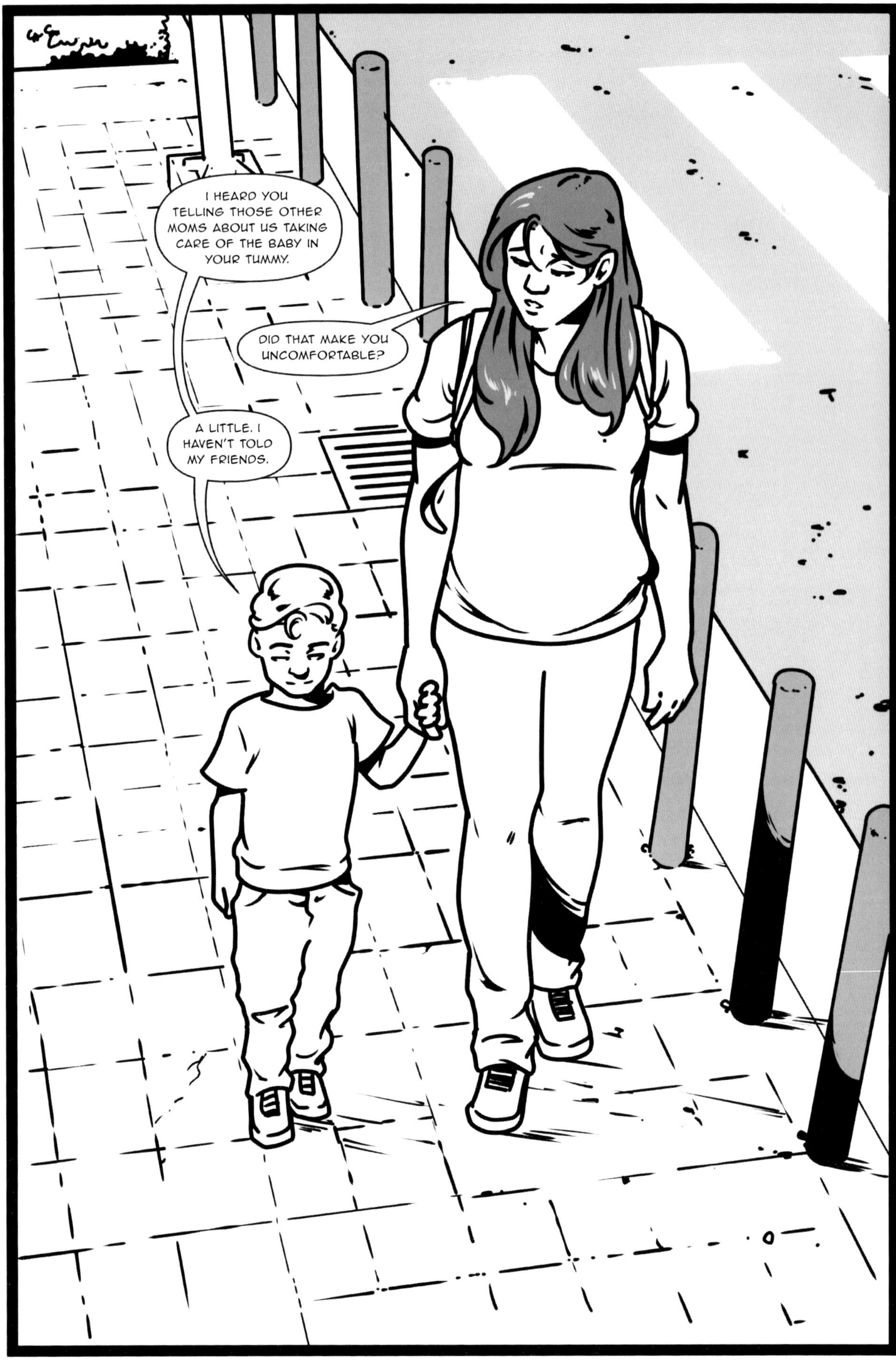
I HEARD YOU TELLING THOSE OTHER MOMS ABOUT US TAKING CARE OF THE BABY IN YOUR TUMMY.
DID THAT MAKE YOU UNCOMFORTABLE?
A LITTLE. I HAVEN'T TOLD MY FRIENDS.

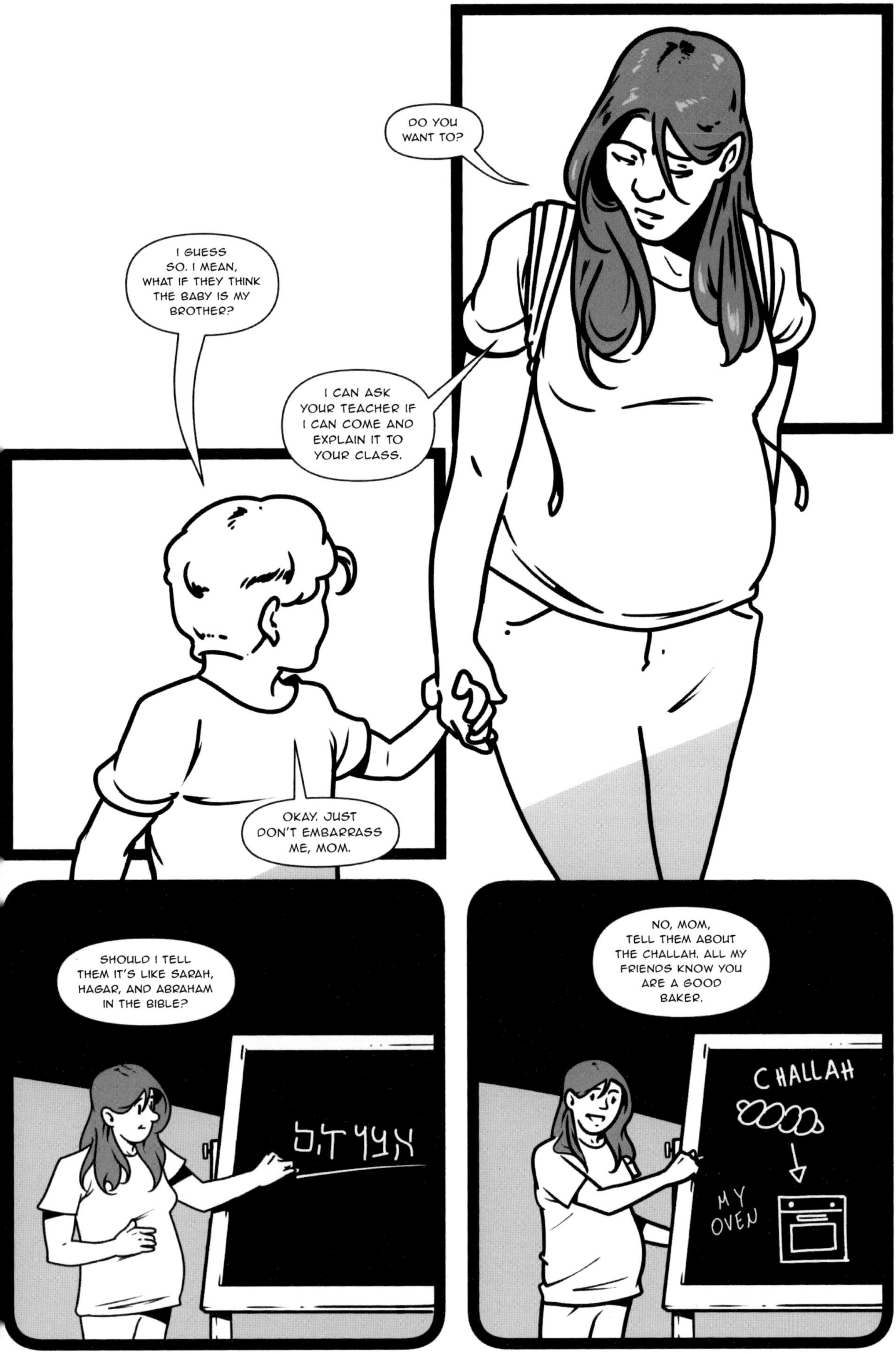
DO YOU WANT TO?
I GUESS SO. I MEAN, WHAT IF THEY THINK THE BABY IS MY BROTHER?
I CAN ASK YOUR TEACHER IF I CAN COME AND EXPLAIN IT TO YOUR CLASS.
OKAY. JUST DON'T EMBARRASS ME, MOM.
SHOULD I TELL THEM IT'S LIKE SARAH, HAGAR, AND ABRAHAM IN THE BIBLE?
NO, MOM, TELL THEM ABOUT THE CHALLAH. ALL MY FRIENDS KNOW YOU ARE A GOOD BAKER.
CHALLAH
MY OVEN

-CHAPTER 14-
BABYSITTING

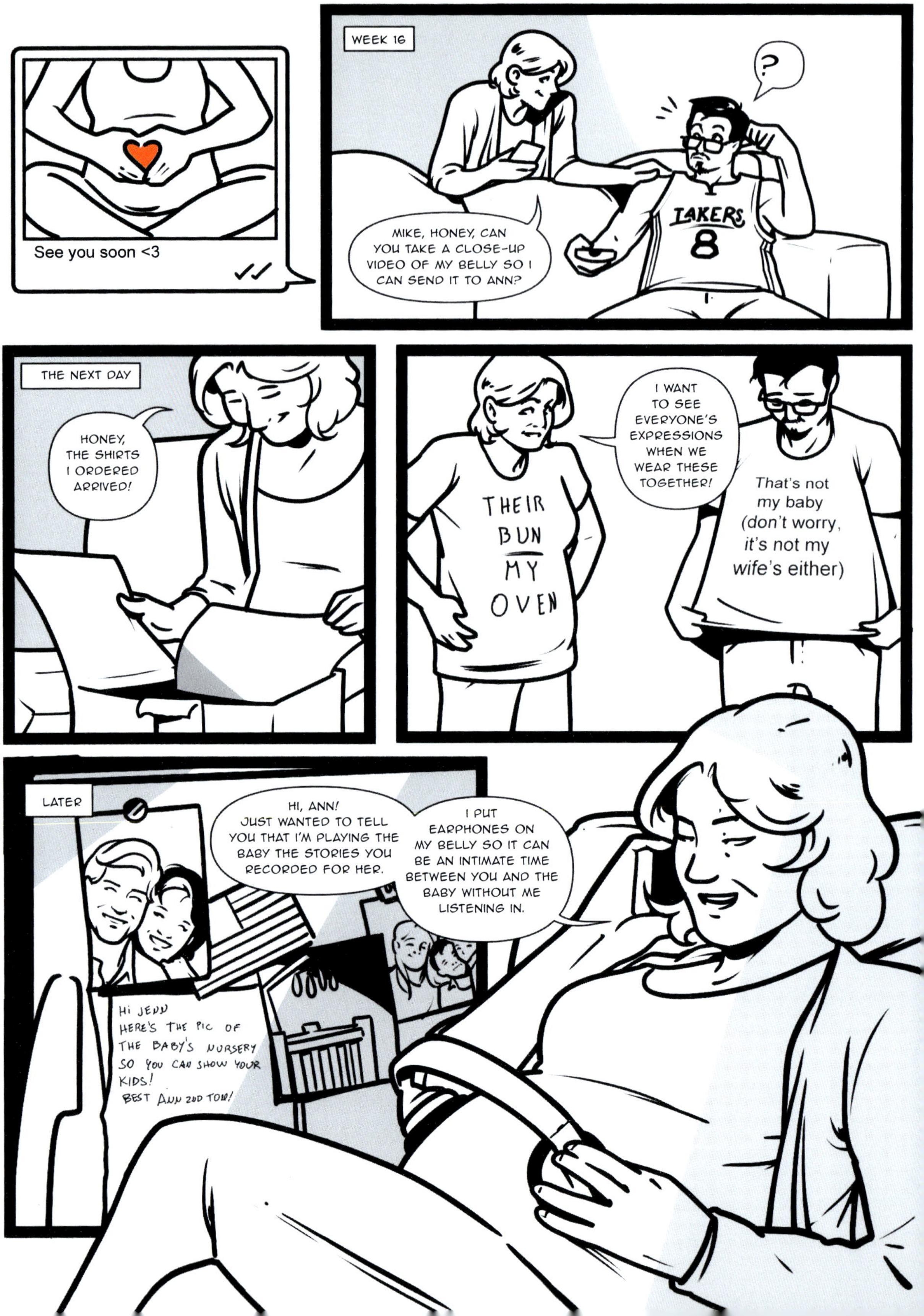
See you soon <3
WEEK 16
?
MIKE, HONEY, CAN YOU TAKE A CLOSE-UP VIDEO OF MY BELLY SO I CAN SEND IT TO ANN?
LAKERS 8
THE NEXT DAY
HONEY, THE SHIRTS I ORDERED ARRIVED!
THEIR BUN MY OVEN
I WANT TO SEE EVERYONE'S EXPRESSIONS WHEN WE WEAR THESE TOGETHER!
That's not my baby (don't worry, it's not my wife's either)
LATER
HI JENN
HERE'S THE PIC OF THE BABY'S NURSERY SO YOU CAN SHOW YOUR KIDS!
BEST ANN AND TOM!
HI, ANN! JUST WANTED TO TELL YOU THAT I'M PLAYING THE BABY THE STORIES YOU RECORDED FOR HER.
I PUT EARPHONES ON MY BELLY SO IT CAN BE AN INTIMATE TIME BETWEEN YOU AND THE BABY WITHOUT ME LISTENING IN.

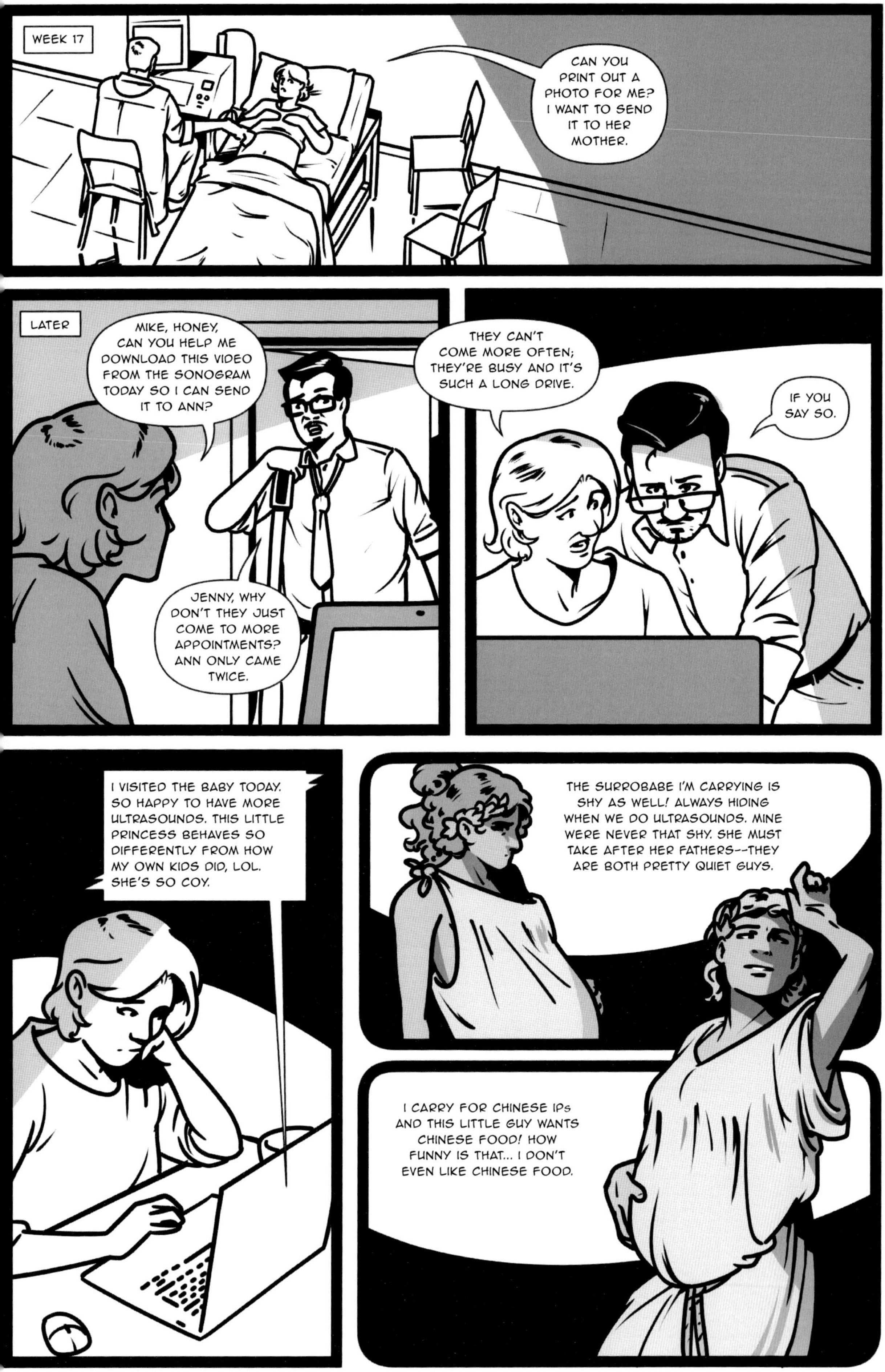
WEEK 17
CAN YOU PRINT OUT A PHOTO FOR ME? I WANT TO SEND IT TO HER MOTHER.
LATER
MIKE, HONEY, CAN YOU HELP ME DOWNLOAD THIS VIDEO FROM THE SONOGRAM TODAY SO I CAN SEND IT TO ANN?
JENNY, WHY DON'T THEY JUST COME TO MORE APPOINTMENTS? ANN ONLY CAME TWICE.
THEY CAN'T COME MORE OFTEN; THEY'RE BUSY AND IT'S SUCH A LONG DRIVE.
IF YOU SAY SO.
I VISITED THE BABY TODAY. SO HAPPY TO HAVE MORE ULTRASOUNDS. THIS LITTLE PRINCESS BEHAVES SO DIFFERENTLY FROM HOW MY OWN KIDS DID, LOL. SHE'S SO COY.
THE SURROBABE I'M CARRYING IS SHY AS WELL! ALWAYS HIDING WHEN WE DO ULTRASOUNDS. MINE WERE NEVER THAT SHY. SHE MUST TAKE AFTER HER FATHERS--THEY ARE BOTH PRETTY QUIET GUYS.
I CARRY FOR CHINESE IPs AND THIS LITTLE GUY WANTS CHINESE FOOD! HOW FUNNY IS THAT... I DON'T EVEN LIKE CHINESE FOOD.

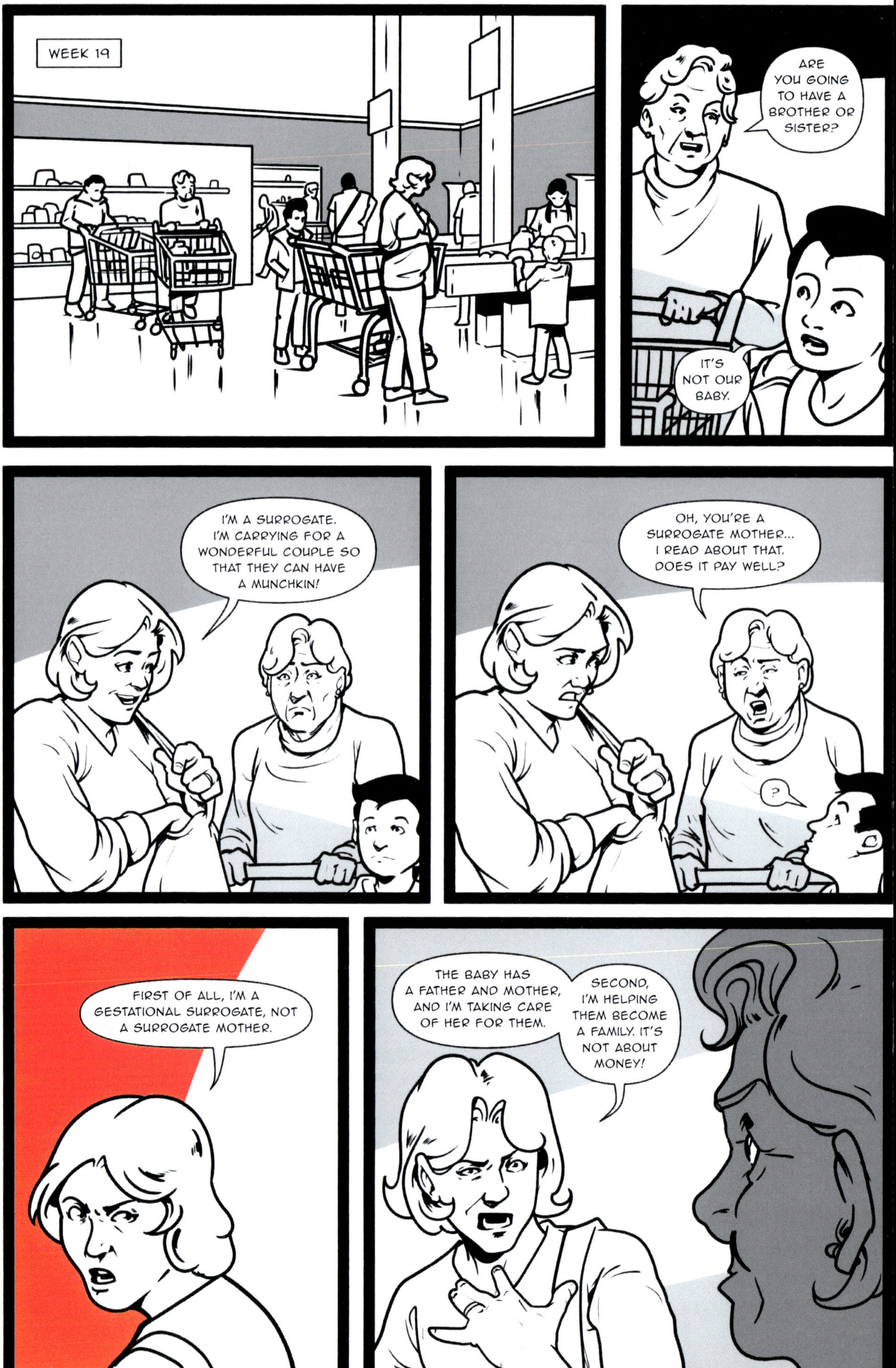
WEEK 19
ARE YOU GOING TO HAVE A BROTHER OR SISTER?
IT'S NOT OUR BABY.
I'M A SURROGATE. I'M CARRYING FOR A WONDERFUL COUPLE SO THAT THEY CAN HAVE A MUNCHKIN!
OH, YOU'RE A SURROGATE MOTHER... I READ ABOUT THAT. DOES IT PAY WELL?
?
FIRST OF ALL, I'M A GESTATIONAL SURROGATE, NOT A SURROGATE MOTHER.
THE BABY HAS A FATHER AND MOTHER, AND I'M TAKING CARE OF HER FOR THEM.
SECOND, I'M HELPING THEM BECOME A FAMILY. IT'S NOT ABOUT MONEY!

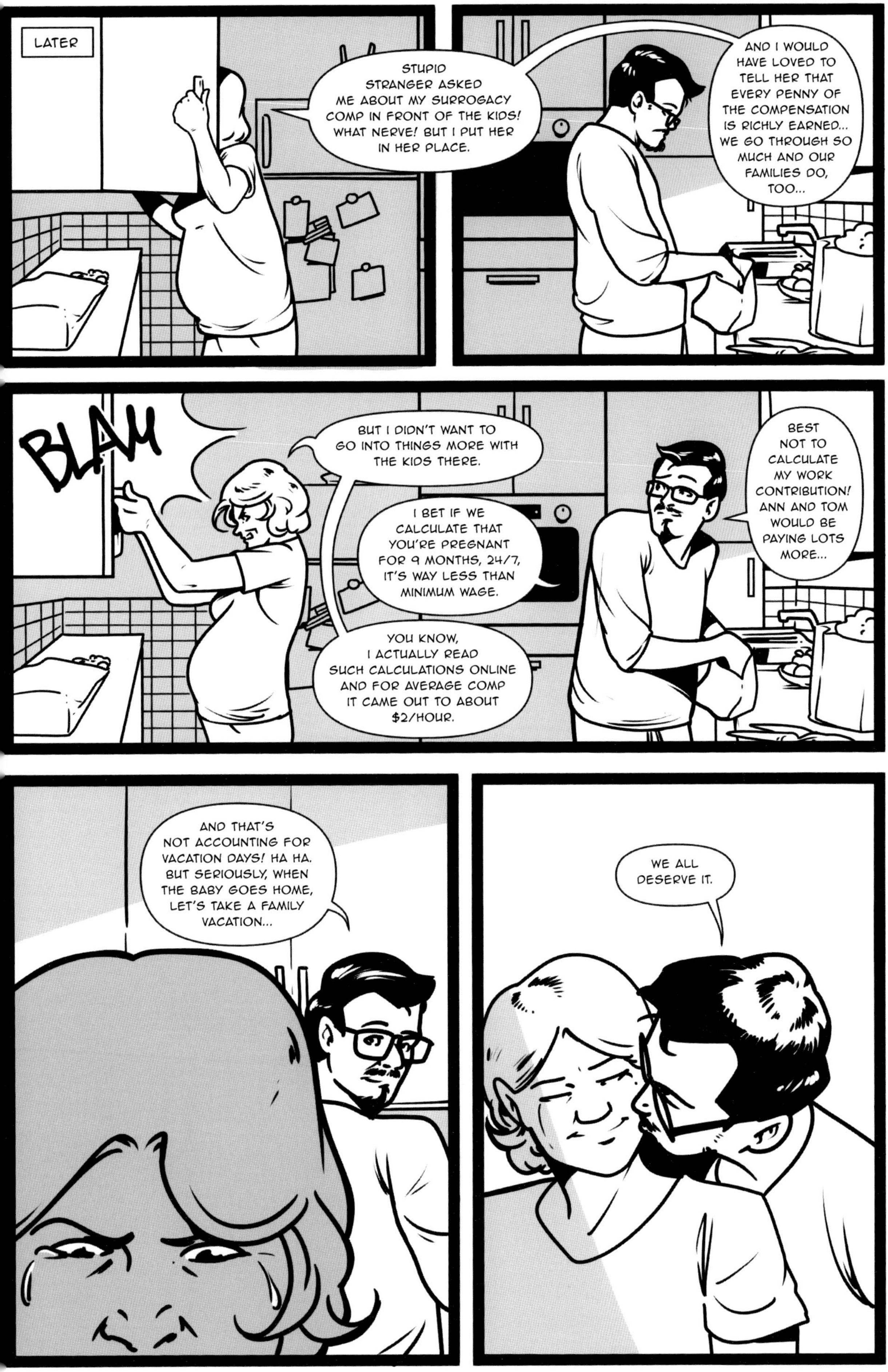
LATER
STUPID STRANGER ASKED ME ABOUT MY SURROGACY COMP IN FRONT OF THE KIDS! WHAT NERVE! BUT I PUT HER IN HER PLACE.
AND I WOULD HAVE LOVED TO TELL HER THAT EVERY PENNY OF THE COMPENSATION IS RICHLY EARNED... WE GO THROUGH SO MUCH AND OUR FAMILIES DO, TOO...
BLAM
BUT I DIDN'T WANT TO GO INTO THINGS MORE WITH THE KIDS THERE.
I BET IF WE CALCULATE THAT YOU'RE PREGNANT FOR 9 MONTHS, 24/7, IT'S WAY LESS THAN MINIMUM WAGE.
YOU KNOW, I ACTUALLY READ SUCH CALCULATIONS ONLINE AND FOR AVERAGE COMP IT CAME OUT TO ABOUT $2/HOUR.
BEST NOT TO CALCULATE MY WORK CONTRIBUTION! ANN AND TOM WOULD BE PAYING LOTS MORE...
AND THAT'S NOT ACCOUNTING FOR VACATION DAYS! HA HA. BUT SERIOUSLY, WHEN THE BABY GOES HOME, LET'S TAKE A FAMILY VACATION...
WE ALL DESERVE IT.

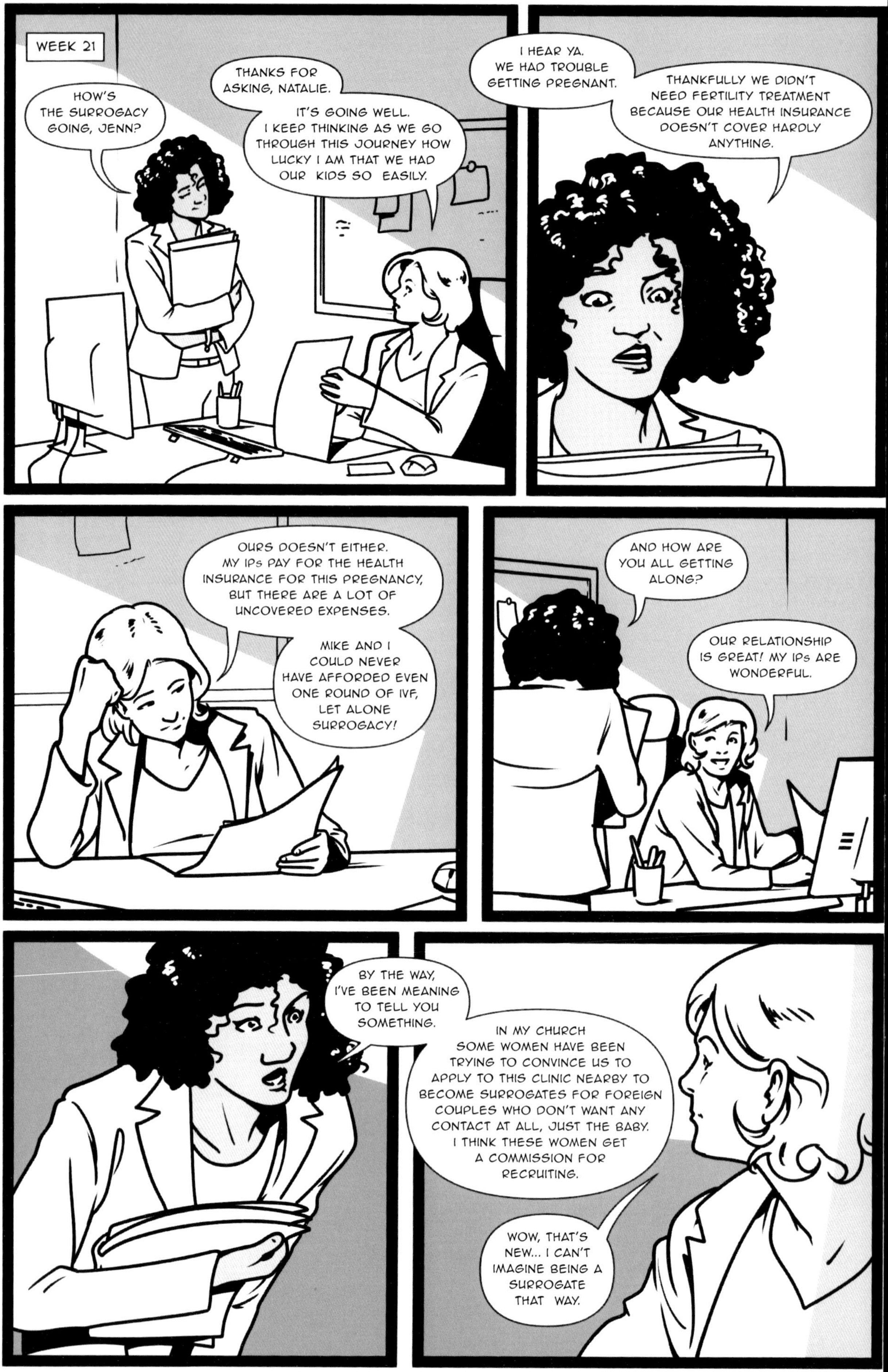
WEEK 21
HOW'S THE SURROGACY GOING, JENN?
THANKS FOR ASKING, NATALIE.
IT'S GOING WELL. I KEEP THINKING AS WE GO THROUGH THIS JOURNEY HOW LUCKY I AM THAT WE HAD OUR KIDS SO EASILY.
I HEAR YA. WE HAD TROUBLE GETTING PREGNANT.
THANKFULLY WE DIDN'T NEED FERTILITY TREATMENT BECAUSE OUR HEALTH INSURANCE DOESN'T COVER HARDLY ANYTHING.
OURS DOESN'T EITHER. MY IPs PAY FOR THE HEALTH INSURANCE FOR THIS PREGNANCY, BUT THERE ARE A LOT OF UNCOVERED EXPENSES.
MIKE AND I COULD NEVER HAVE AFFORDED EVEN ONE ROUND OF IVF, LET ALONE SURROGACY!
AND HOW ARE YOU ALL GETTING ALONG?
OUR RELATIONSHIP IS GREAT! MY IPs ARE WONDERFUL.
BY THE WAY, I'VE BEEN MEANING TO TELL YOU SOMETHING.
IN MY CHURCH SOME WOMEN HAVE BEEN TRYING TO CONVINCE US TO APPLY TO THIS CLINIC NEARBY TO BECOME SURROGATES FOR FOREIGN COUPLES WHO DON'T WANT ANY CONTACT AT ALL, JUST THE BABY. I THINK THESE WOMEN GET A COMMISSION FOR RECRUITING.
WOW, THAT'S NEW... I CAN'T IMAGINE BEING A SURROGATE THAT WAY.

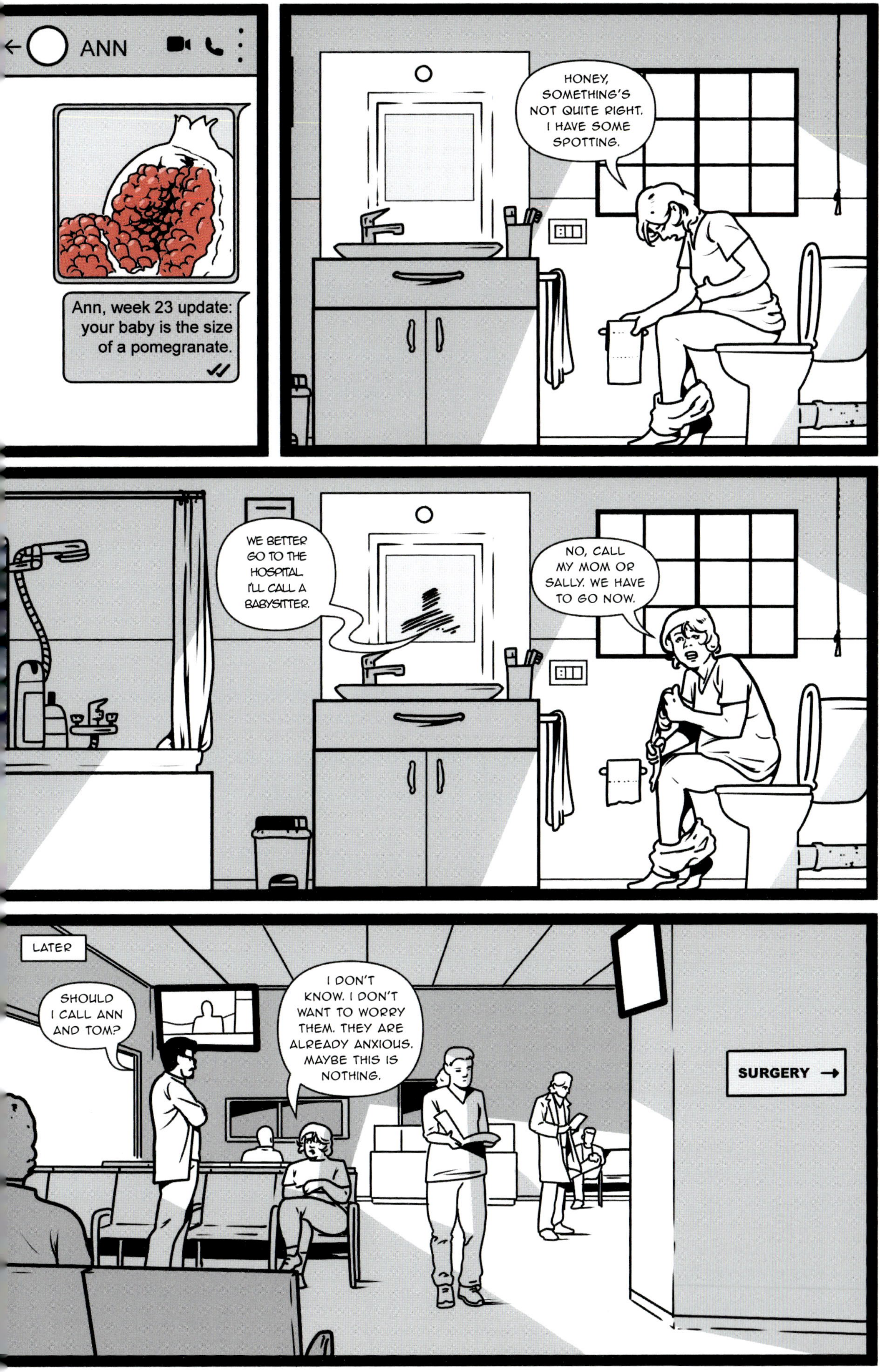
ANN
Ann, week 23 update: your baby is the size of a pomegranate.
HONEY, SOMETHING'S NOT QUITE RIGHT. I HAVE SOME SPOTTING.
WE BETTER GO TO THE HOSPITAL. I'LL CALL A BABYSITTER.
NO, CALL MY MOM OR SALLY. WE HAVE TO GO NOW.
LATER
SHOULD I CALL ANN AND TOM?
I DON'T KNOW. I DON'T WANT TO WORRY THEM. THEY ARE ALREADY ANXIOUS. MAYBE THIS IS NOTHING.
SURGERY →

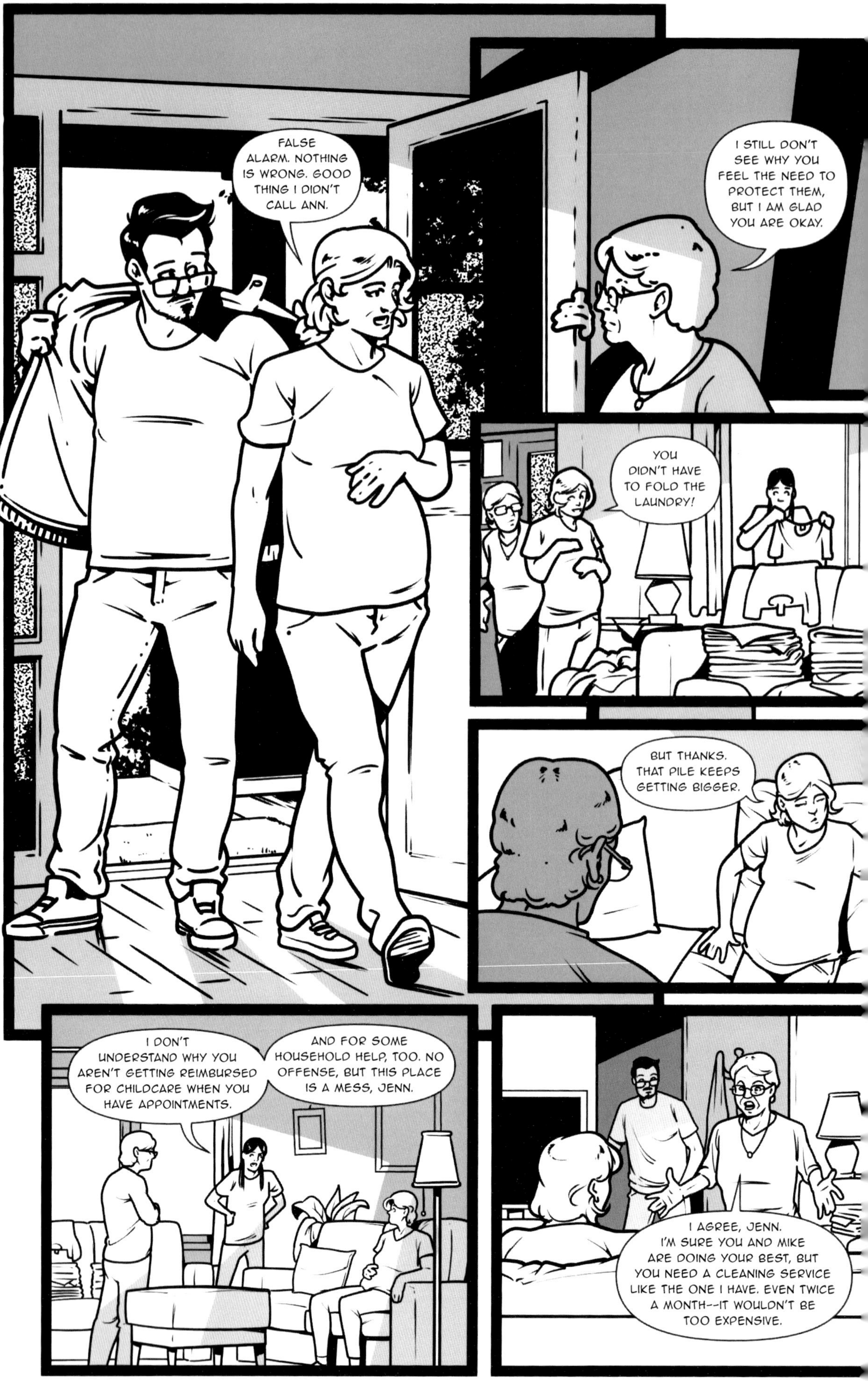
FALSE ALARM. NOTHING IS WRONG. GOOD THING I DIDN'T CALL ANN.
I STILL DON'T SEE WHY YOU FEEL THE NEED TO PROTECT THEM, BUT I AM GLAD YOU ARE OKAY.
YOU DIDN'T HAVE TO FOLD THE LAUNDRY!
BUT THANKS. THAT PILE KEEPS GETTING BIGGER.
I DON'T UNDERSTAND WHY YOU AREN'T GETTING REIMBURSED FOR CHILDCARE WHEN YOU HAVE APPOINTMENTS.
AND FOR SOME HOUSEHOLD HELP, TOO. NO OFFENSE, BUT THIS PLACE IS A MESS, JENN.
I AGREE, JENN. I'M SURE YOU AND MIKE ARE DOING YOUR BEST, BUT YOU NEED A CLEANING SERVICE LIKE THE ONE I HAVE. EVEN TWICE A MONTH--IT WOULDN'T BE TOO EXPENSIVE.

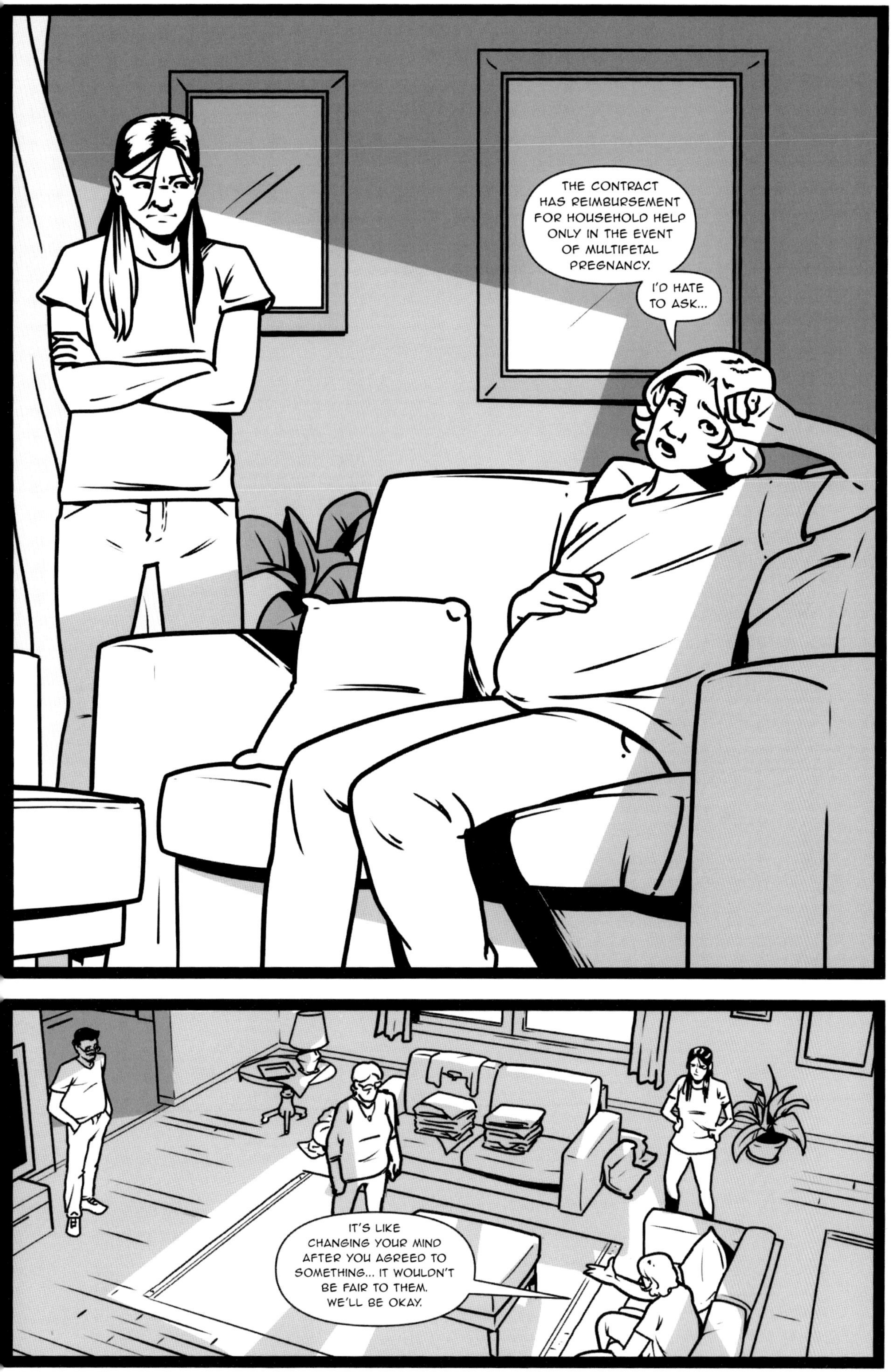
THE CONTRACT HAS REIMBURSEMENT FOR HOUSEHOLD HELP ONLY IN THE EVENT OF MULTIFETAL PREGNANCY.
I'D HATE TO ASK...
IT'S LIKE CHANGING YOUR MIND AFTER YOU AGREED TO SOMETHING... IT WOULDN'T BE FAIR TO THEM. WE'LL BE OKAY.

INTERLUDE: JARUWAN, SURROGATE IN BANGKOK, THAILAND

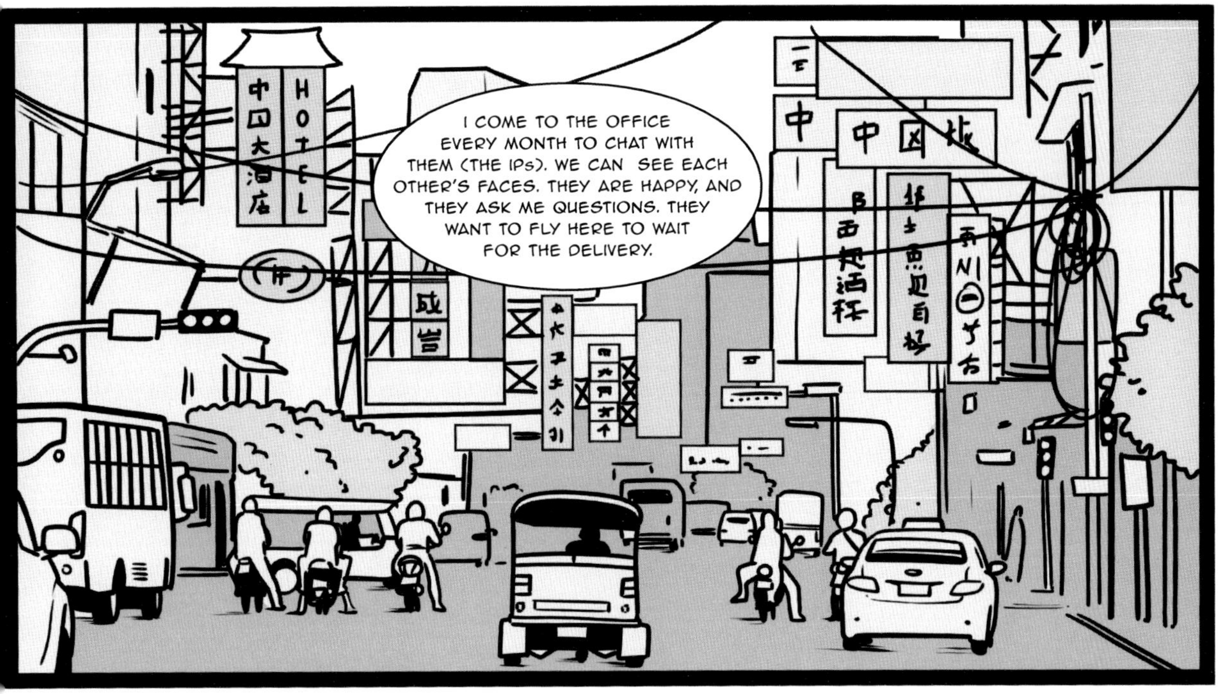
HOTEL
I COME TO THE OFFICE EVERY MONTH TO CHAT WITH THEM (THE IPs). WE CAN SEE EACH OTHER'S FACES. THEY ARE HAPPY, AND THEY ASK ME QUESTIONS. THEY WANT TO FLY HERE TO WAIT FOR THE DELIVERY.

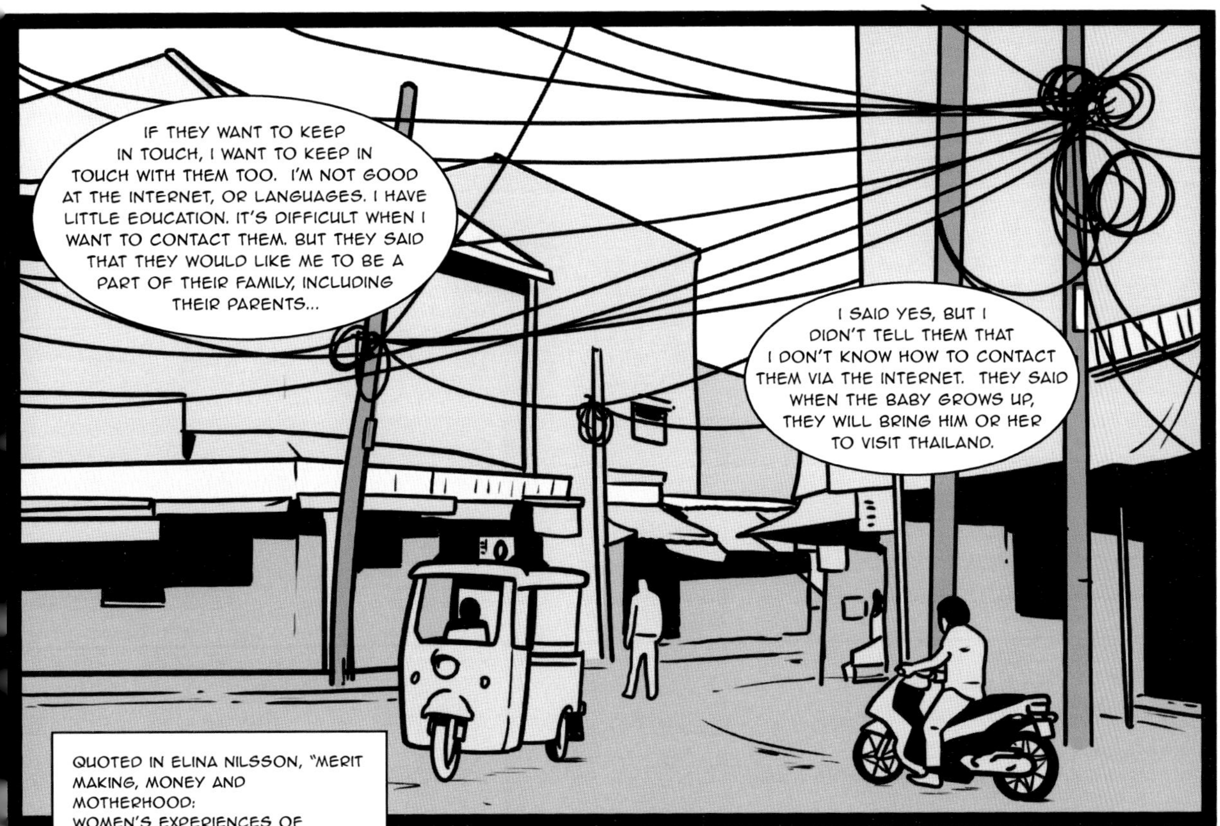
IF THEY WANT TO KEEP IN TOUCH, I WANT TO KEEP IN TOUCH WITH THEM TOO. I'M NOT GOOD AT THE INTERNET, OR LANGUAGES. I HAVE LITTLE EDUCATION. IT'S DIFFICULT WHEN I WANT TO CONTACT THEM. BUT THEY SAID THAT THEY WOULD LIKE ME TO BE A PART OF THEIR FAMILY, INCLUDING THEIR PARENTS...
I SAID YES, BUT I DIDN'T TELL THEM THAT I DON'T KNOW HOW TO CONTACT THEM VIA THE INTERNET. THEY SAID WHEN THE BABY GROWS UP, THEY WILL BRING HIM OR HER TO VISIT THAILAND.

QUOTED IN ELINA NILSSON, "MERIT MAKING, MONEY AND MOTHERHOOD: WOMEN'S EXPERIENCES OF COMMERCIAL SURROGACY IN THAILAND" (MA THESIS, CENTER FOR GENDER STUDIES, UPPSALA UNIVERSITY), 59.

-CHAPTER 15-
BIRTH PLAN

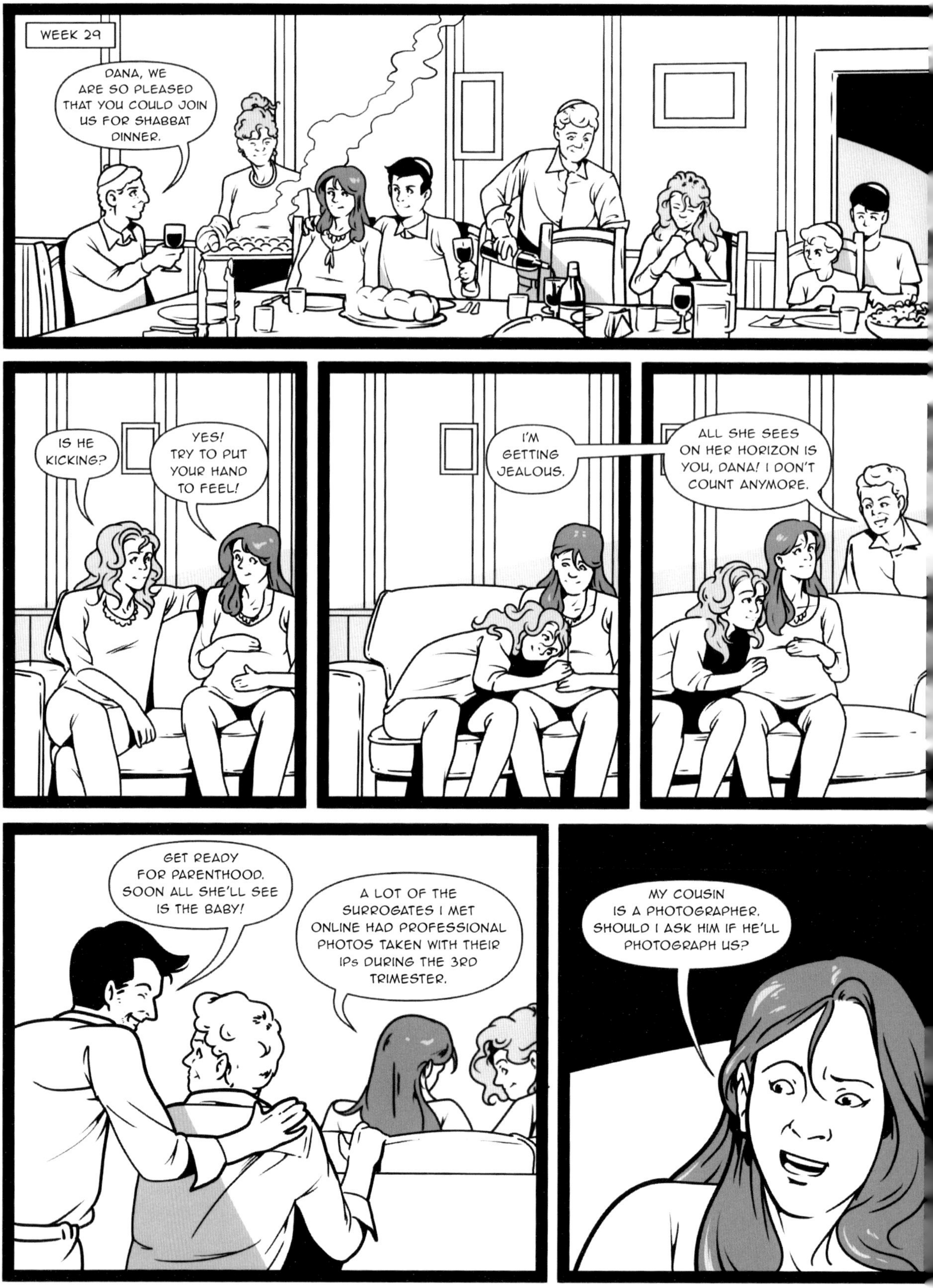
WEEK 29
DANA, WE ARE SO PLEASED THAT YOU COULD JOIN US FOR SHABBAT DINNER.
IS HE KICKING?
YES! TRY TO PUT YOUR HAND TO FEEL!
I'M GETTING JEALOUS.
ALL SHE SEES ON HER HORIZON IS YOU, DANA! I DON'T COUNT ANYMORE.
GET READY FOR PARENTHOOD. SOON ALL SHE'LL SEE IS THE BABY!
A LOT OF THE SURROGATES I MET ONLINE HAD PROFESSIONAL PHOTOS TAKEN WITH THEIR IPs DURING THE 3RD TRIMESTER.
MY COUSIN IS A PHOTOGRAPHER. SHOULD I ASK HIM IF HE'LL PHOTOGRAPH US?

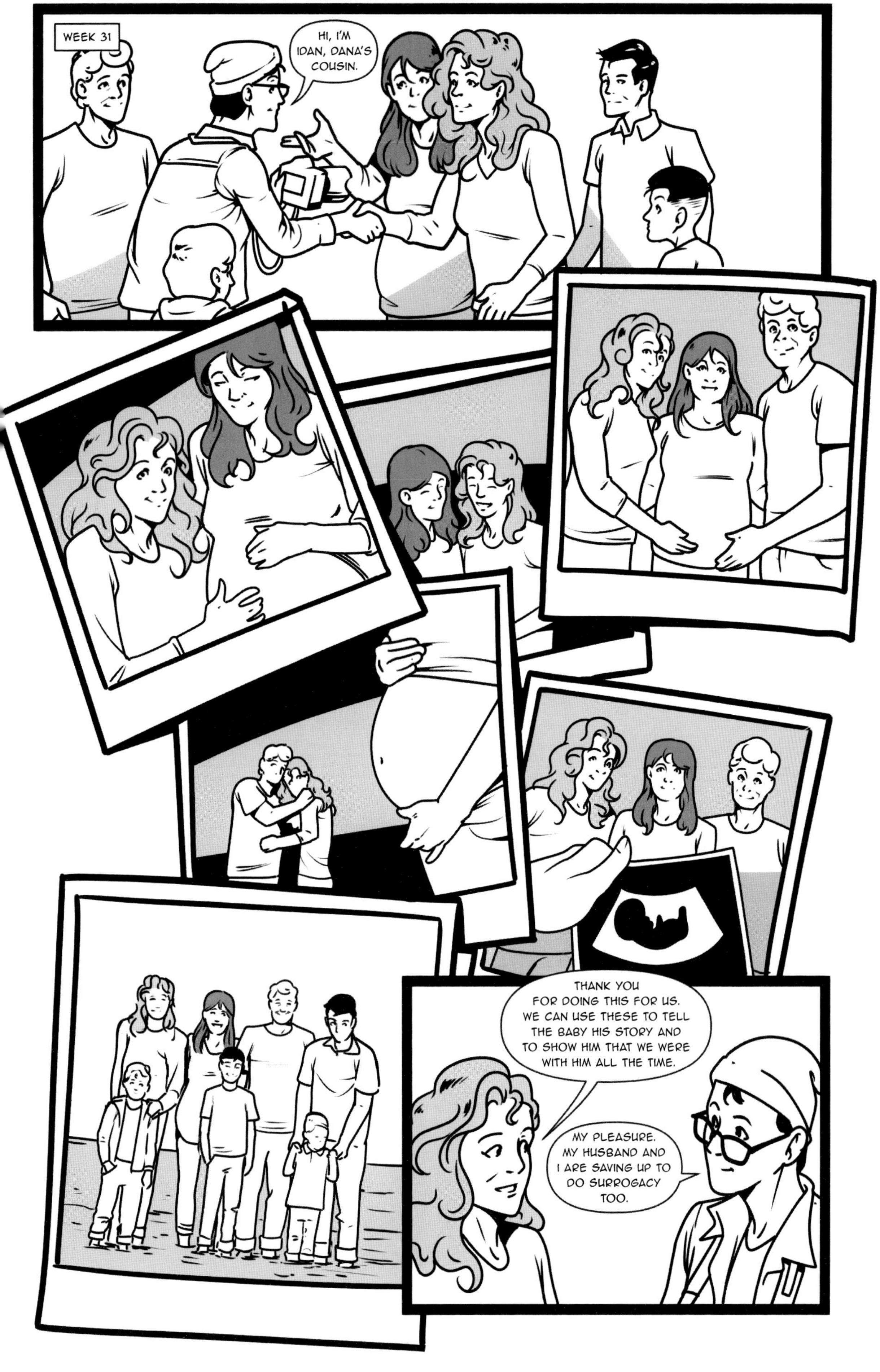
WEEK 31
HI, I'M IDAN, DANA'S COUSIN.
THANK YOU FOR DOING THIS FOR US. WE CAN USE THESE TO TELL THE BABY HIS STORY AND TO SHOW HIM THAT WE WERE WITH HIM ALL THE TIME.
MY PLEASURE. MY HUSBAND AND I ARE SAVING UP TO DO SURROGACY TOO.

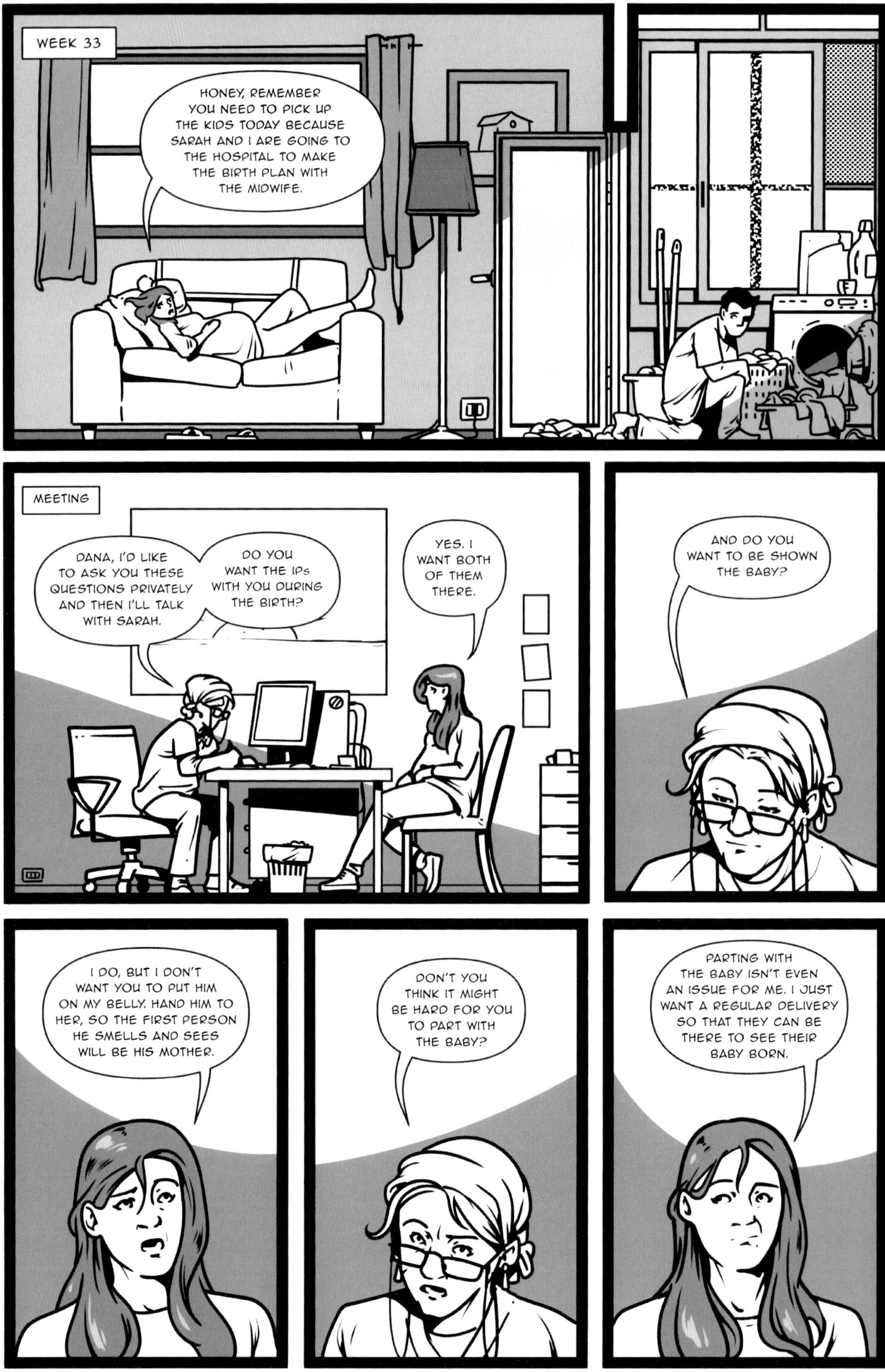
WEEK 33
HONEY, REMEMBER YOU NEED TO PICK UP THE KIDS TODAY BECAUSE SARAH AND I ARE GOING TO THE HOSPITAL TO MAKE THE BIRTH PLAN WITH THE MIDWIFE.
MEETING
DANA, I'D LIKE TO ASK YOU THESE QUESTIONS PRIVATELY AND THEN I'LL TALK WITH SARAH.
DO YOU WANT THE IPs WITH YOU DURING THE BIRTH?
YES. I WANT BOTH OF THEM THERE.
AND DO YOU WANT TO BE SHOWN THE BABY?
I DO, BUT I DON'T WANT YOU TO PUT HIM ON MY BELLY. HAND HIM TO HER, SO THE FIRST PERSON HE SMELLS AND SEES WILL BE HIS MOTHER.
DON'T YOU THINK IT MIGHT BE HARD FOR YOU TO PART WITH THE BABY?
PARTING WITH THE BABY ISN'T EVEN AN ISSUE FOR ME. I JUST WANT A REGULAR DELIVERY SO THAT THEY CAN BE THERE TO SEE THEIR BABY BORN.

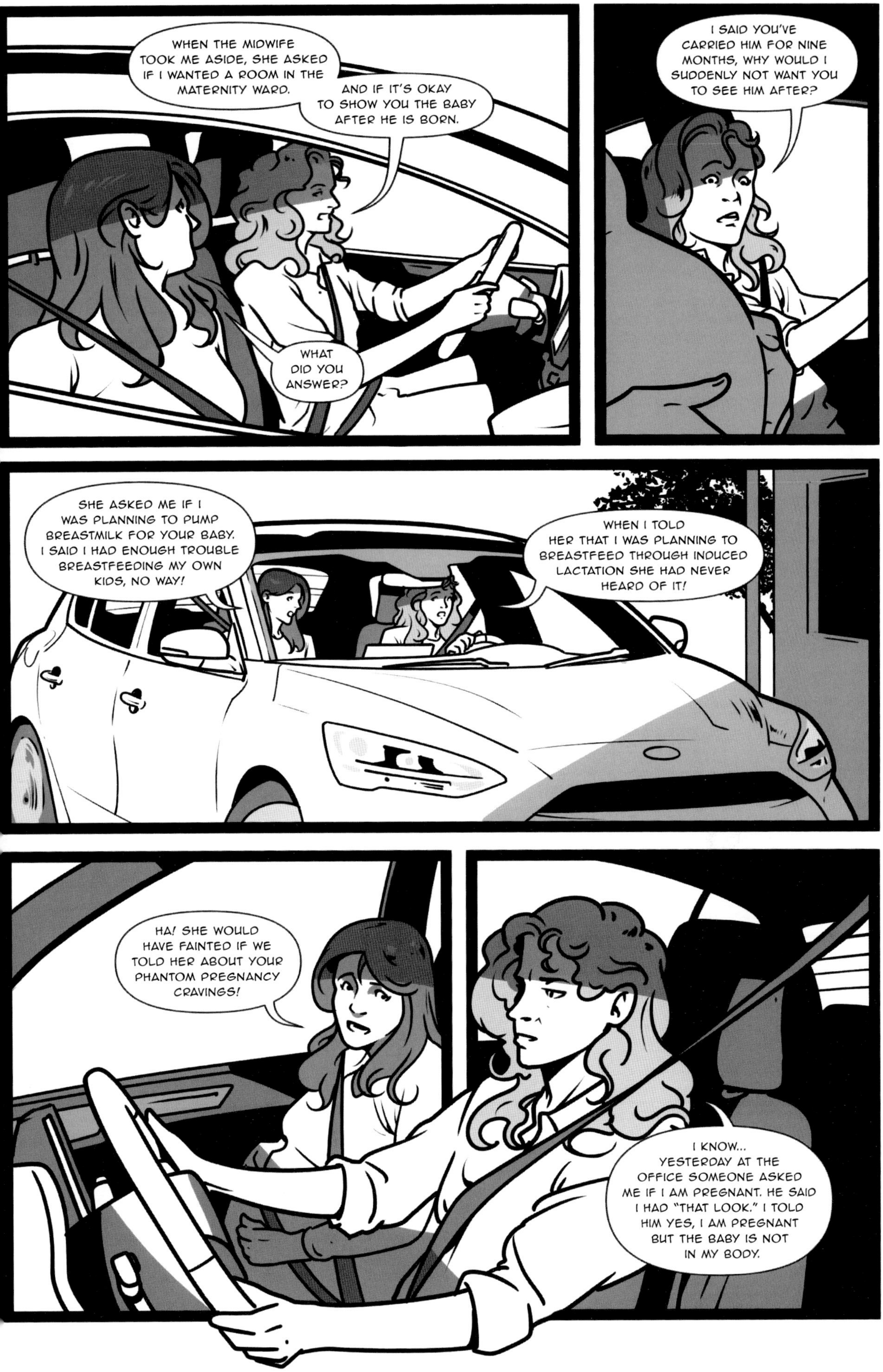
WHEN THE MIDWIFE TOOK ME ASIDE, SHE ASKED IF I WANTED A ROOM IN THE MATERNITY WARD.
AND IF IT'S OKAY TO SHOW YOU THE BABY AFTER HE IS BORN.
WHAT DID YOU ANSWER?
I SAID YOU'VE CARRIED HIM FOR NINE MONTHS, WHY WOULD I SUDDENLY NOT WANT YOU TO SEE HIM AFTER?
SHE ASKED ME IF I WAS PLANNING TO PUMP BREASTMILK FOR YOUR BABY. I SAID I HAD ENOUGH TROUBLE BREASTFEEDING MY OWN KIDS, NO WAY!
WHEN I TOLD HER THAT I WAS PLANNING TO BREASTFEED THROUGH INDUCED LACTATION SHE HAD NEVER HEARD OF IT!
HA! SHE WOULD HAVE FAINTED IF WE TOLD HER ABOUT YOUR PHANTOM PREGNANCY CRAVINGS!
I KNOW... YESTERDAY AT THE OFFICE SOMEONE ASKED ME IF I AM PREGNANT. HE SAID I HAD "THAT LOOK." I TOLD HIM YES, I AM PREGNANT BUT THE BABY IS NOT IN MY BODY.

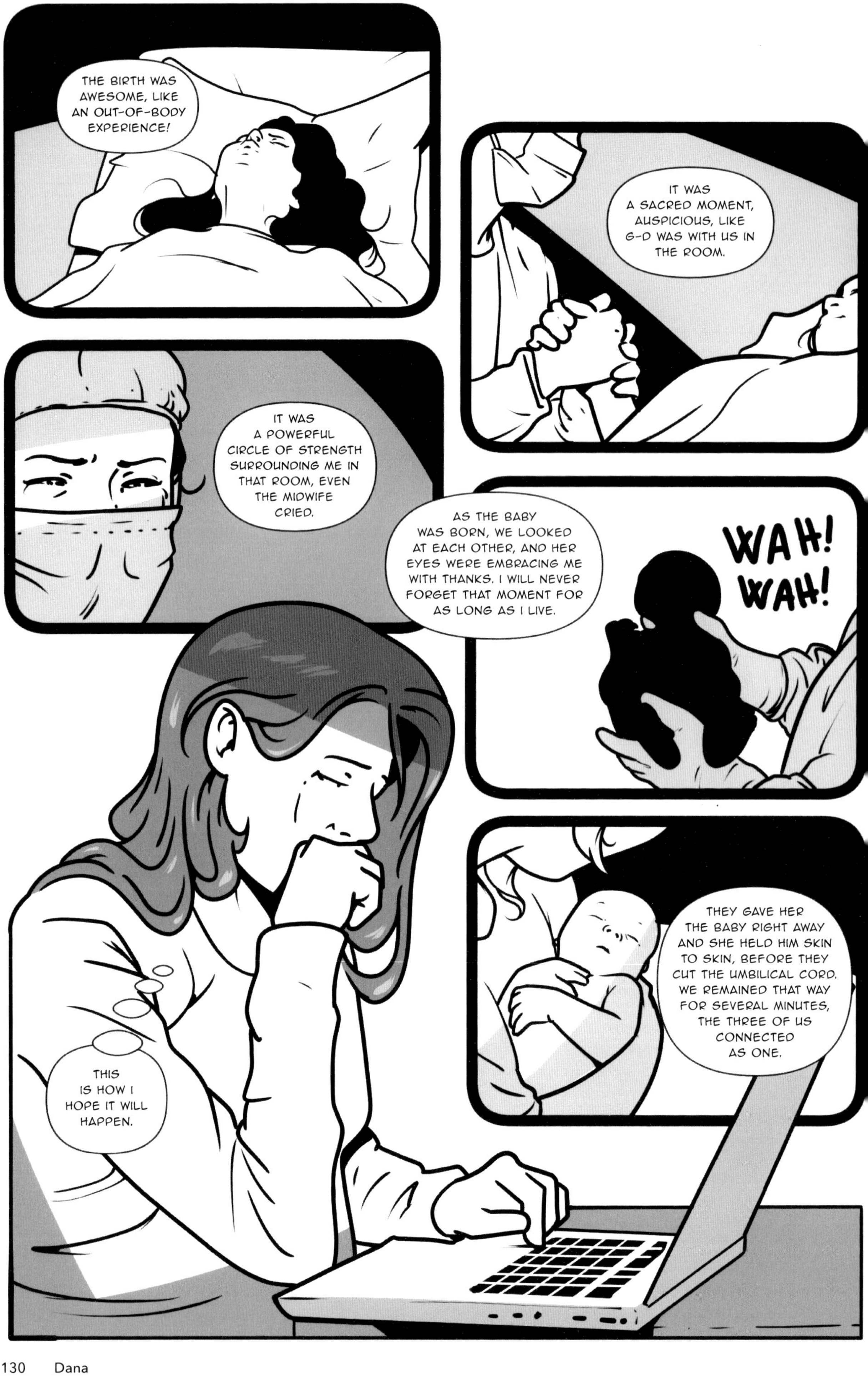
THE BIRTH WAS AWESOME, LIKE AN OUT-OF-BODY EXPERIENCE!
IT WAS A SACRED MOMENT, AUSPICIOUS, LIKE G-D WAS WITH US IN THE ROOM.
IT WAS A POWERFUL CIRCLE OF STRENGTH SURROUNDING ME IN THAT ROOM, EVEN THE MIDWIFE CRIED.
AS THE BABY WAS BORN, WE LOOKED AT EACH OTHER, AND HER EYES WERE EMBRACING ME WITH THANKS. I WILL NEVER FORGET THAT MOMENT FOR AS LONG AS I LIVE.
WAH! WAH!
THEY GAVE HER THE BABY RIGHT AWAY AND SHE HELD HIM SKIN TO SKIN, BEFORE THEY CUT THE UMBILICAL CORD. WE REMAINED THAT WAY FOR SEVERAL MINUTES, THE THREE OF US CONNECTED AS ONE.
THIS IS HOW I HOPE IT WILL HAPPEN.

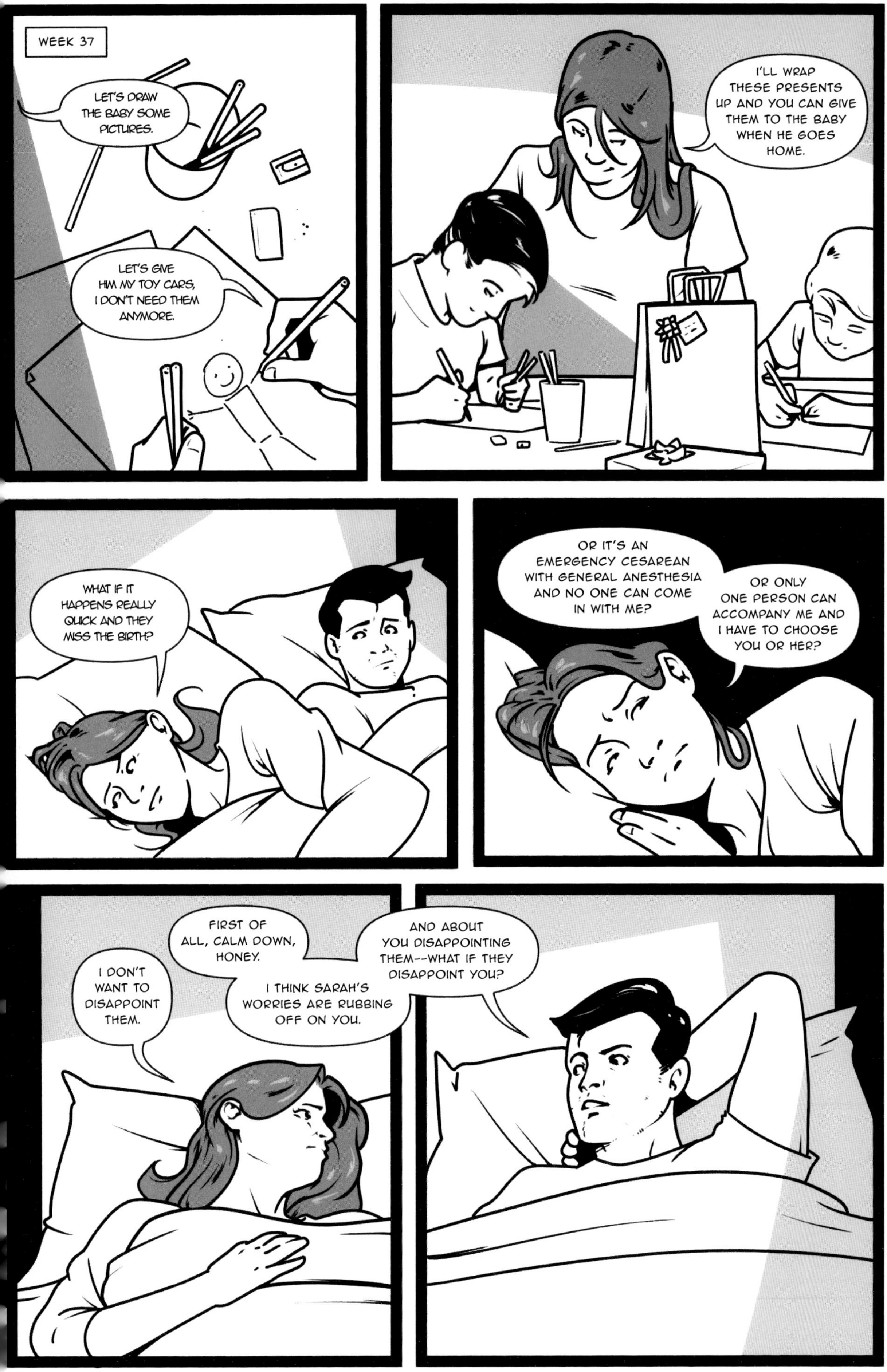
WEEK 37
LET'S DRAW THE BABY SOME PICTURES.
LET'S GIVE HIM MY TOY CARS, I DON'T NEED THEM ANYMORE.
I'LL WRAP THESE PRESENTS UP AND YOU CAN GIVE THEM TO THE BABY WHEN HE GOES HOME.
WHAT IF IT HAPPENS REALLY QUICK AND THEY MISS THE BIRTH?
OR IT'S AN EMERGENCY CESAREAN WITH GENERAL ANESTHESIA AND NO ONE CAN COME IN WITH ME?
OR ONLY ONE PERSON CAN ACCOMPANY ME AND I HAVE TO CHOOSE YOU OR HER?
I DON'T WANT TO DISAPPOINT THEM.
FIRST OF ALL, CALM DOWN, HONEY.
I THINK SARAH'S WORRIES ARE RUBBING OFF ON YOU.
AND ABOUT YOU DISAPPOINTING THEM--WHAT IF THEY DISAPPOINT YOU?

-CHAPTER 16-
THE GIFT

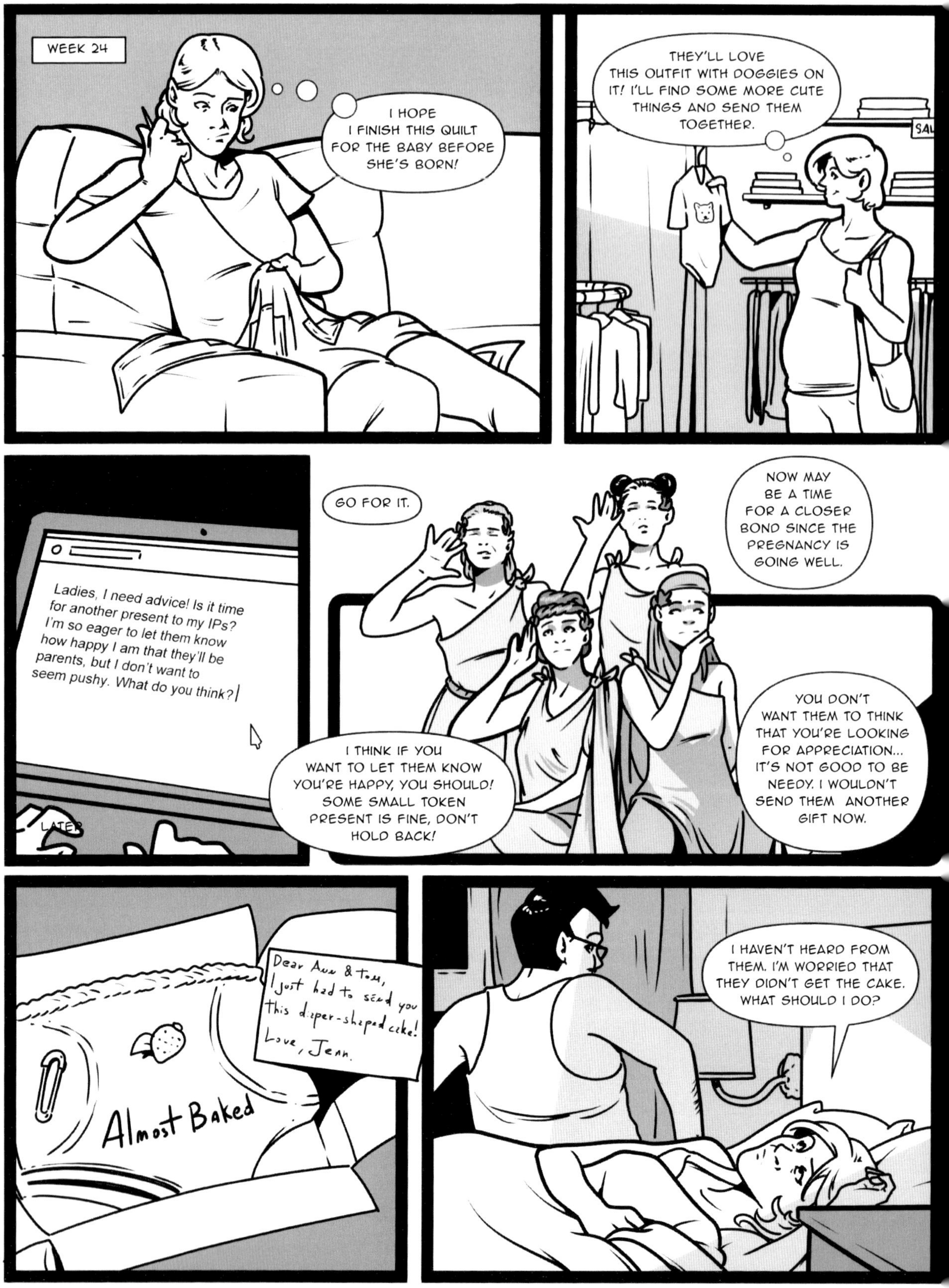

WEEK 24
I HOPE I FINISH THIS QUILT FOR THE BABY BEFORE SHE'S BORN!
THEY'LL LOVE THIS OUTFIT WITH DOGGIES ON IT! I'LL FIND SOME MORE CUTE THINGS AND SEND THEM TOGETHER.
Ladies, I need advice! Is it time for another present to my IPs? I'm so eager to let them know how happy I am that they'll be parents, but I don't want to seem pushy. What do you think?
LATER
GO FOR IT.
NOW MAY BE A TIME FOR A CLOSER BOND SINCE THE PREGNANCY IS GOING WELL.
I THINK IF YOU WANT TO LET THEM KNOW YOU'RE HAPPY, YOU SHOULD! SOME SMALL TOKEN PRESENT IS FINE, DON'T HOLD BACK!
YOU DON'T WANT THEM TO THINK THAT YOU'RE LOOKING FOR APPRECIATION... IT'S NOT GOOD TO BE NEEDY. I WOULDN'T SEND THEM ANOTHER GIFT NOW.
Almost Baked
Dear Ann & Tom, I just had to send you this diaper-shaped cake! Love, Jenn.
I HAVEN'T HEARD FROM THEM. I'M WORRIED THAT THEY DIDN'T GET THE CAKE. WHAT SHOULD I DO?

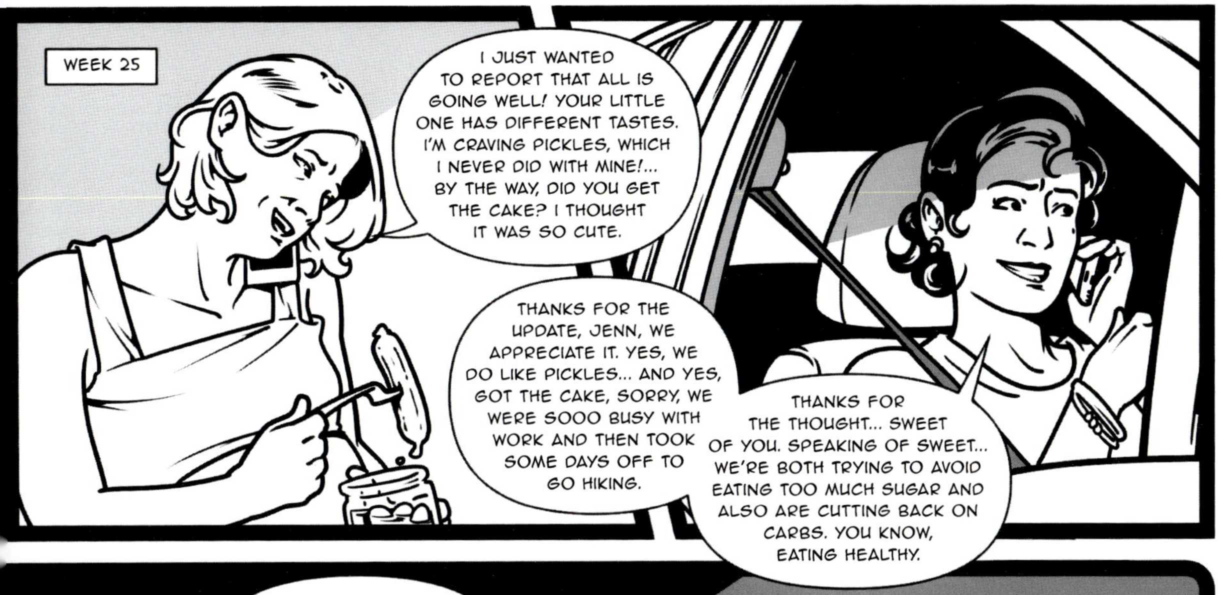
WEEK 25
I JUST WANTED TO REPORT THAT ALL IS GOING WELL! YOUR LITTLE ONE HAS DIFFERENT TASTES. I'M CRAVING PICKLES, WHICH I NEVER DID WITH MINE!... BY THE WAY, DID YOU GET THE CAKE? I THOUGHT IT WAS SO CUTE.
THANKS FOR THE UPDATE, JENN, WE APPRECIATE IT. YES, WE DO LIKE PICKLES... AND YES, GOT THE CAKE, SORRY, WE WERE SOOO BUSY WITH WORK AND THEN TOOK SOME DAYS OFF TO GO HIKING.
THANKS FOR THE THOUGHT... SWEET OF YOU. SPEAKING OF SWEET... WE'RE BOTH TRYING TO AVOID EATING TOO MUCH SUGAR AND ALSO ARE CUTTING BACK ON CARBS. YOU KNOW, EATING HEALTHY.

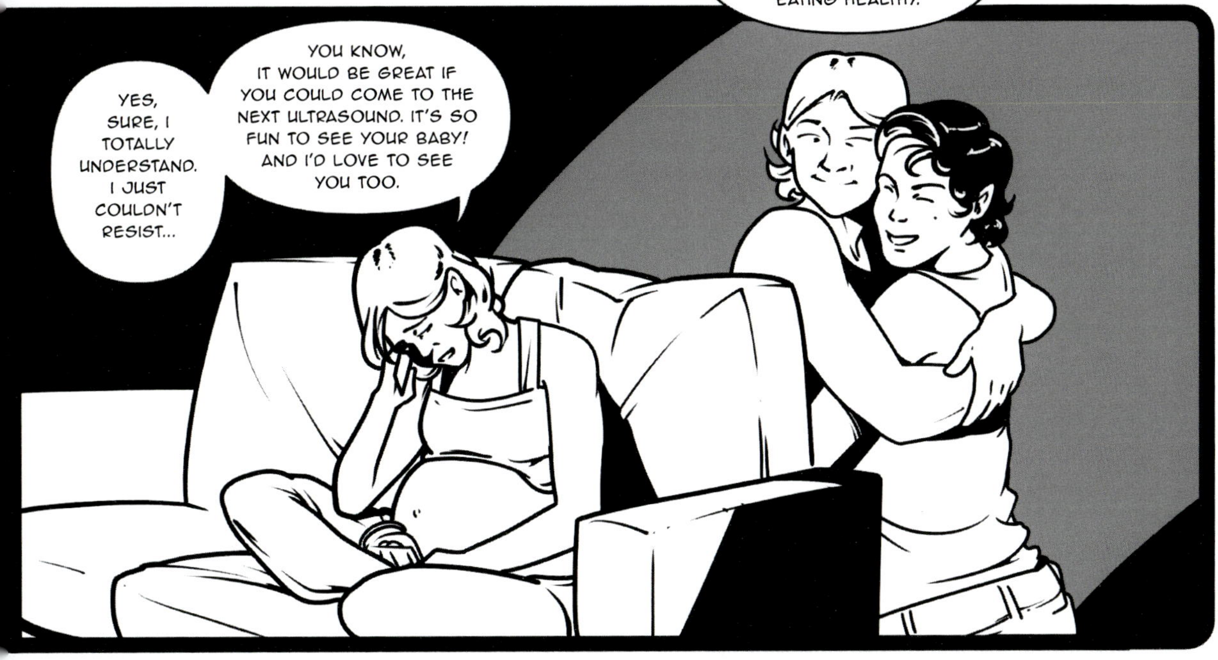
YES, SURE, I TOTALLY UNDERSTAND. I JUST COULDN'T RESIST...
YOU KNOW, IT WOULD BE GREAT IF YOU COULD COME TO THE NEXT ULTRASOUND. IT'S SO FUN TO SEE YOUR BABY! AND I'D LOVE TO SEE YOU TOO.

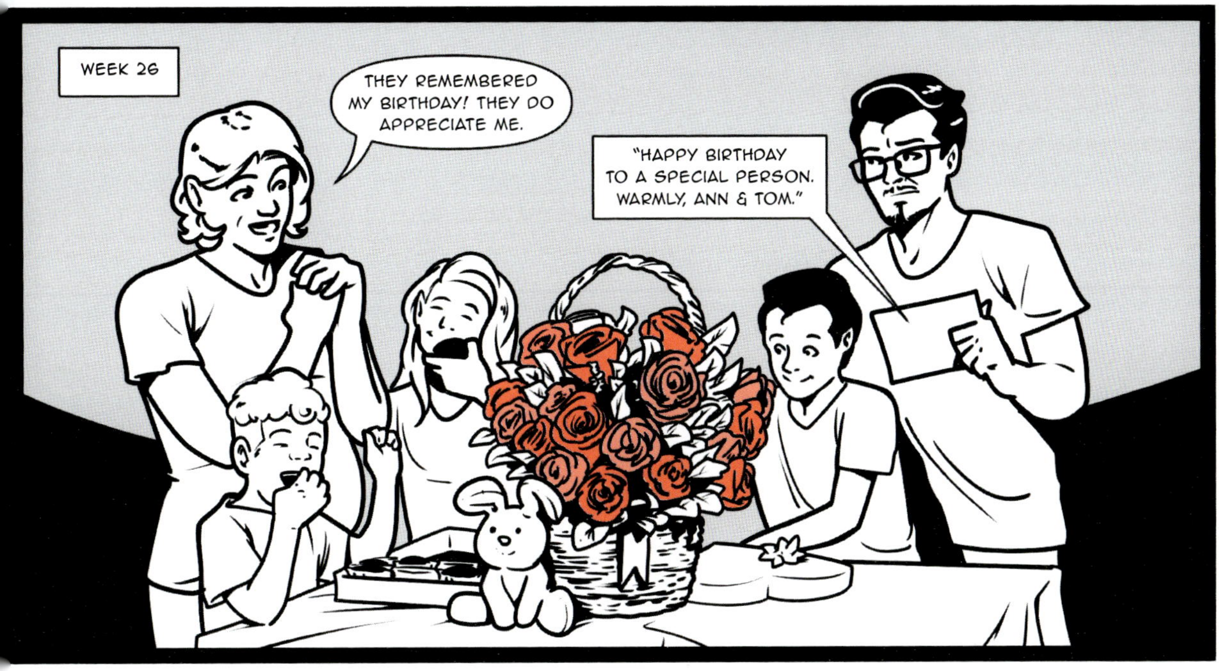
WEEK 26
THEY REMEMBERED MY BIRTHDAY! THEY DO APPRECIATE ME.
"HAPPY BIRTHDAY TO A SPECIAL PERSON. WARMLY, ANN & TOM."

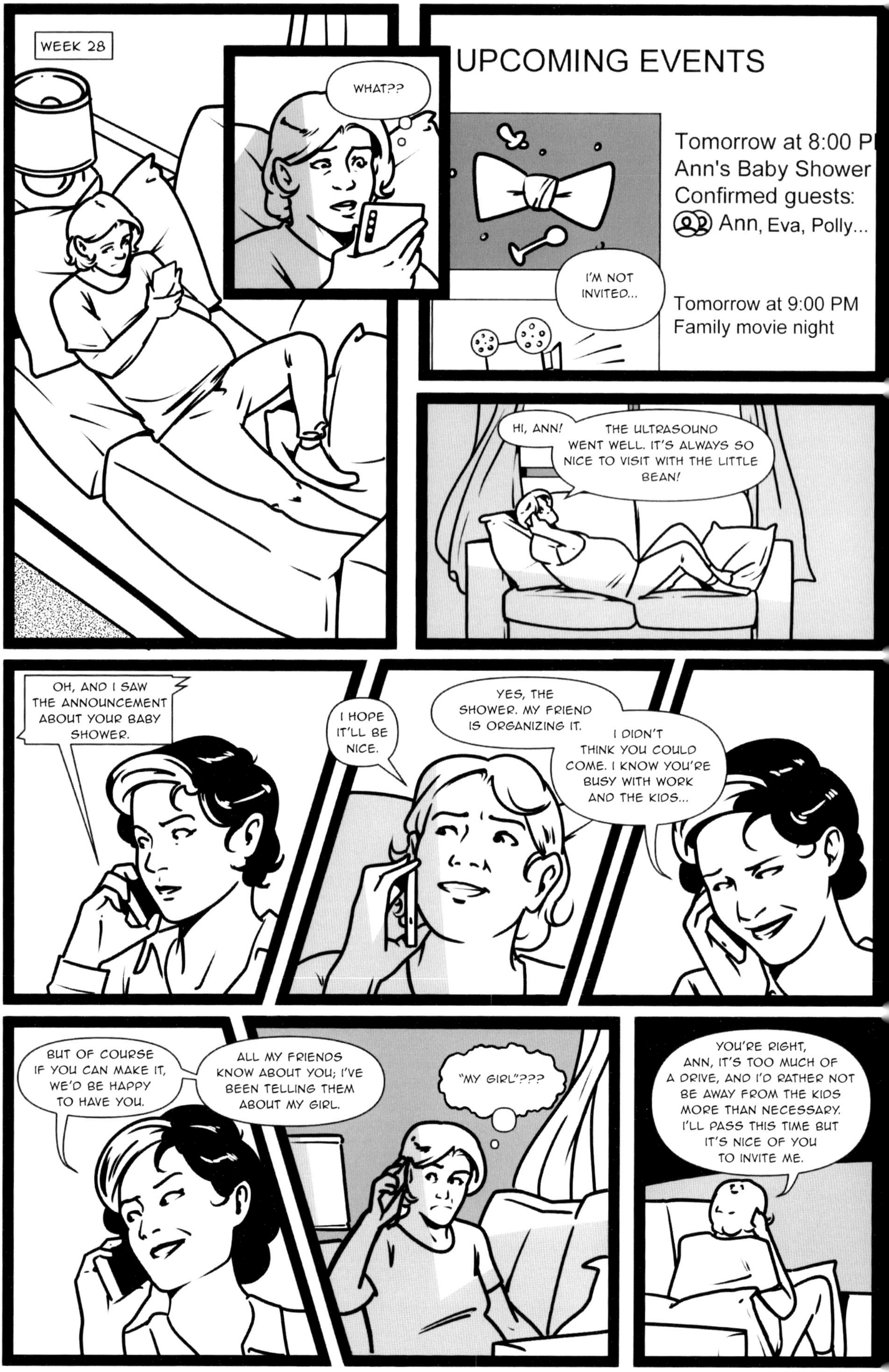
WEEK 28
WHAT??
UPCOMING EVENTS
Tomorrow at 8:00 P
Ann's Baby Shower
Confirmed guests:
Ann, Eva, Polly...
I'M NOT INVITED...
Tomorrow at 9:00 PM
Family movie night
HI, ANN!
THE ULTRASOUND WENT WELL. IT'S ALWAYS SO NICE TO VISIT WITH THE LITTLE BEAN!
OH, AND I SAW THE ANNOUNCEMENT ABOUT YOUR BABY SHOWER.
I HOPE IT'LL BE NICE.
YES, THE SHOWER. MY FRIEND IS ORGANIZING IT.
I DIDN'T THINK YOU COULD COME. I KNOW YOU'RE BUSY WITH WORK AND THE KIDS...
BUT OF COURSE IF YOU CAN MAKE IT, WE'D BE HAPPY TO HAVE YOU.
ALL MY FRIENDS KNOW ABOUT YOU; I'VE BEEN TELLING THEM ABOUT MY GIRL.
"MY GIRL"???
YOU'RE RIGHT, ANN, IT'S TOO MUCH OF A DRIVE, AND I'D RATHER NOT BE AWAY FROM THE KIDS MORE THAN NECESSARY. I'LL PASS THIS TIME BUT IT'S NICE OF YOU TO INVITE ME.

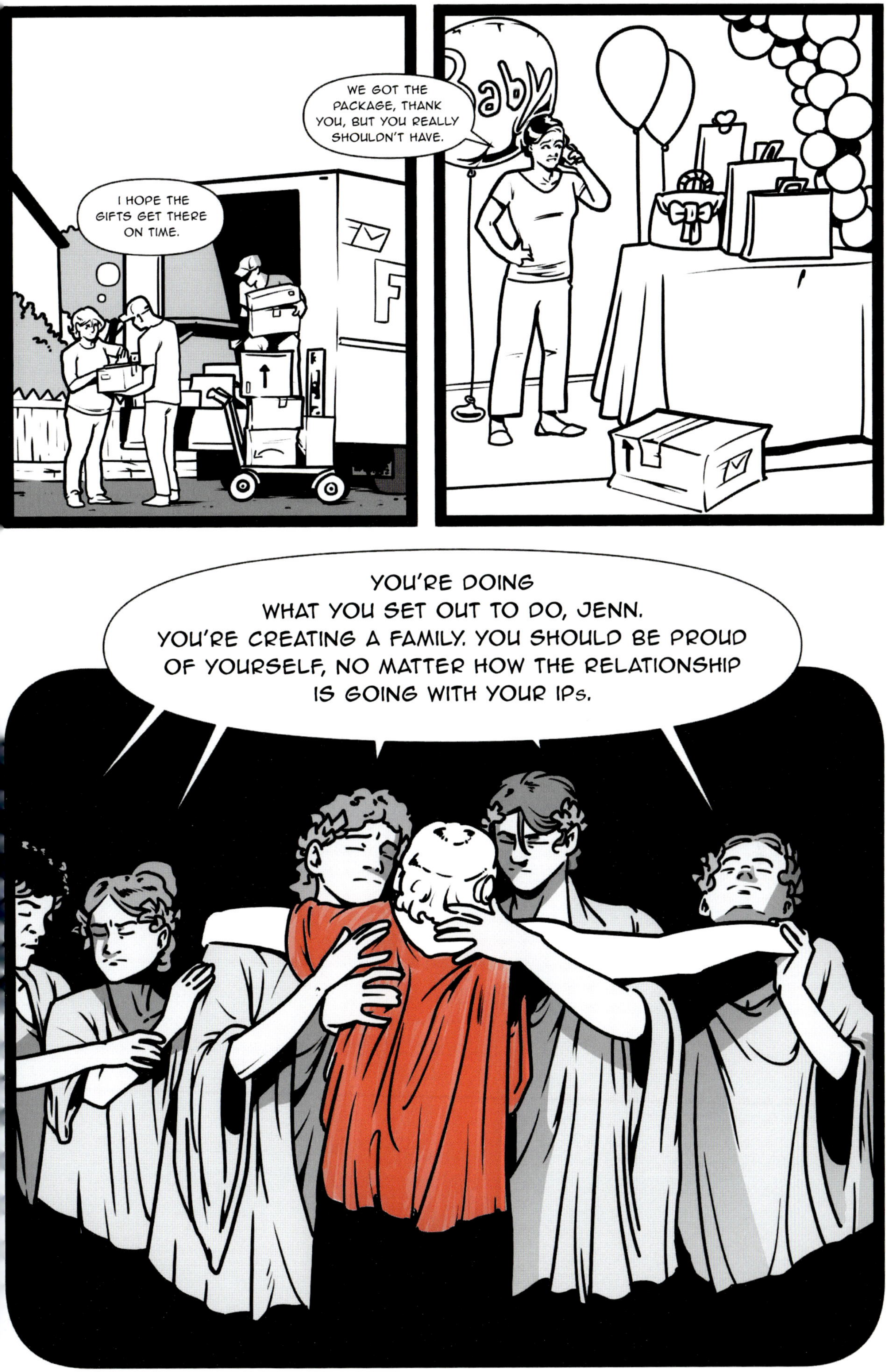
I HOPE THE GIFTS GET THERE ON TIME.
WE GOT THE PACKAGE, THANK YOU, BUT YOU REALLY SHOULDN'T HAVE.
YOU'RE DOING WHAT YOU SET OUT TO DO, JENN. YOU'RE CREATING A FAMILY. YOU SHOULD BE PROUD OF YOURSELF, NO MATTER HOW THE RELATIONSHIP IS GOING WITH YOUR IPs.

NTERLUDE: DR. VERMA, DOCTOR AT SURROGACY CLINIC IN DELHI

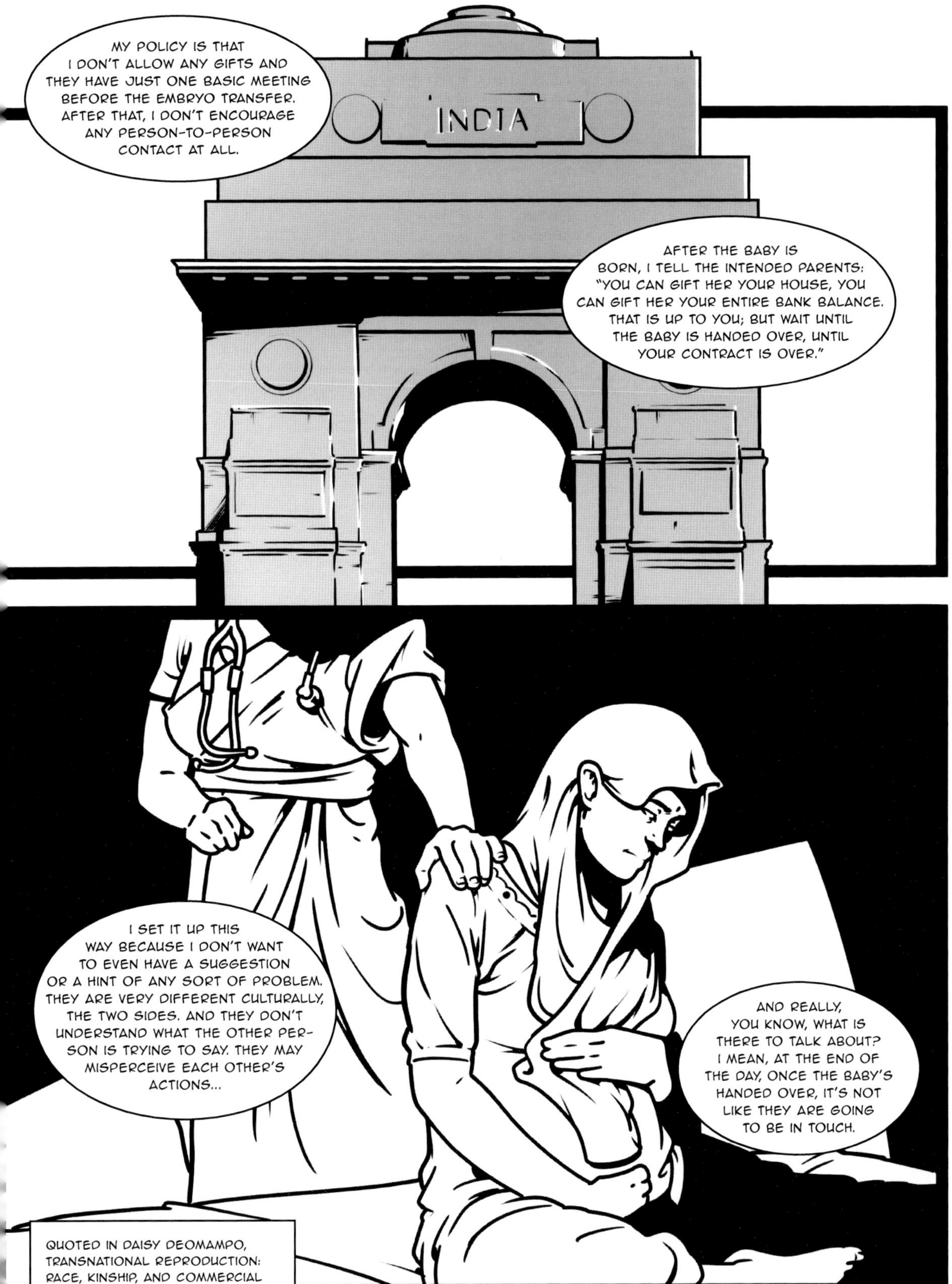

MY POLICY IS THAT I DON'T ALLOW ANY GIFTS AND THEY HAVE JUST ONE BASIC MEETING BEFORE THE EMBRYO TRANSFER. AFTER THAT, I DON'T ENCOURAGE ANY PERSON-TO-PERSON CONTACT AT ALL.
INDIA
AFTER THE BABY IS BORN, I TELL THE INTENDED PARENTS: "YOU CAN GIFT HER YOUR HOUSE, YOU CAN GIFT HER YOUR ENTIRE BANK BALANCE. THAT IS UP TO YOU; BUT WAIT UNTIL THE BABY IS HANDED OVER, UNTIL YOUR CONTRACT IS OVER."
I SET IT UP THIS WAY BECAUSE I DON'T WANT TO EVEN HAVE A SUGGESTION OR A HINT OF ANY SORT OF PROBLEM. THEY ARE VERY DIFFERENT CULTURALLY, THE TWO SIDES. AND THEY DON'T UNDERSTAND WHAT THE OTHER PER-SON IS TRYING TO SAY. THEY MAY MISPERCEIVE EACH OTHER'S ACTIONS...
AND REALLY, YOU KNOW, WHAT IS THERE TO TALK ABOUT? I MEAN, AT THE END OF THE DAY, ONCE THE BABY'S HANDED OVER, IT'S NOT LIKE THEY ARE GOING TO BE IN TOUCH.

QUOTED IN DAISY DEOMAMPO, TRANSNATIONAL REPRODUCTION: RACE, KINSHIP, AND COMMERCIAL SURROGACY IN INDIA (NYU PRESS, 2016), 160.

-CHAPTER 17-
THE CHOICE

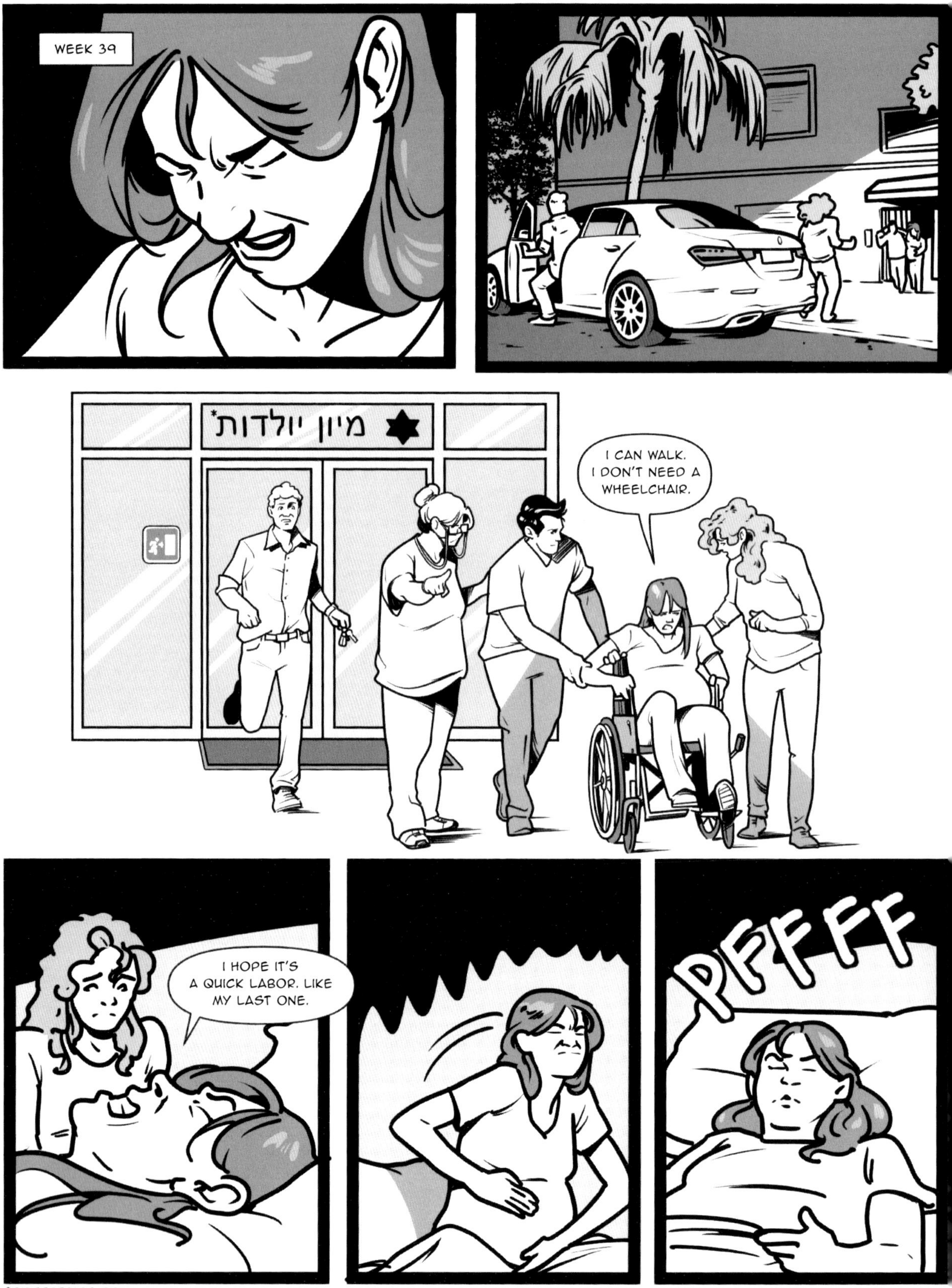
WEEK 39
מיון יולדות*
I CAN WALK. I DON'T NEED A WHEELCHAIR.
I HOPE IT'S A QUICK LABOR. LIKE MY LAST ONE.
PFFFF

*OBSTETRICS ER

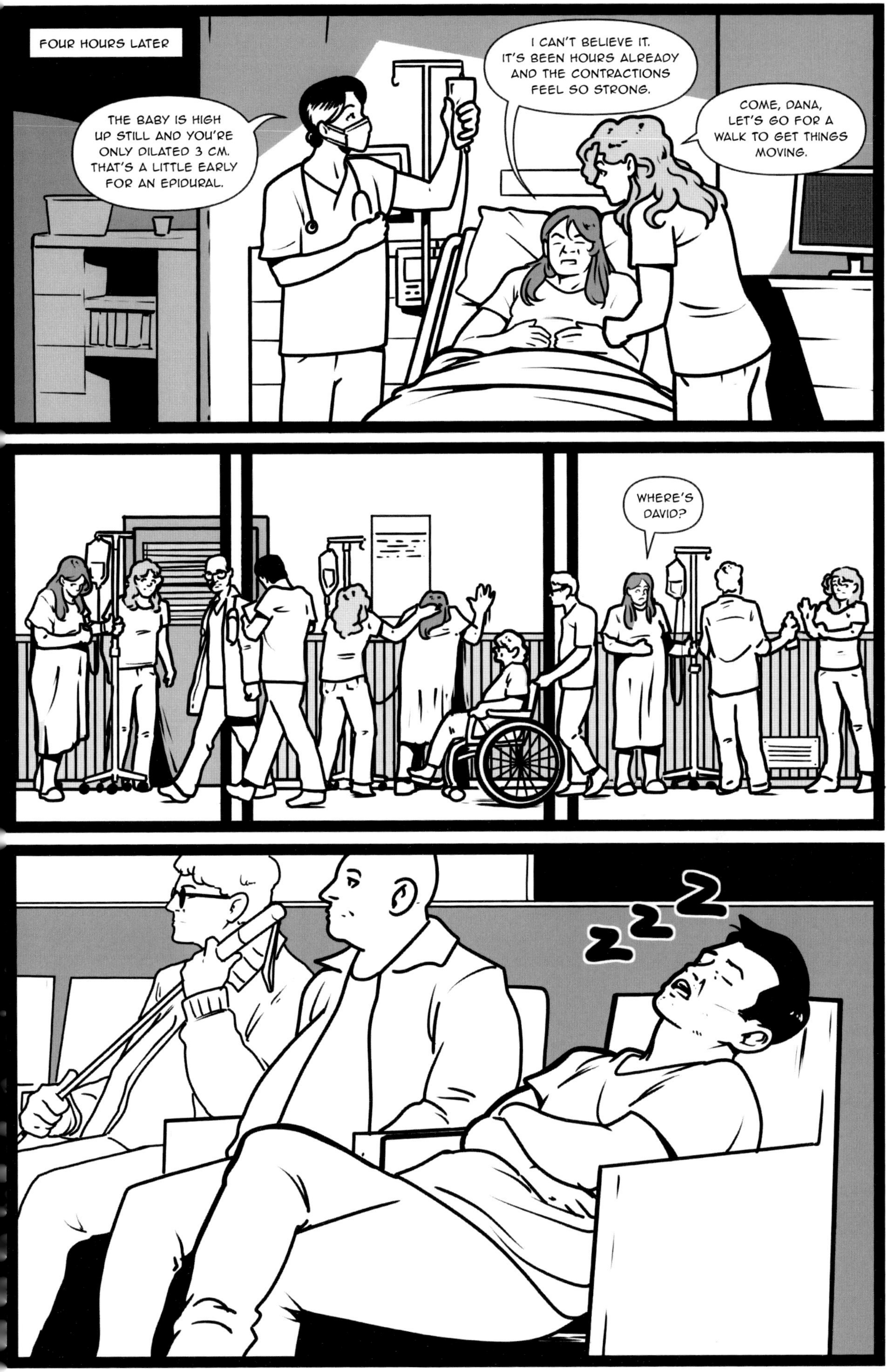
FOUR HOURS LATER
THE BABY IS HIGH UP STILL AND YOU'RE ONLY DILATED 3 CM. THAT'S A LITTLE EARLY FOR AN EPIDURAL.
I CAN'T BELIEVE IT. IT'S BEEN HOURS ALREADY AND THE CONTRACTIONS FEEL SO STRONG.
COME, DANA, LET'S GO FOR A WALK TO GET THINGS MOVING.
WHERE'S DAVID?
ZZZ

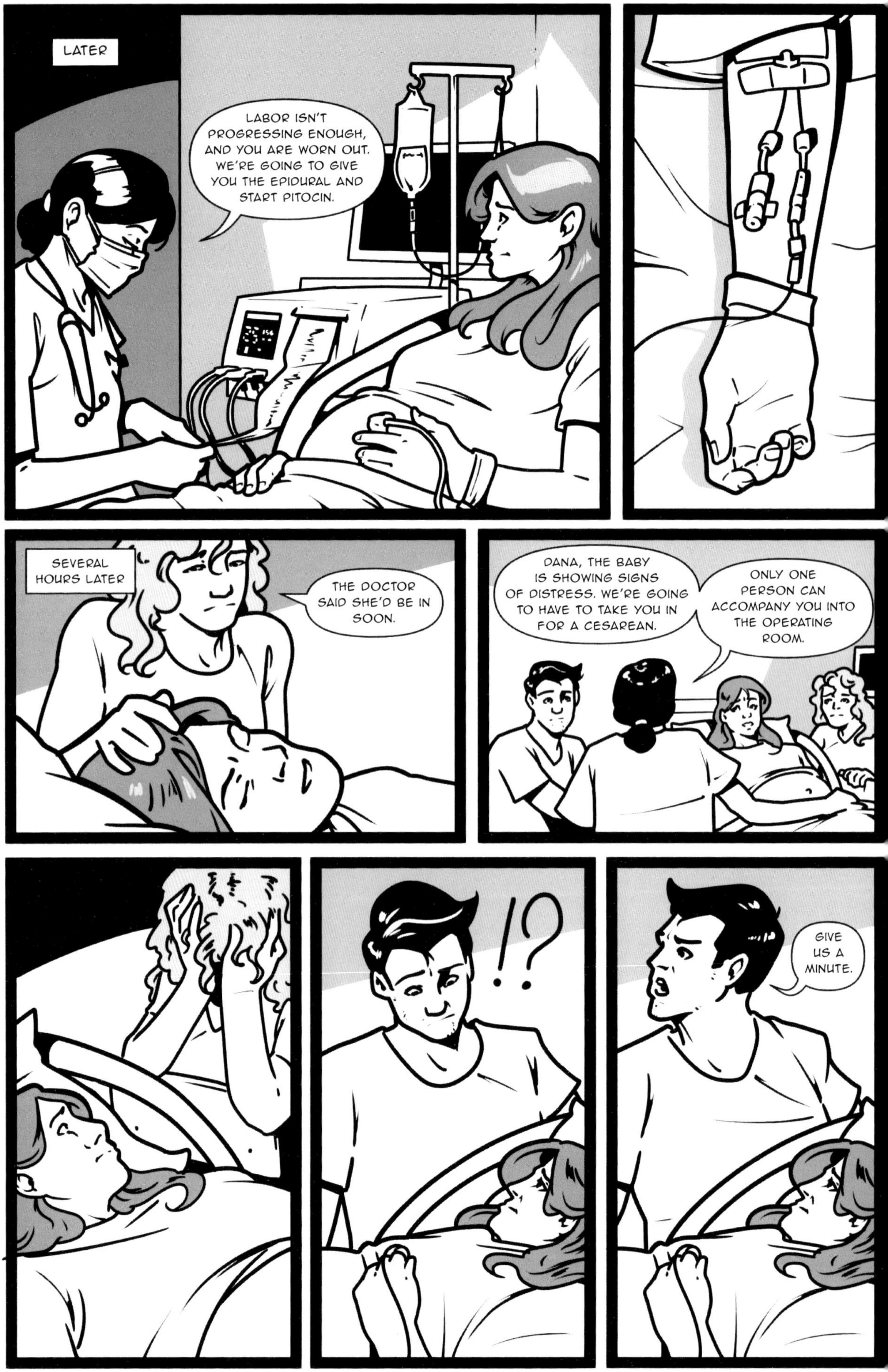
LATER
LABOR ISN'T PROGRESSING ENOUGH, AND YOU ARE WORN OUT. WE'RE GOING TO GIVE YOU THE EPIDURAL AND START PITOCIN.
SEVERAL HOURS LATER
THE DOCTOR SAID SHE'D BE IN SOON.
DANA, THE BABY IS SHOWING SIGNS OF DISTRESS. WE'RE GOING TO HAVE TO TAKE YOU IN FOR A CESAREAN.
ONLY ONE PERSON CAN ACCOMPANY YOU INTO THE OPERATING ROOM.
!?
GIVE US A MINUTE.

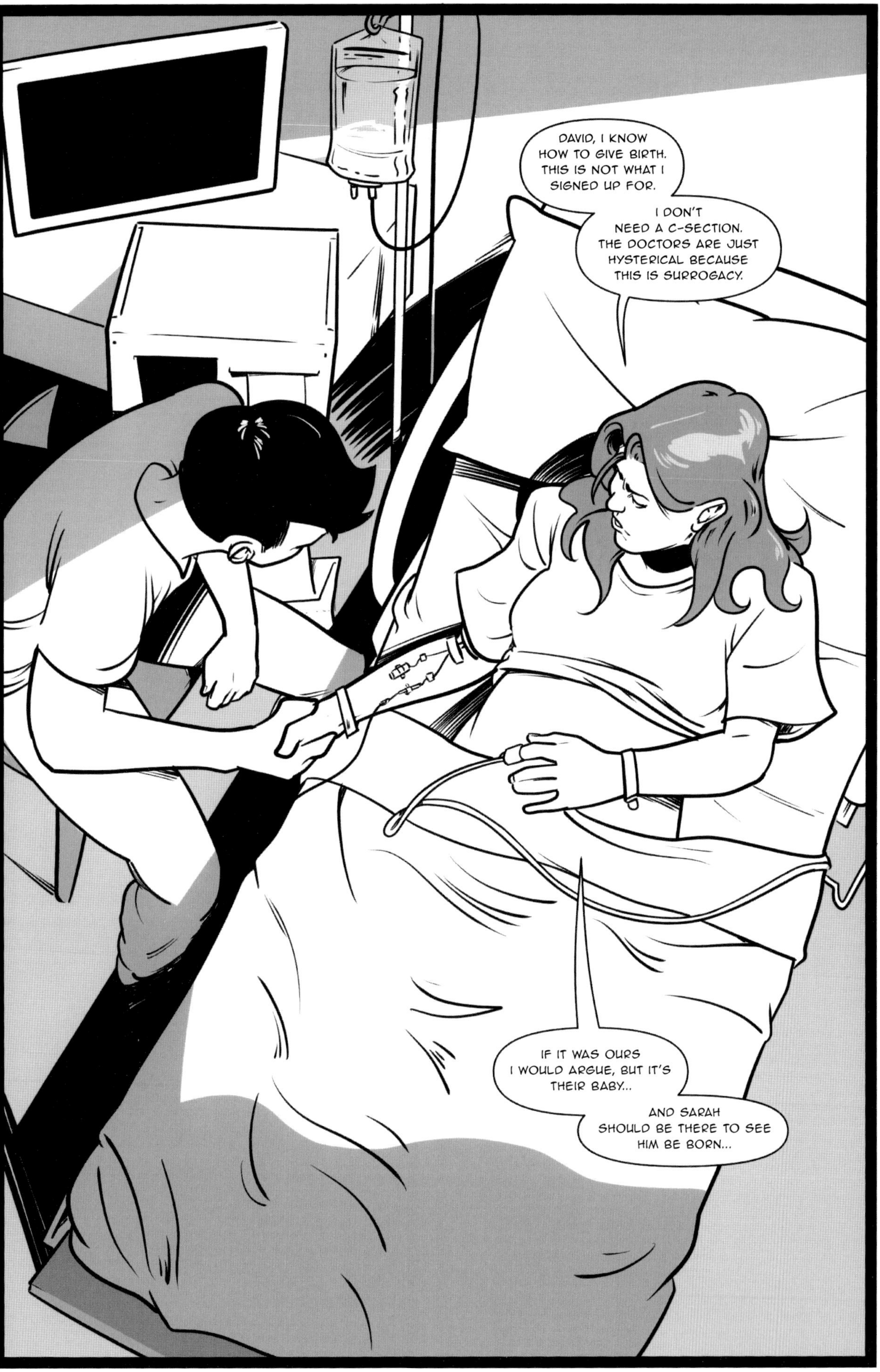
DAVID, I KNOW HOW TO GIVE BIRTH. THIS IS NOT WHAT I SIGNED UP FOR.
I DON'T NEED A C-SECTION. THE DOCTORS ARE JUST HYSTERICAL BECAUSE THIS IS SURROGACY.
IF IT WAS OURS I WOULD ARGUE, BUT IT'S THEIR BABY...
AND SARAH SHOULD BE THERE TO SEE HIM BE BORN...

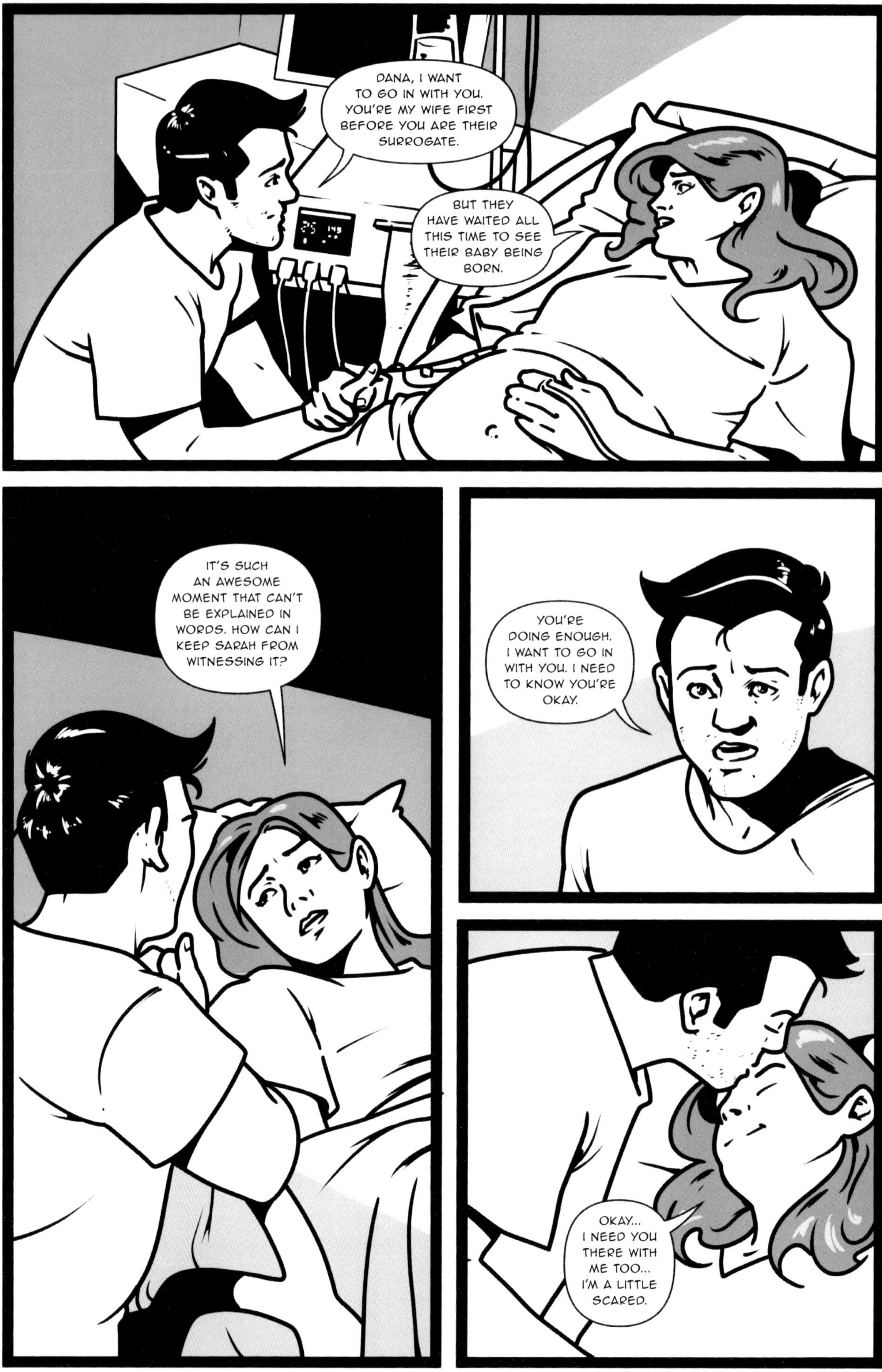
DANA, I WANT TO GO IN WITH YOU. YOU'RE MY WIFE FIRST BEFORE YOU ARE THEIR SURROGATE.
BUT THEY HAVE WAITED ALL THIS TIME TO SEE THEIR BABY BEING BORN.
IT'S SUCH AN AWESOME MOMENT THAT CAN'T BE EXPLAINED IN WORDS. HOW CAN I KEEP SARAH FROM WITNESSING IT?
YOU'RE DOING ENOUGH. I WANT TO GO IN WITH YOU. I NEED TO KNOW YOU'RE OKAY.
OKAY... I NEED YOU THERE WITH ME TOO... I'M A LITTLE SCARED.

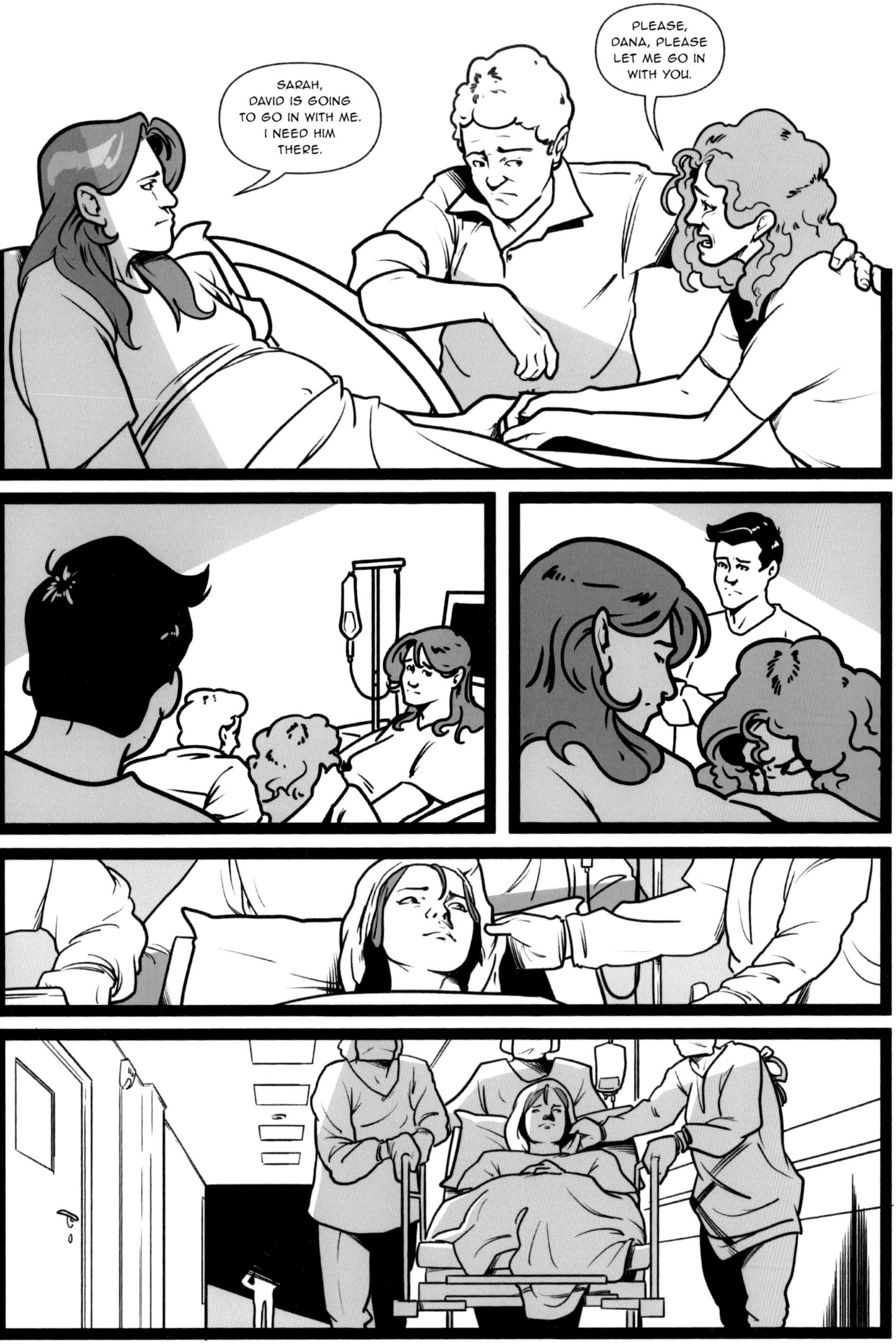
SARAH, DAVID IS GOING TO GO IN WITH ME. I NEED HIM THERE.
PLEASE, DANA, PLEASE LET ME GO IN WITH YOU.

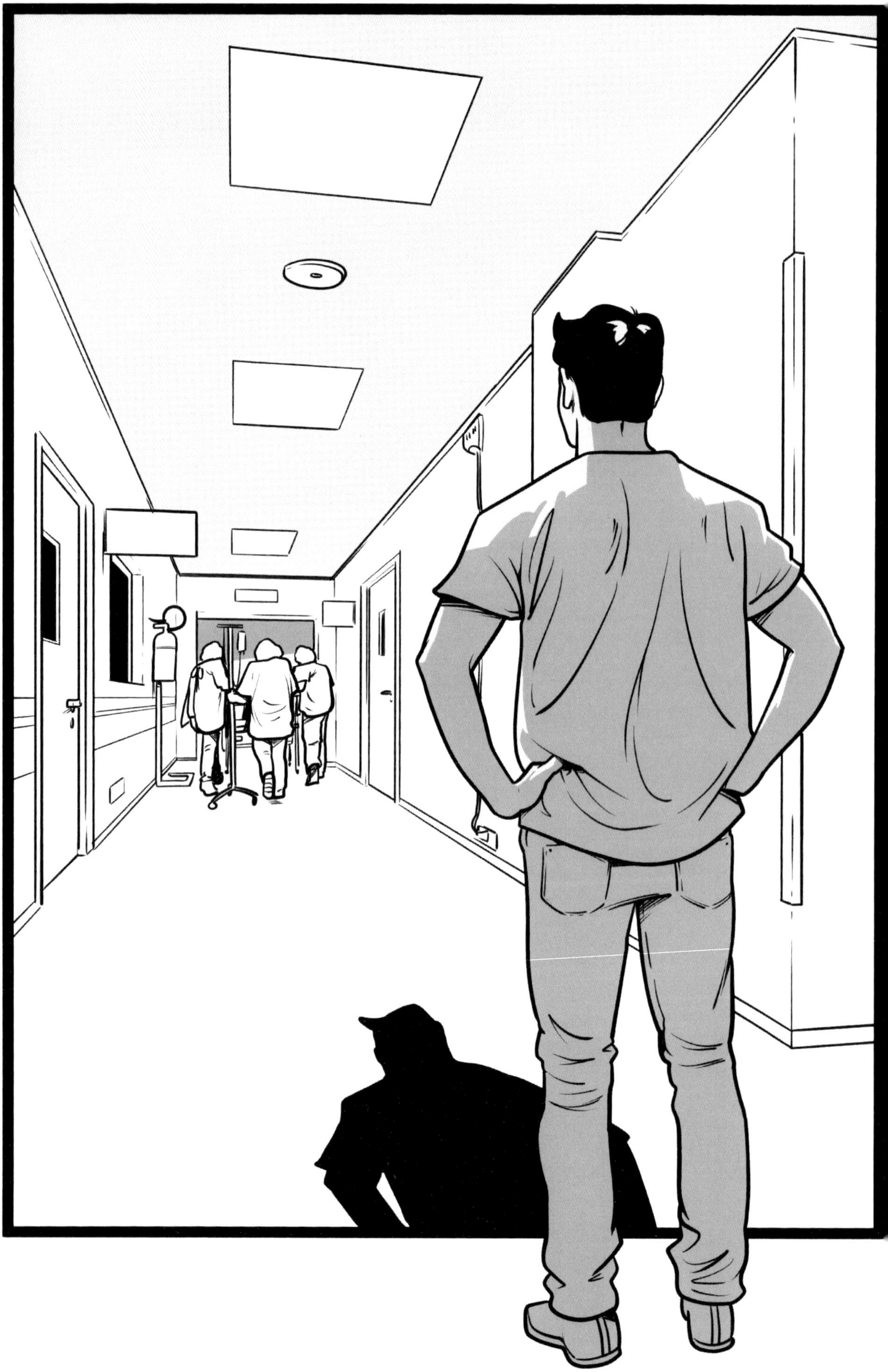

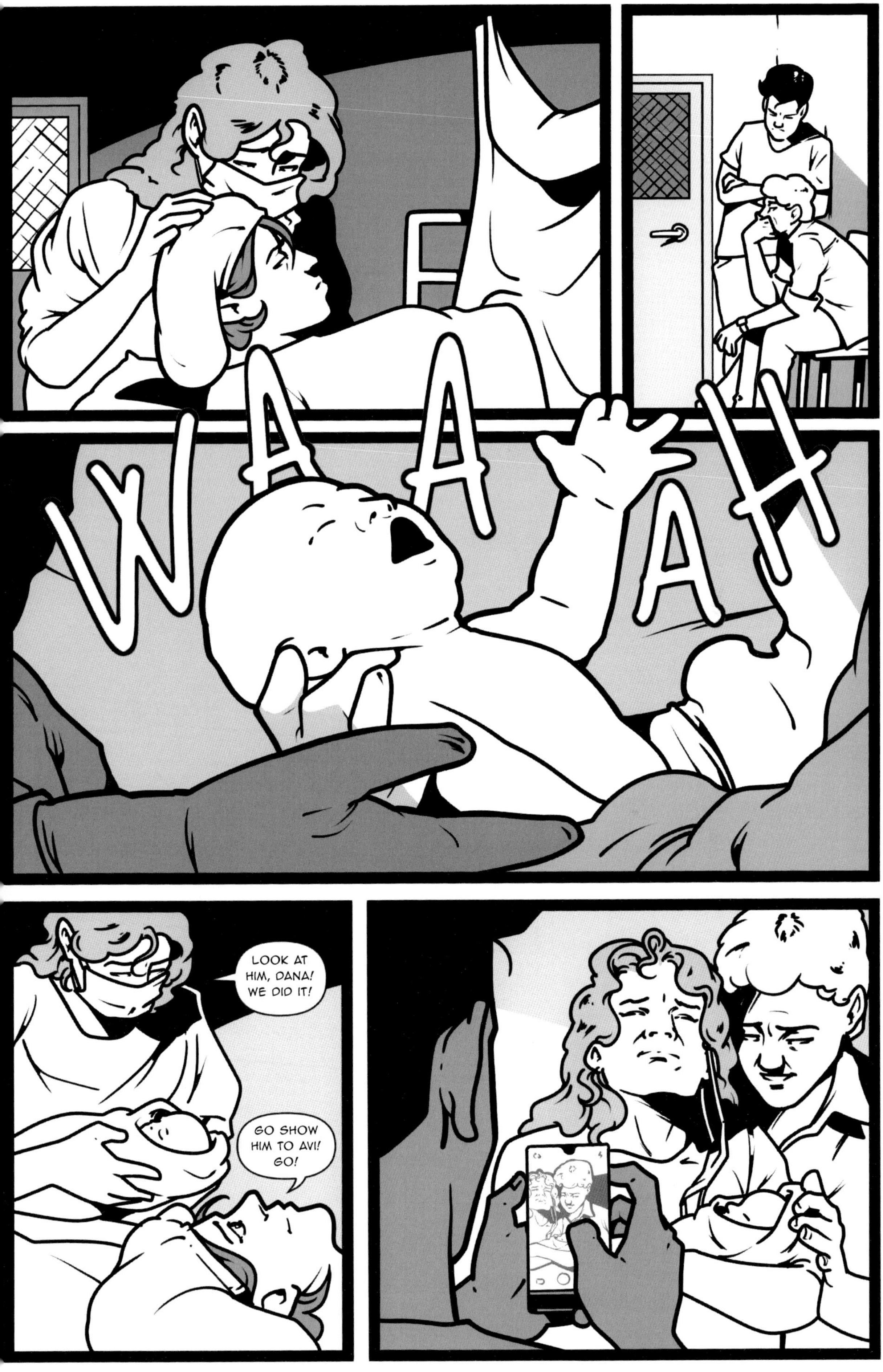
WAAAH
LOOK AT HIM, DANA! WE DID IT!
GO SHOW HIM TO AVI! GO!

-CHAPTER 18-
DELIVERY

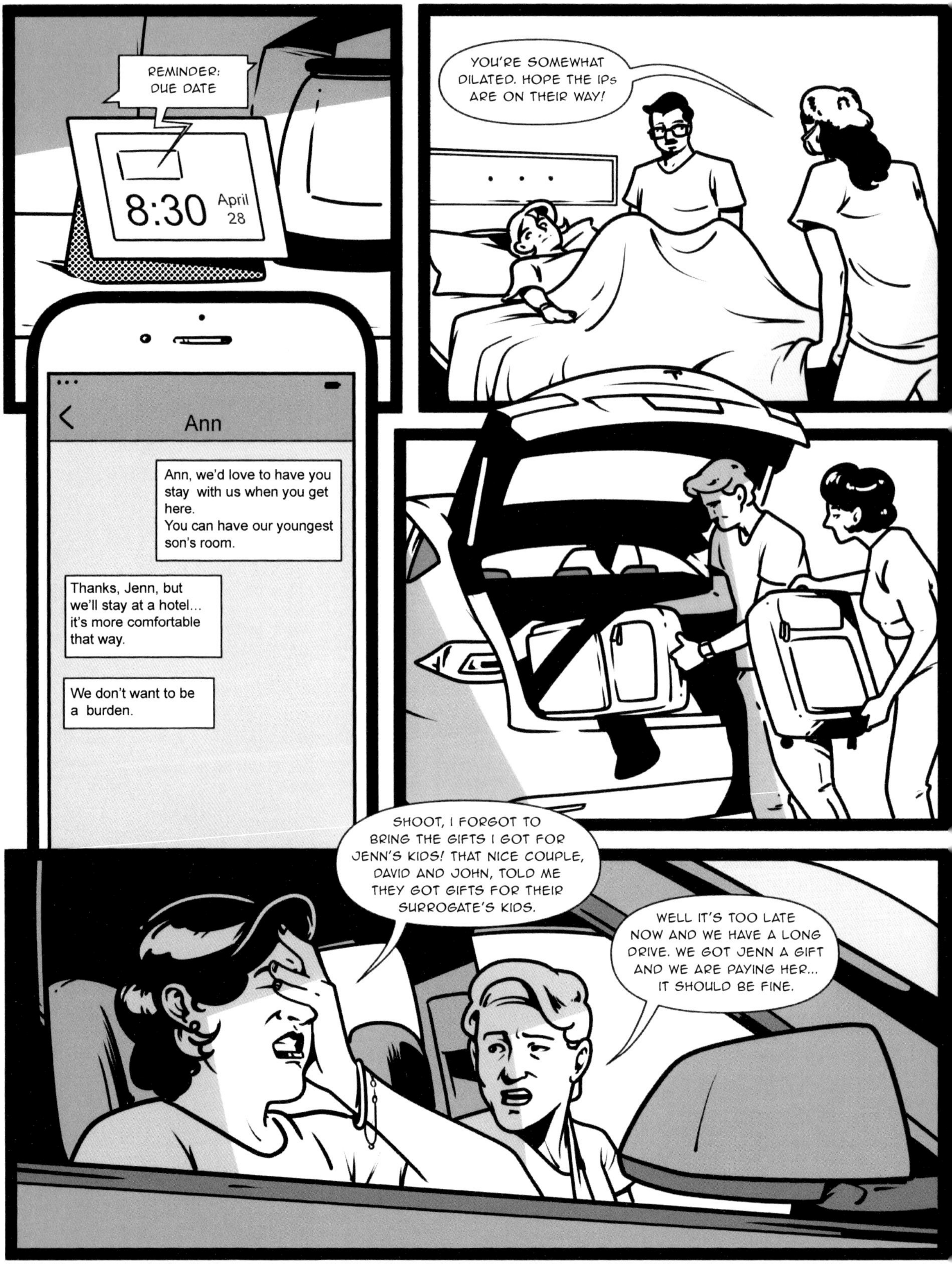
REMINDER: DUE DATE
8:30 April 28
Ann
Ann, we'd love to have you stay with us when you get here.
You can have our youngest son's room.
Thanks, Jenn, but we'll stay at a hotel... it's more comfortable that way.
We don't want to be a burden.
YOU'RE SOMEWHAT DILATED. HOPE THE IPs ARE ON THEIR WAY!
SHOOT, I FORGOT TO BRING THE GIFTS I GOT FOR JENN'S KIDS! THAT NICE COUPLE, DAVID AND JOHN, TOLD ME THEY GOT GIFTS FOR THEIR SURROGATE'S KIDS.
WELL IT'S TOO LATE NOW AND WE HAVE A LONG DRIVE. WE GOT JENN A GIFT AND WE ARE PAYING HER... IT SHOULD BE FINE.

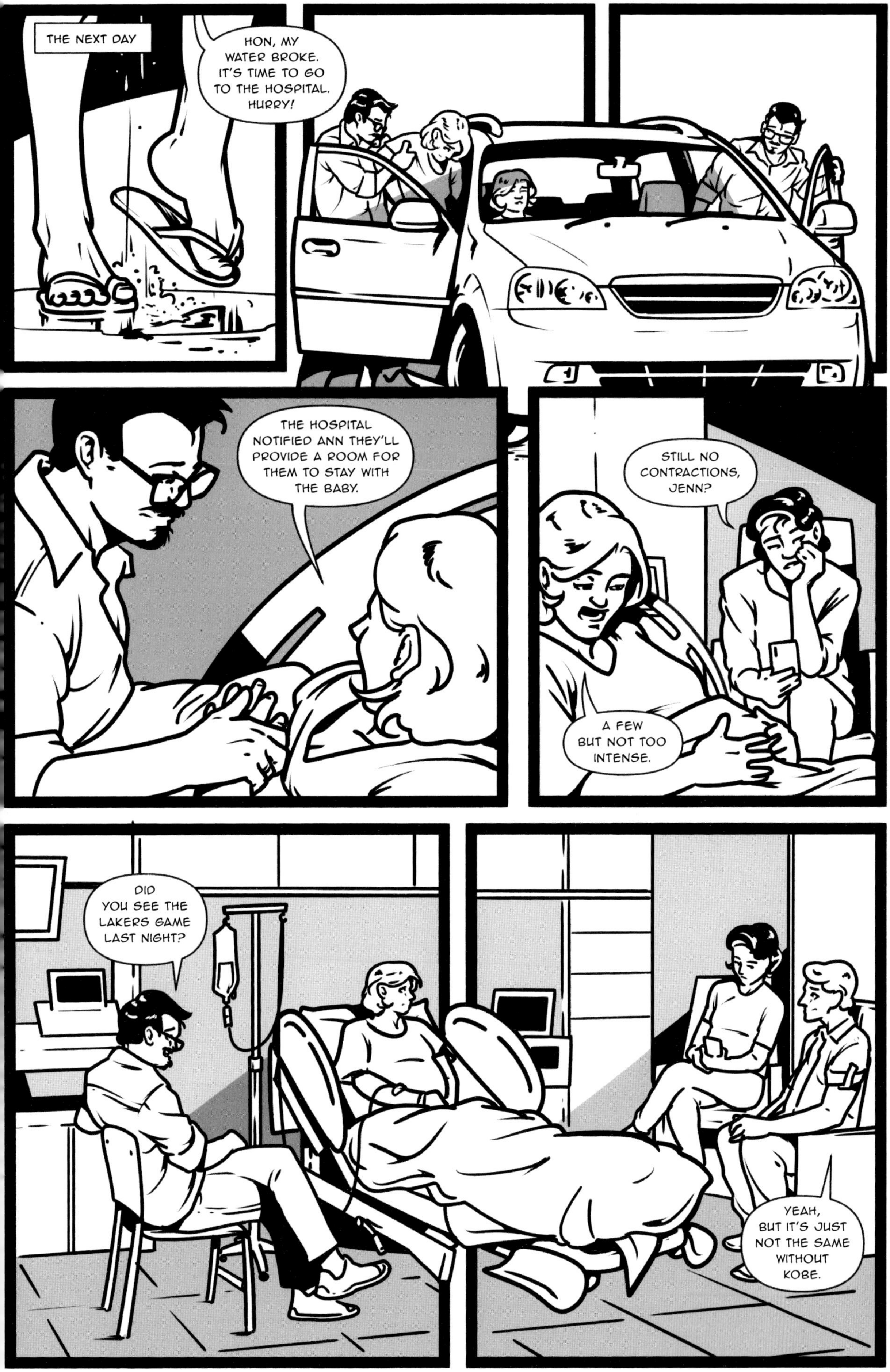
THE NEXT DAY
HON, MY WATER BROKE. IT'S TIME TO GO TO THE HOSPITAL. HURRY!
THE HOSPITAL NOTIFIED ANN THEY'LL PROVIDE A ROOM FOR THEM TO STAY WITH THE BABY.
STILL NO CONTRACTIONS, JENN?
A FEW BUT NOT TOO INTENSE.
DID YOU SEE THE LAKERS GAME LAST NIGHT?
YEAH, BUT IT'S JUST NOT THE SAME WITHOUT KOBE.

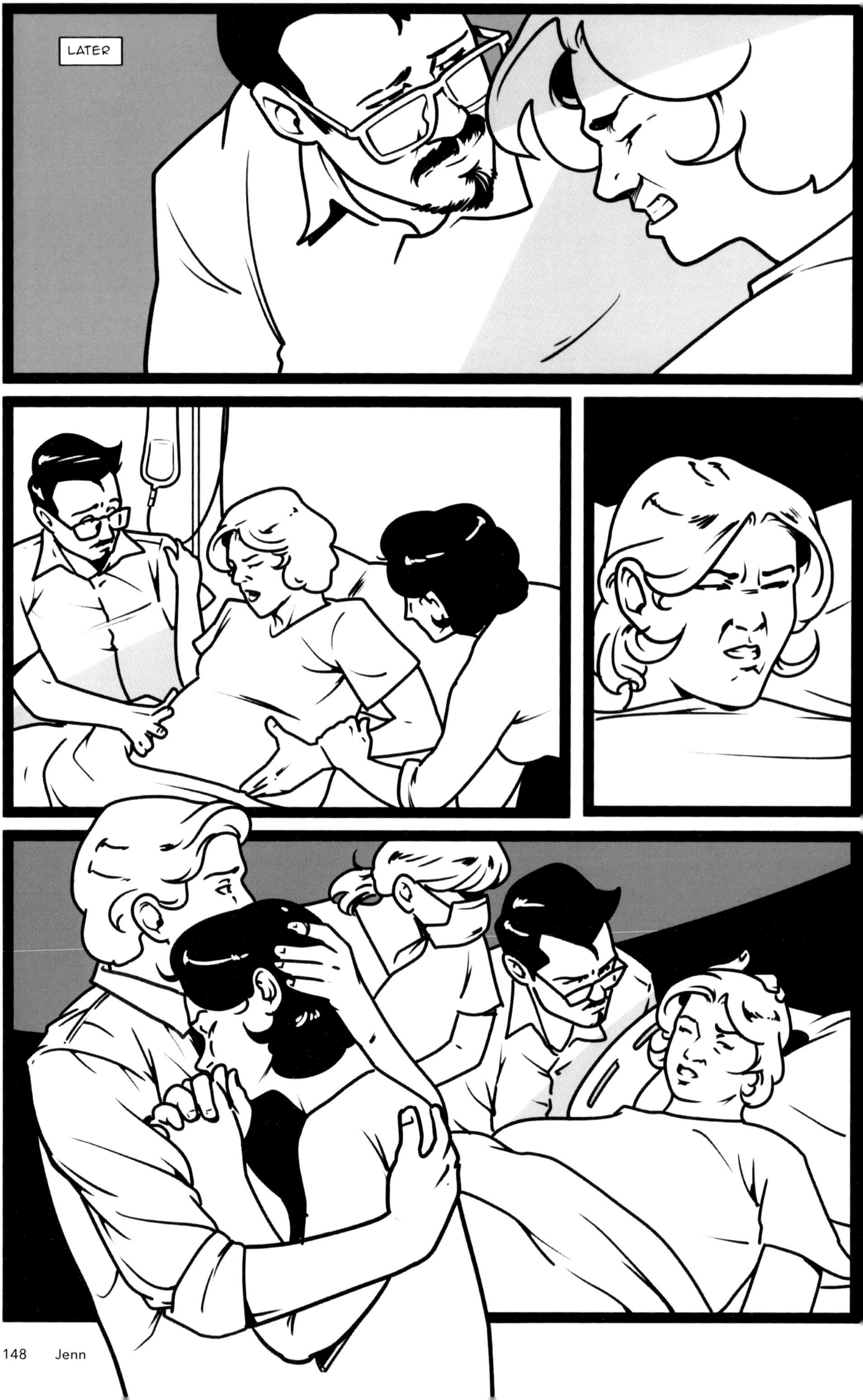
LATER

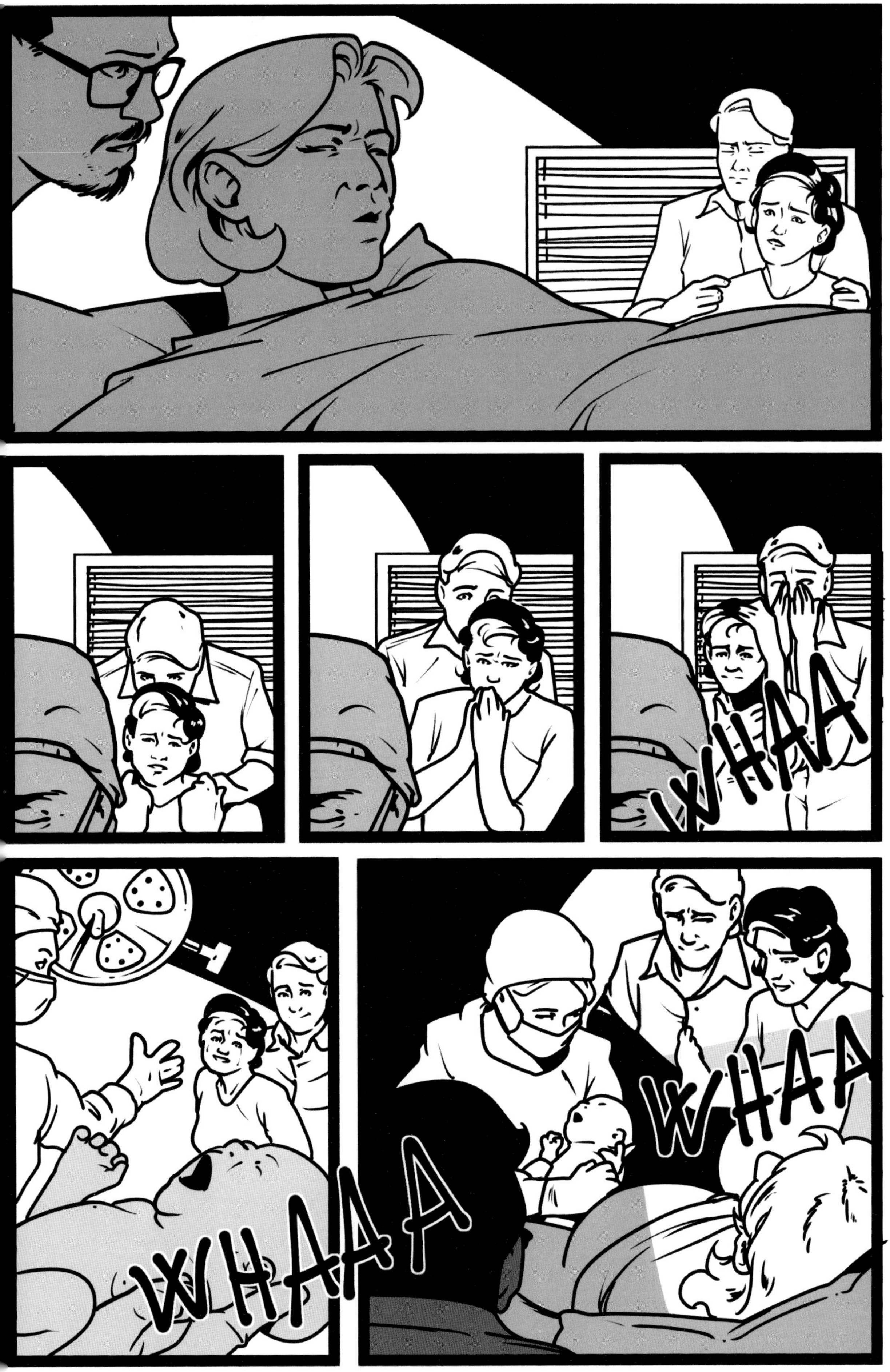
WHAA
WHAAA
WHAA

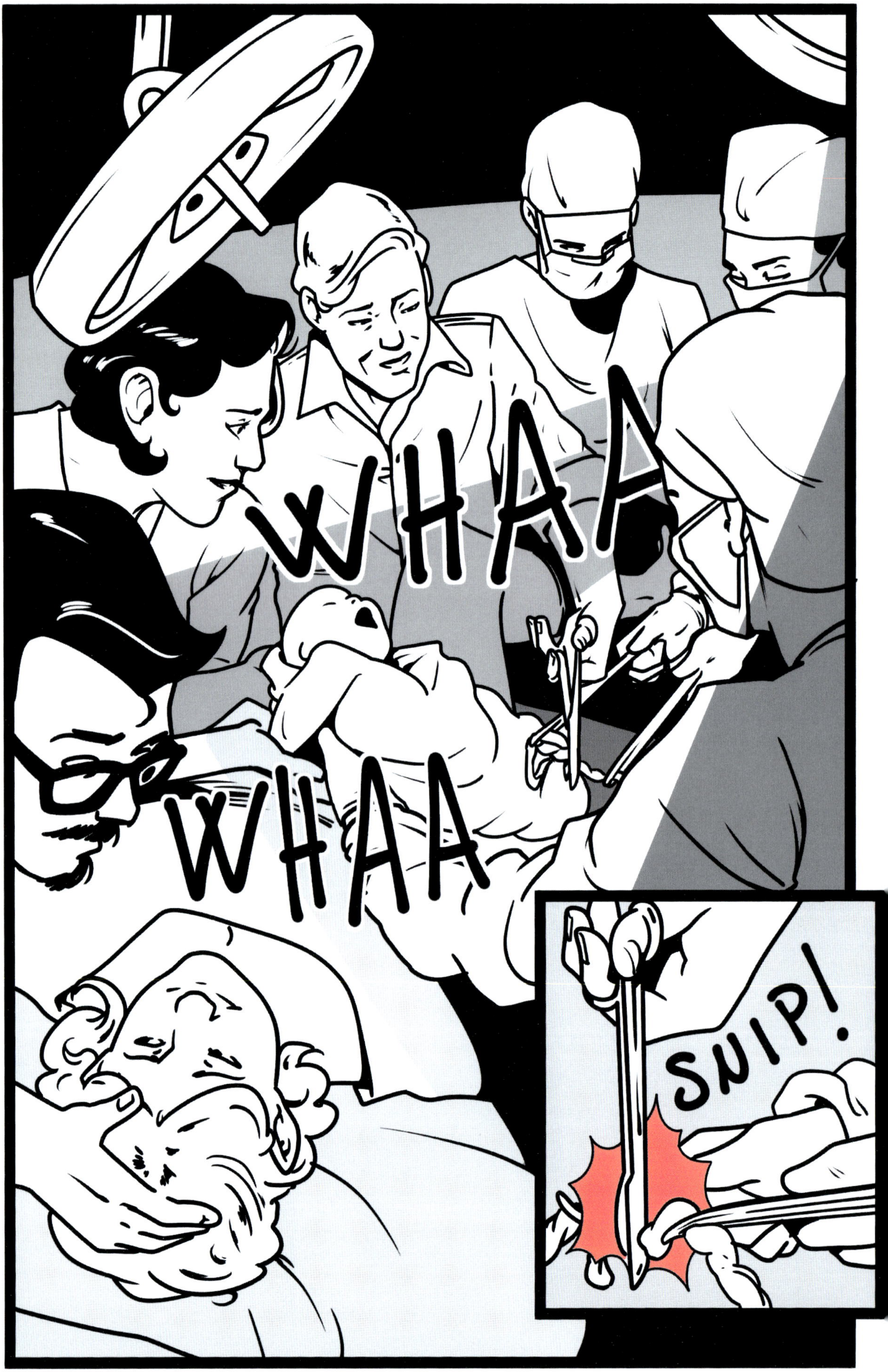
WHAA
WHAA
SNIP!

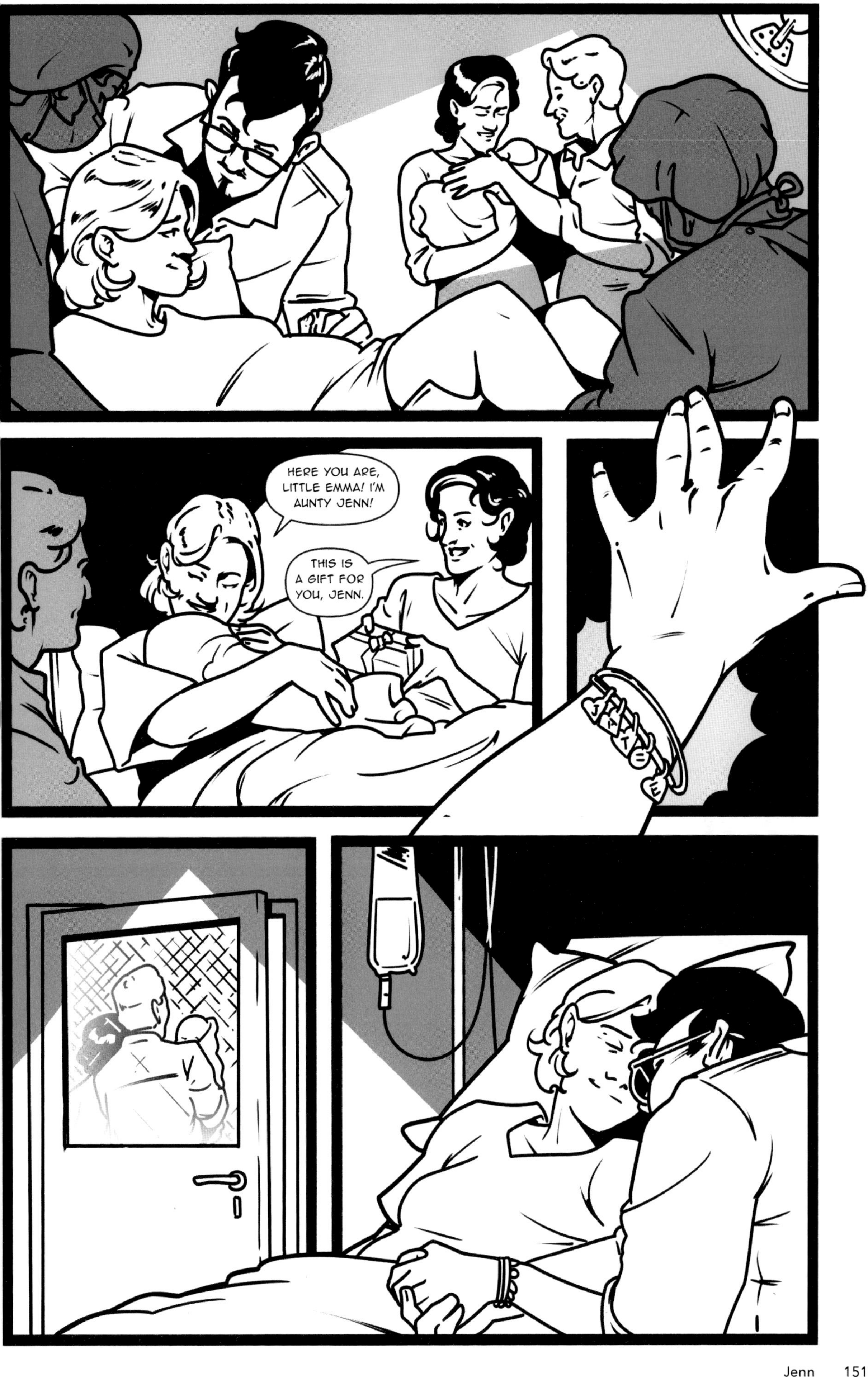
HERE YOU ARE, LITTLE EMMA! I'M AUNTY JENN!
THIS IS A GIFT FOR YOU, JENN.

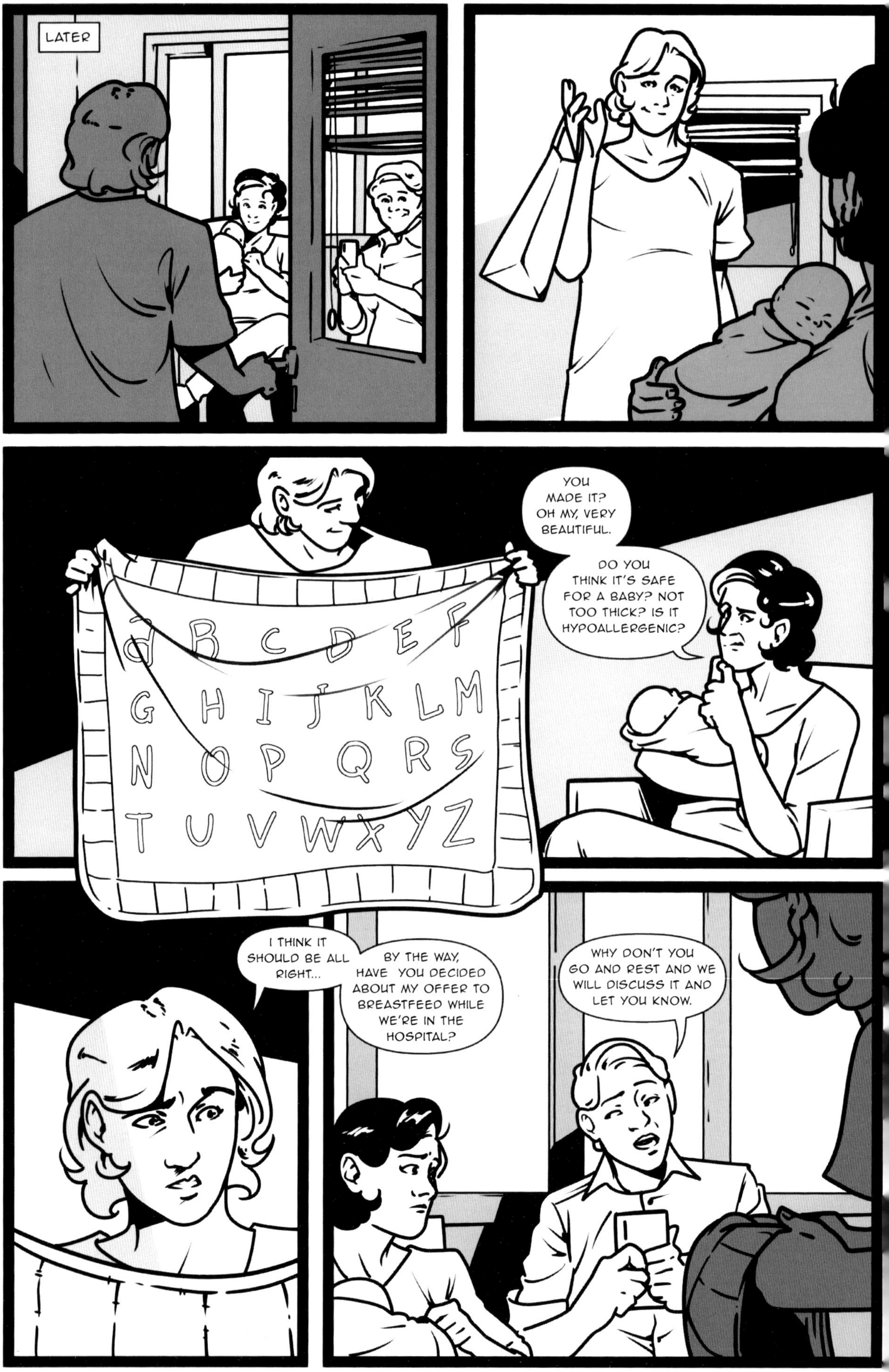
LATER
YOU MADE IT? OH MY, VERY BEAUTIFUL.
DO YOU THINK IT'S SAFE FOR A BABY? NOT TOO THICK? IS IT HYPOALLERGENIC?
ABCDEF GHIJKLM NOPQRS TUVWXYZ
I THINK IT SHOULD BE ALL RIGHT...
BY THE WAY, HAVE YOU DECIDED ABOUT MY OFFER TO BREASTFEED WHILE WE'RE IN THE HOSPITAL?
WHY DON'T YOU GO AND REST AND WE WILL DISCUSS IT AND LET YOU KNOW.

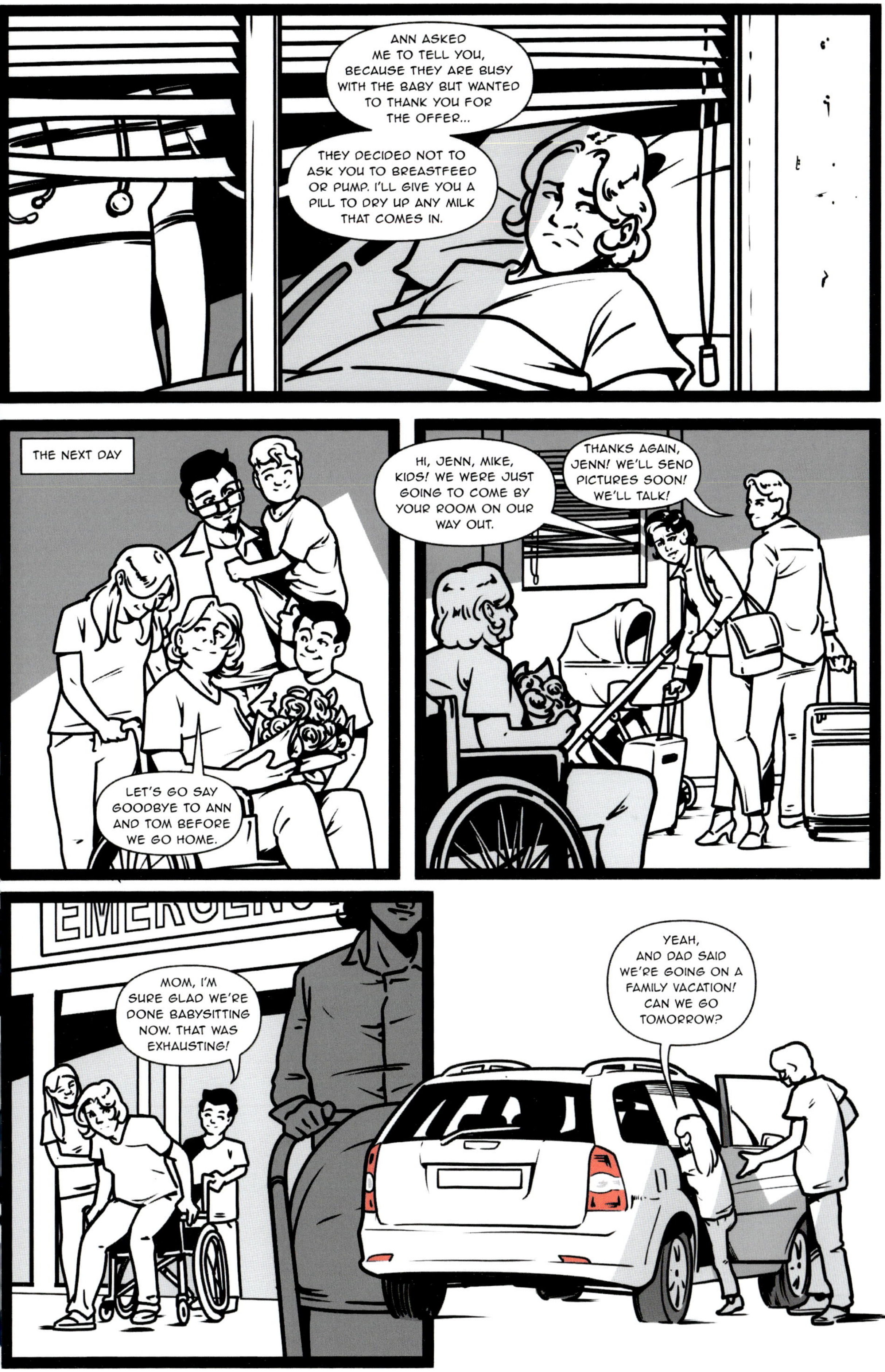
ANN ASKED ME TO TELL YOU, BECAUSE THEY ARE BUSY WITH THE BABY BUT WANTED TO THANK YOU FOR THE OFFER...
THEY DECIDED NOT TO ASK YOU TO BREASTFEED OR PUMP. I'LL GIVE YOU A PILL TO DRY UP ANY MILK THAT COMES IN.
THE NEXT DAY
LET'S GO SAY GOODBYE TO ANN AND TOM BEFORE WE GO HOME.
HI, JENN, MIKE, KIDS! WE WERE JUST GOING TO COME BY YOUR ROOM ON OUR WAY OUT.
THANKS AGAIN, JENN! WE'LL SEND PICTURES SOON! WE'LL TALK!
EMERGENCY
MOM, I'M SURE GLAD WE'RE DONE BABYSITTING NOW. THAT WAS EXHAUSTING!
YEAH, AND DAD SAID WE'RE GOING ON A FAMILY VACATION! CAN WE GO TOMORROW?

INTERLUDE: TABASCO, MEXICO

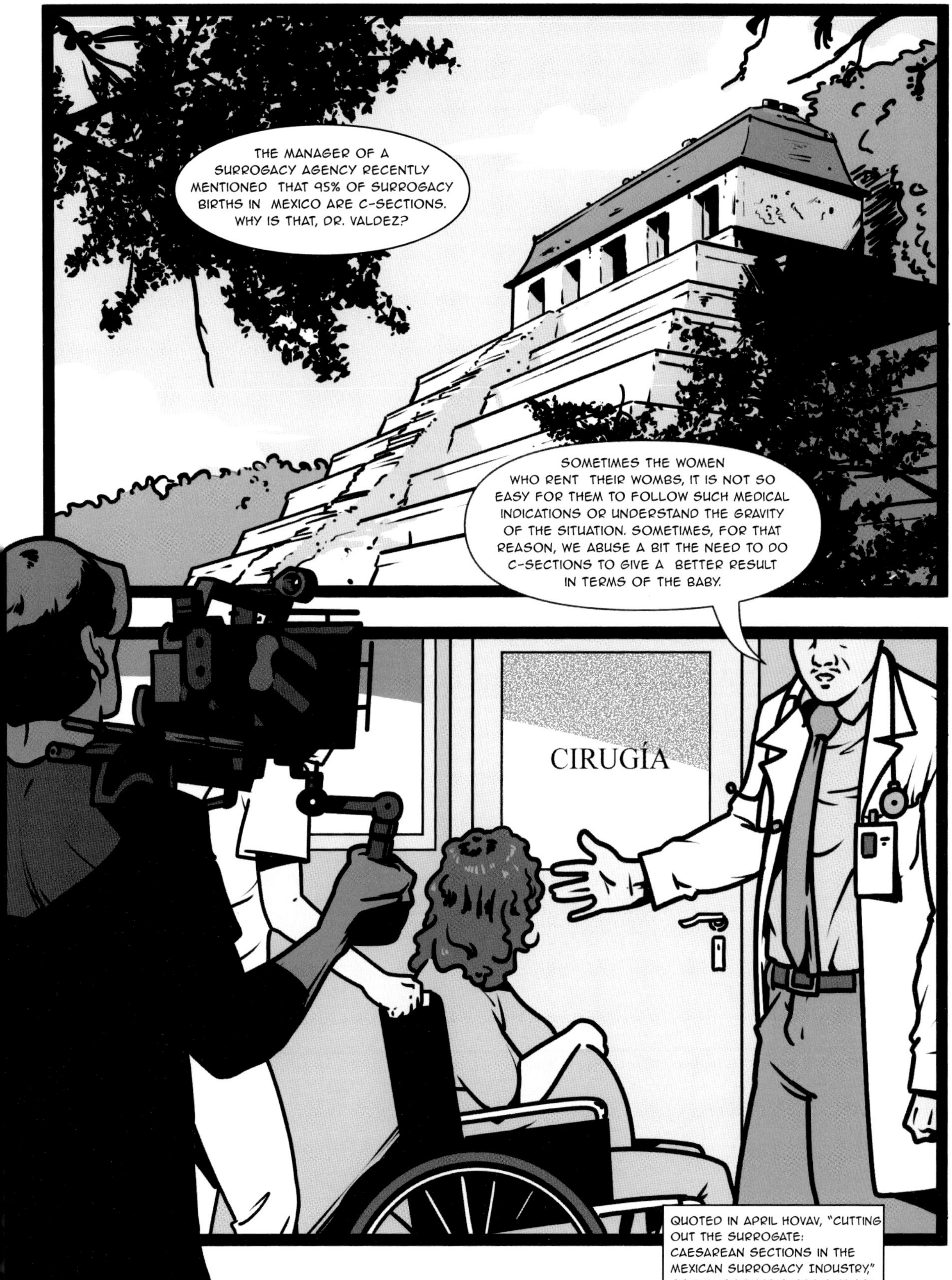
THE MANAGER OF A SURROGACY AGENCY RECENTLY MENTIONED THAT 95% OF SURROGACY BIRTHS IN MEXICO ARE C-SECTIONS. WHY IS THAT, DR. VALDEZ?
SOMETIMES THE WOMEN WHO RENT THEIR WOMBS, IT IS NOT SO EASY FOR THEM TO FOLLOW SUCH MEDICAL INDICATIONS OR UNDERSTAND THE GRAVITY OF THE SITUATION. SOMETIMES, FOR THAT REASON, WE ABUSE A BIT THE NEED TO DO C-SECTIONS TO GIVE A BETTER RESULT IN TERMS OF THE BABY.
CIRUGÍA

QUOTED IN APRIL HOVAV, "CUTTING OUT THE SURROGATE: CAESAREAN SECTIONS IN THE MEXICAN SURROGACY INDUSTRY," SOCIAL SCIENCE & MEDICINE 256 (2020): 113063.

-CHAPTER 19-
ACKNOWLEDGMENT

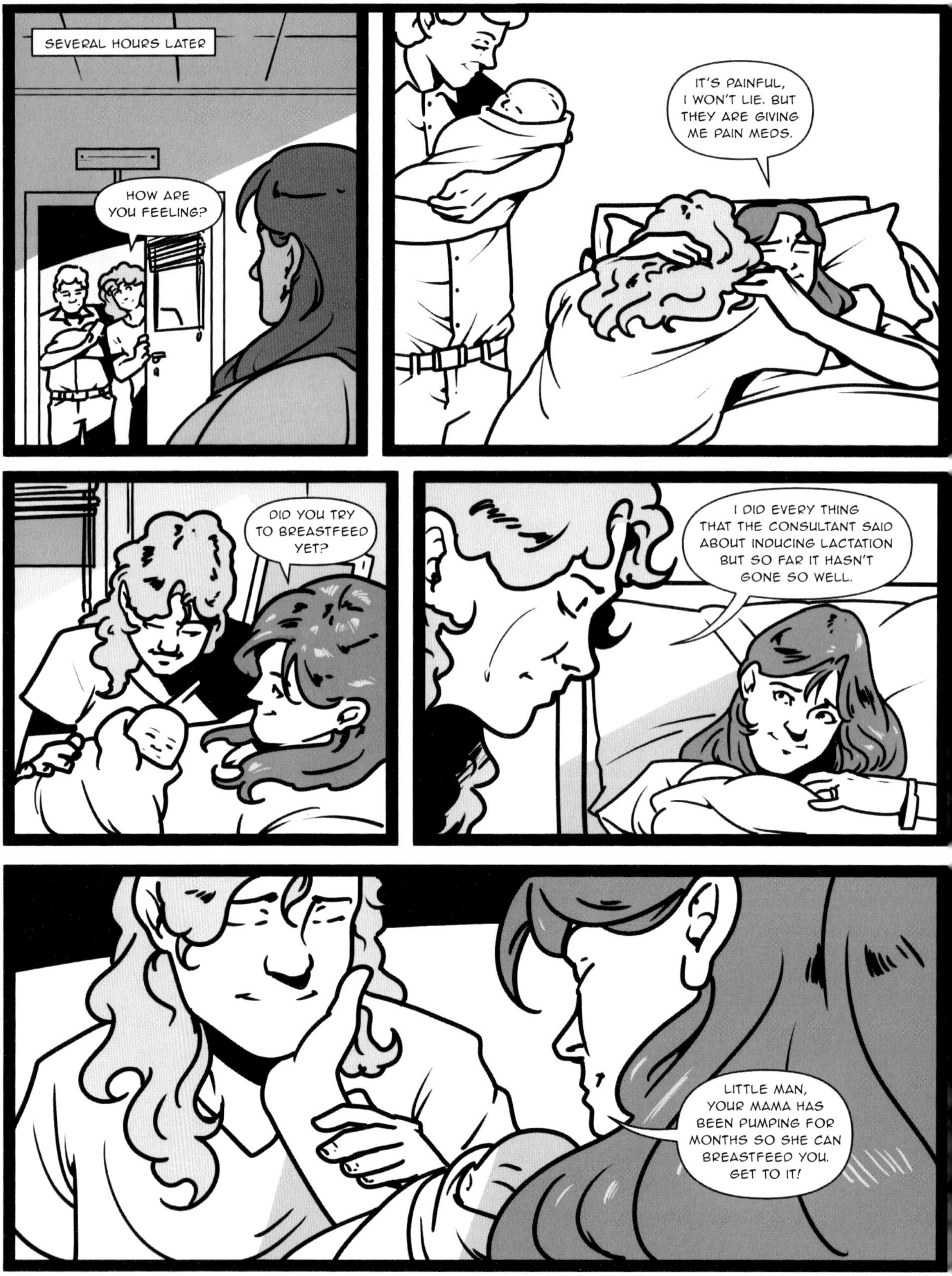
SEVERAL HOURS LATER
HOW ARE YOU FEELING?
IT'S PAINFUL, I WON'T LIE. BUT THEY ARE GIVING ME PAIN MEDS.
DID YOU TRY TO BREASTFEED YET?
I DID EVERY THING THAT THE CONSULTANT SAID ABOUT INDUCING LACTATION BUT SO FAR IT HASN'T GONE SO WELL.
LITTLE MAN, YOUR MAMA HAS BEEN PUMPING FOR MONTHS SO SHE CAN BREASTFEED YOU. GET TO IT!

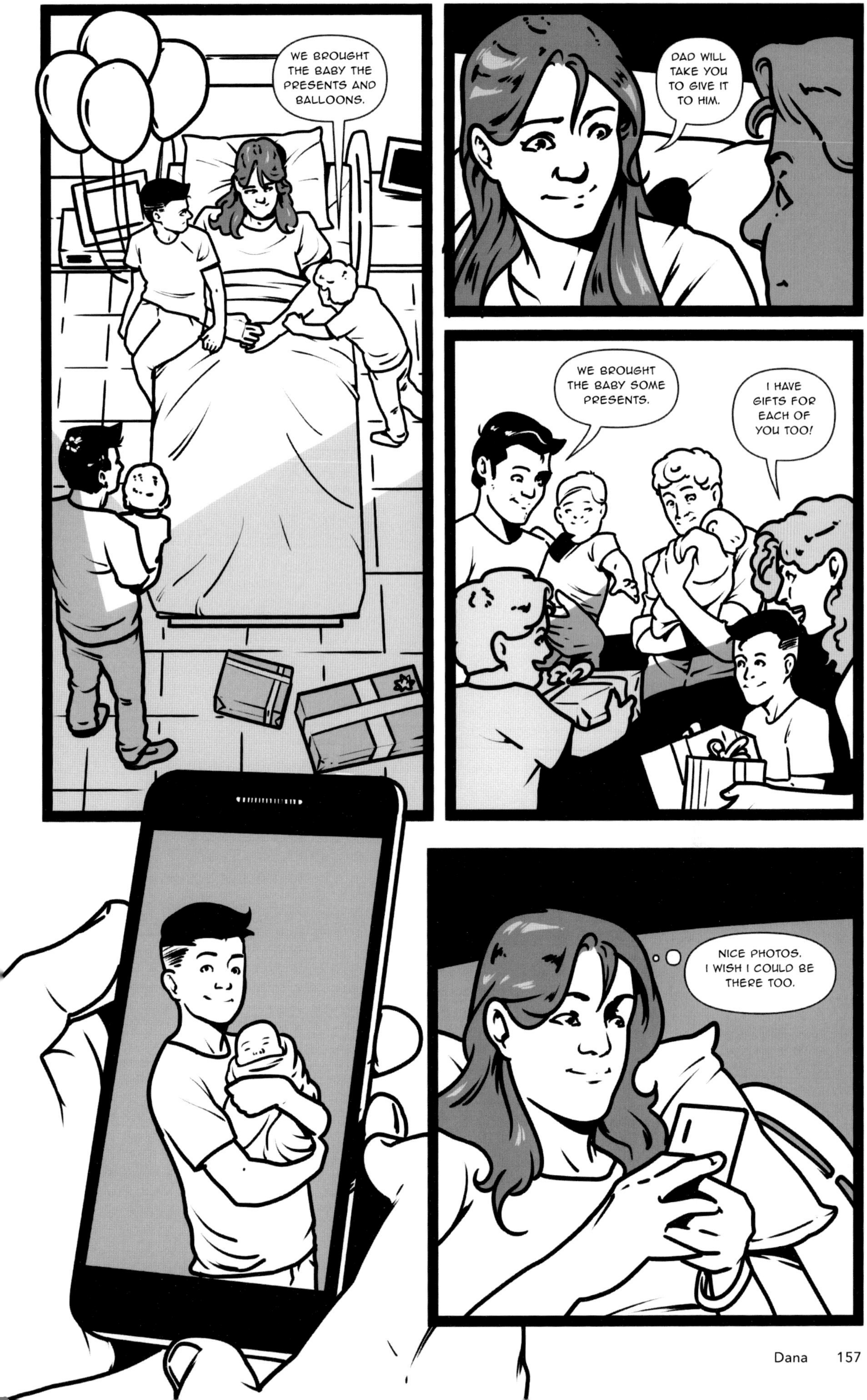
WE BROUGHT THE BABY THE PRESENTS AND BALLOONS.
DAD WILL TAKE YOU TO GIVE IT TO HIM.
WE BROUGHT THE BABY SOME PRESENTS.
I HAVE GIFTS FOR EACH OF YOU TOO!
NICE PHOTOS. I WISH I COULD BE THERE TOO.

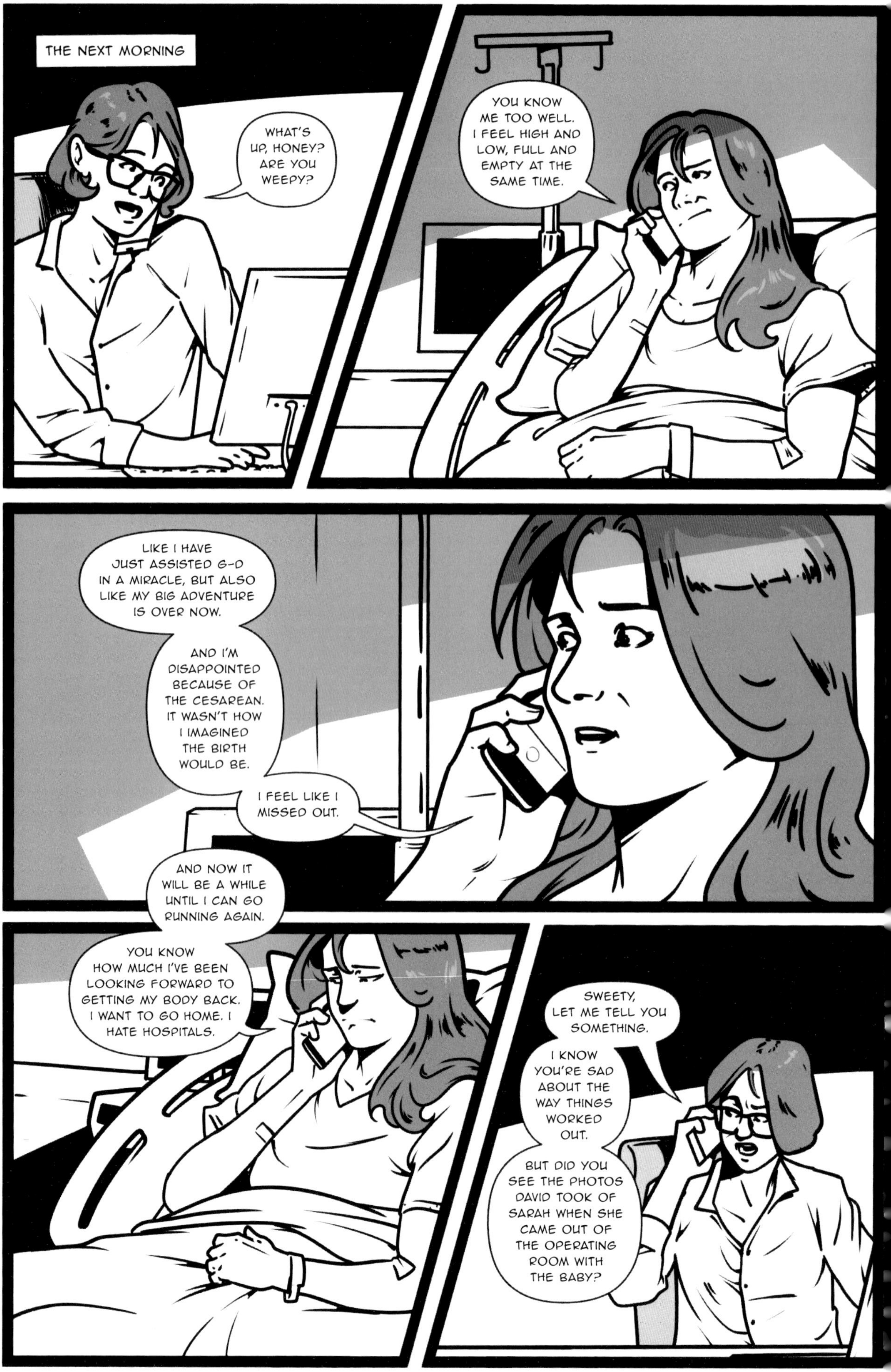
THE NEXT MORNING
WHAT'S UP, HONEY? ARE YOU WEEPY?
YOU KNOW ME TOO WELL. I FEEL HIGH AND LOW, FULL AND EMPTY AT THE SAME TIME.
LIKE I HAVE JUST ASSISTED G-D IN A MIRACLE, BUT ALSO LIKE MY BIG ADVENTURE IS OVER NOW.
AND I'M DISAPPOINTED BECAUSE OF THE CESAREAN. IT WASN'T HOW I IMAGINED THE BIRTH WOULD BE.
I FEEL LIKE I MISSED OUT.
AND NOW IT WILL BE A WHILE UNTIL I CAN GO RUNNING AGAIN.
YOU KNOW HOW MUCH I'VE BEEN LOOKING FORWARD TO GETTING MY BODY BACK. I WANT TO GO HOME. I HATE HOSPITALS.
SWEETY, LET ME TELL YOU SOMETHING.
I KNOW YOU'RE SAD ABOUT THE WAY THINGS WORKED OUT.
BUT DID YOU SEE THE PHOTOS DAVID TOOK OF SARAH WHEN SHE CAME OUT OF THE OPERATING ROOM WITH THE BABY?

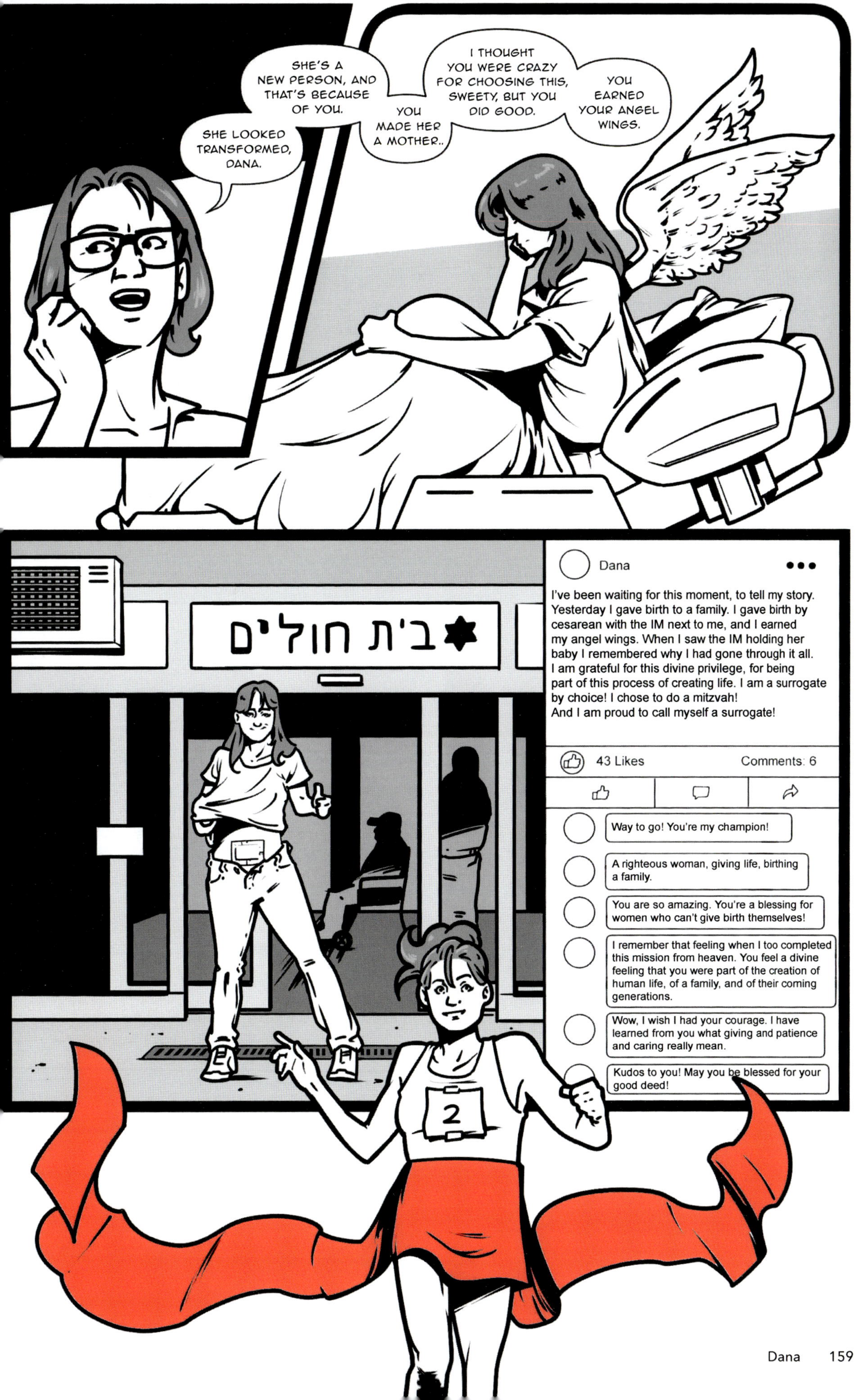
SHE LOOKED TRANSFORMED, DANA.
SHE'S A NEW PERSON, AND THAT'S BECAUSE OF YOU.
YOU MADE HER A MOTHER..
I THOUGHT YOU WERE CRAZY FOR CHOOSING THIS, SWEETY, BUT YOU DID GOOD.
YOU EARNED YOUR ANGEL WINGS.
בית חולים
Dana
I've been waiting for this moment, to tell my story. Yesterday I gave birth to a family. I gave birth by cesarean with the IM next to me, and I earned my angel wings. When I saw the IM holding her baby I remembered why I had gone through it all. I am grateful for this divine privilege, for being part of this process of creating life. I am a surrogate by choice! I chose to do a mitzvah! And I am proud to call myself a surrogate!
43 Likes
Comments: 6
Way to go! You're my champion!
A righteous woman, giving life, birthing a family.
You are so amazing. You're a blessing for women who can't give birth themselves!
I remember that feeling when I too completed this mission from heaven. You feel a divine feeling that you were part of the creation of human life, of a family, and of their coming generations.
Wow, I wish I had your courage. I have learned from you what giving and patience and caring really mean.
Kudos to you! May you be blessed for your good deed!
2

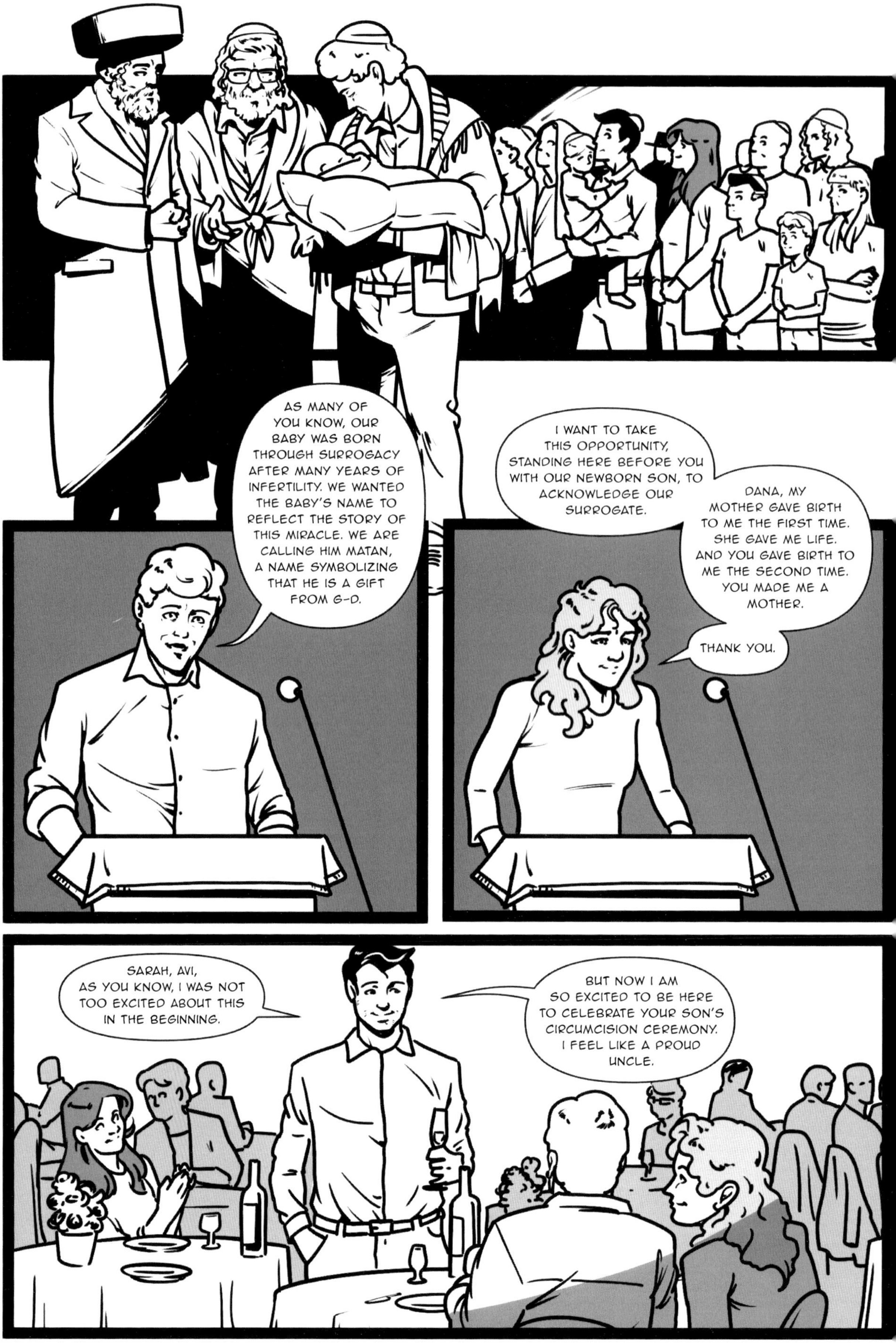
AS MANY OF YOU KNOW, OUR BABY WAS BORN THROUGH SURROGACY AFTER MANY YEARS OF INFERTILITY. WE WANTED THE BABY'S NAME TO REFLECT THE STORY OF THIS MIRACLE. WE ARE CALLING HIM MATAN, A NAME SYMBOLIZING THAT HE IS A GIFT FROM G-D.
I WANT TO TAKE THIS OPPORTUNITY, STANDING HERE BEFORE YOU WITH OUR NEWBORN SON, TO ACKNOWLEDGE OUR SURROGATE.
DANA, MY MOTHER GAVE BIRTH TO ME THE FIRST TIME. SHE GAVE ME LIFE. AND YOU GAVE BIRTH TO ME THE SECOND TIME. YOU MADE ME A MOTHER.
THANK YOU.
SARAH, AVI, AS YOU KNOW, I WAS NOT TOO EXCITED ABOUT THIS IN THE BEGINNING.
BUT NOW I AM SO EXCITED TO BE HERE TO CELEBRATE YOUR SON'S CIRCUMCISION CEREMONY. I FEEL LIKE A PROUD UNCLE.

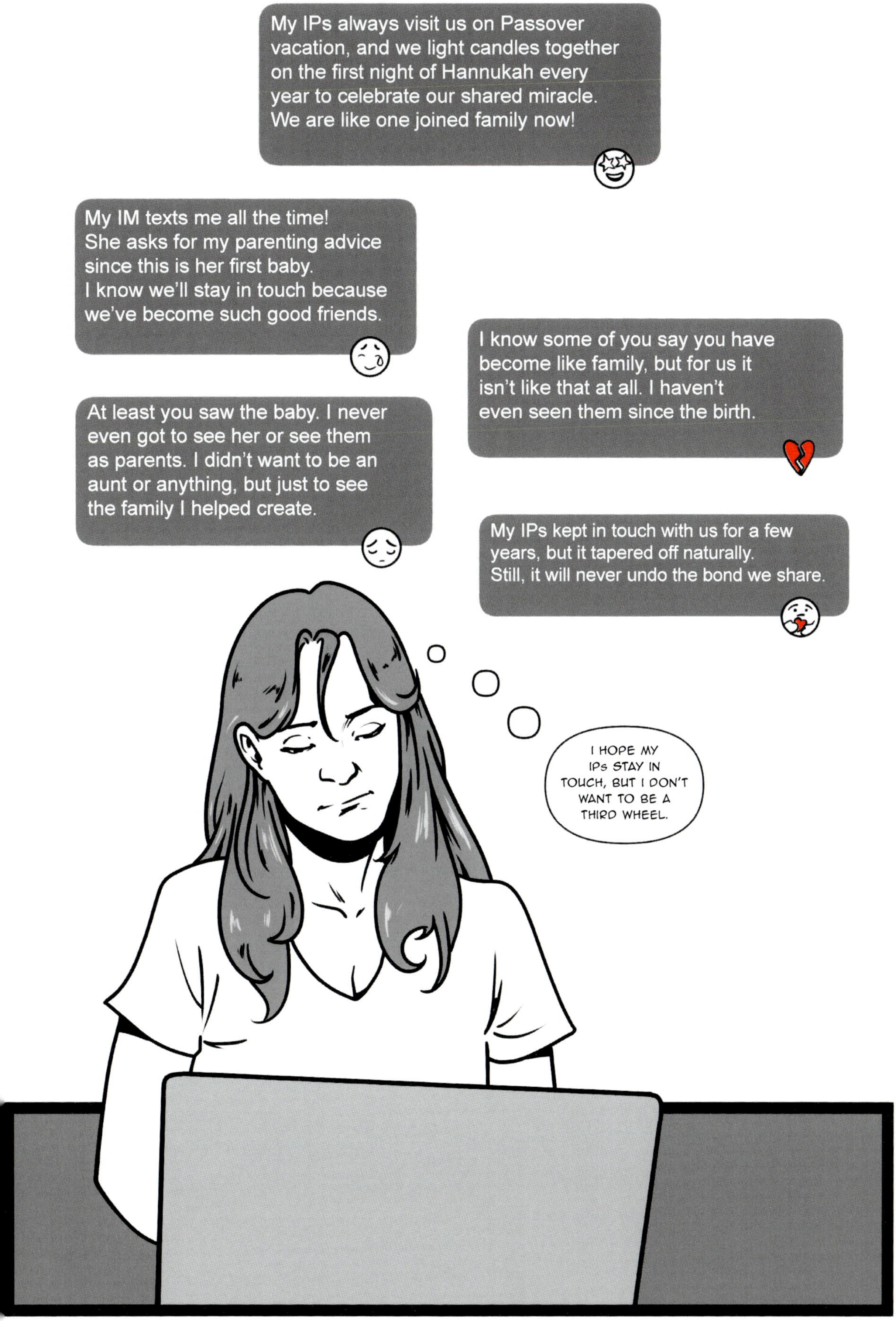

My IPs always visit us on Passover vacation, and we light candles together on the first night of Hannukah every year to celebrate our shared miracle. We are like one joined family now!
My IM texts me all the time! She asks for my parenting advice since this is her first baby. I know we'll stay in touch because we've become such good friends.
I know some of you say you have become like family, but for us it isn't like that at all. I haven't even seen them since the birth.
At least you saw the baby. I never even got to see her or see them as parents. I didn't want to be an aunt or anything, but just to see the family I helped create.
My IPs kept in touch with us for a few years, but it tapered off naturally. Still, it will never undo the bond we share.
I HOPE MY IPs STAY IN TOUCH, BUT I DON'T WANT TO BE A THIRD WHEEL.

-CHAPTER 20-
POSTPARTUM

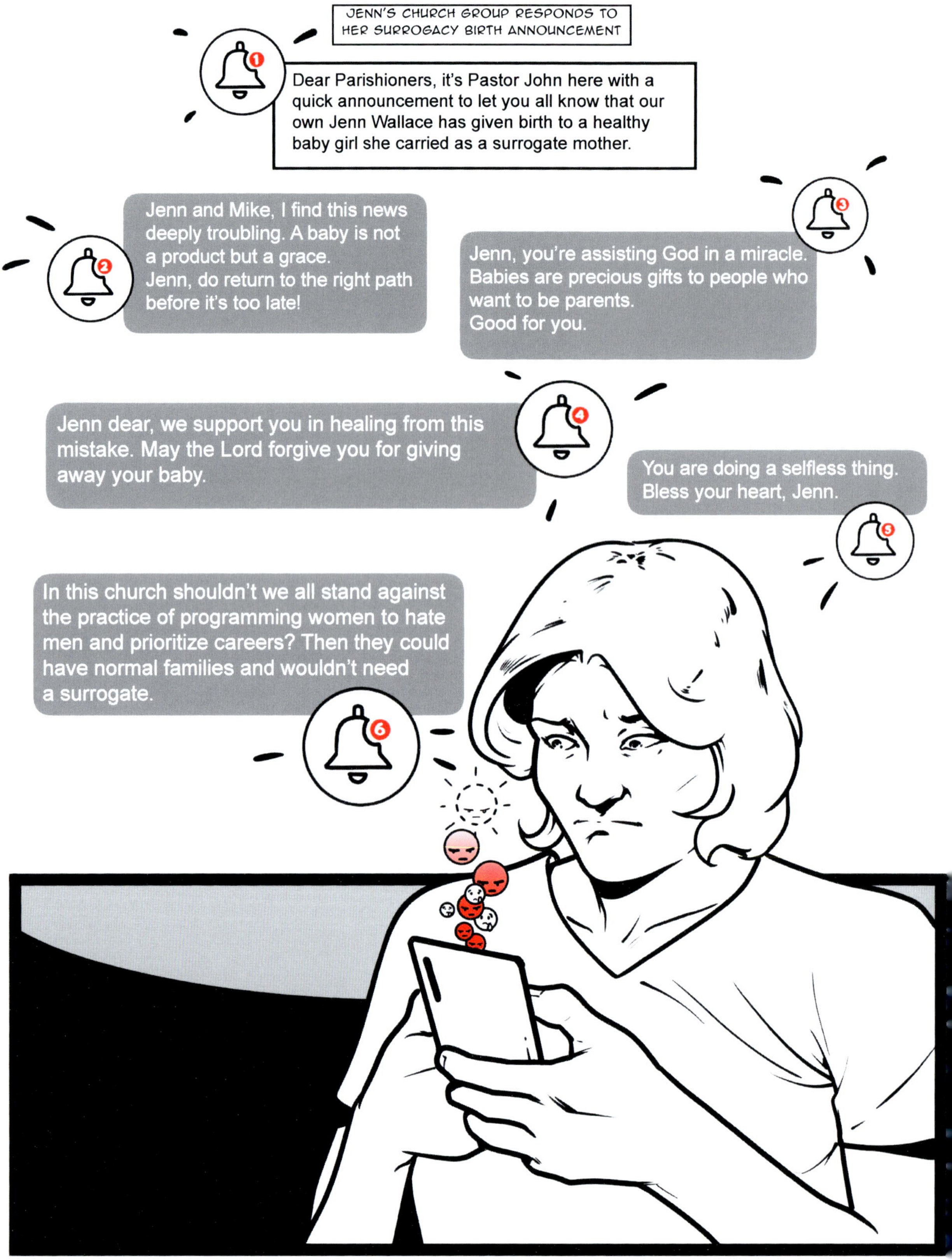

JENN'S CHURCH GROUP RESPONDS TO HER SURROGACY BIRTH ANNOUNCEMENT
Dear Parishioners, it's Pastor John here with a quick announcement to let you all know that our own Jenn Wallace has given birth to a healthy baby girl she carried as a surrogate mother.
Jenn and Mike, I find this news deeply troubling. A baby is not a product but a grace. Jenn, do return to the right path before it's too late!
Jenn, you're assisting God in a miracle. Babies are precious gifts to people who want to be parents. Good for you.
Jenn dear, we support you in healing from this mistake. May the Lord forgive you for giving away your baby.
You are doing a selfless thing. Bless your heart, Jenn.
In this church shouldn't we all stand against the practice of programming women to hate men and prioritize careers? Then they could have normal families and wouldn't need a surrogate.

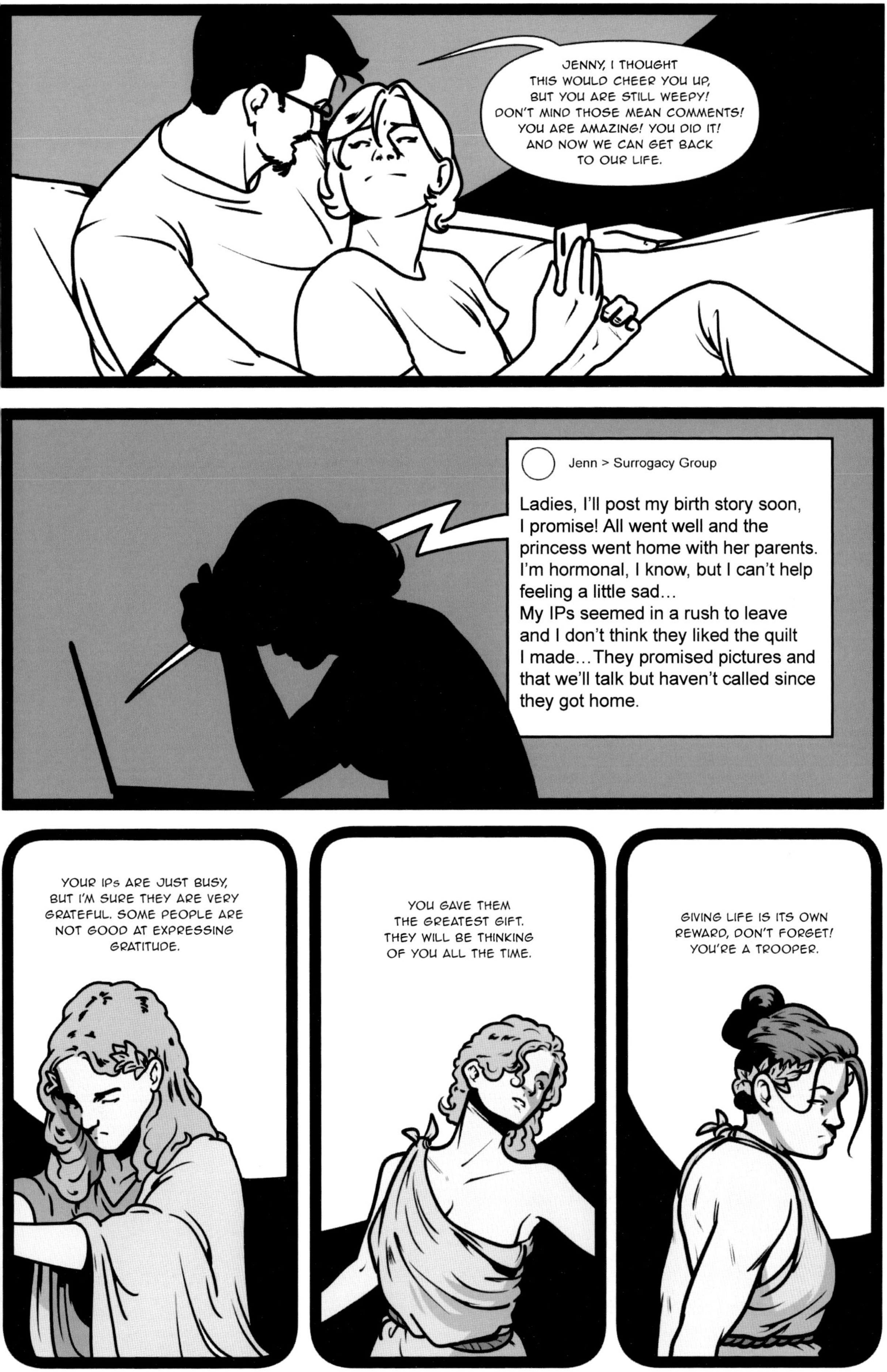
JENNY, I THOUGHT THIS WOULD CHEER YOU UP, BUT YOU ARE STILL WEEPY! DON'T MIND THOSE MEAN COMMENTS! YOU ARE AMAZING! YOU DID IT! AND NOW WE CAN GET BACK TO OUR LIFE.
Jenn > Surrogacy Group
Ladies, I'll post my birth story soon, I promise! All went well and the princess went home with her parents. I'm hormonal, I know, but I can't help feeling a little sad…
My IPs seemed in a rush to leave and I don't think they liked the quilt I made…They promised pictures and that we'll talk but haven't called since they got home.
YOUR IPs ARE JUST BUSY, BUT I'M SURE THEY ARE VERY GRATEFUL. SOME PEOPLE ARE NOT GOOD AT EXPRESSING GRATITUDE.
YOU GAVE THEM THE GREATEST GIFT. THEY WILL BE THINKING OF YOU ALL THE TIME.
GIVING LIFE IS ITS OWN REWARD, DON'T FORGET! YOU'RE A TROOPER.

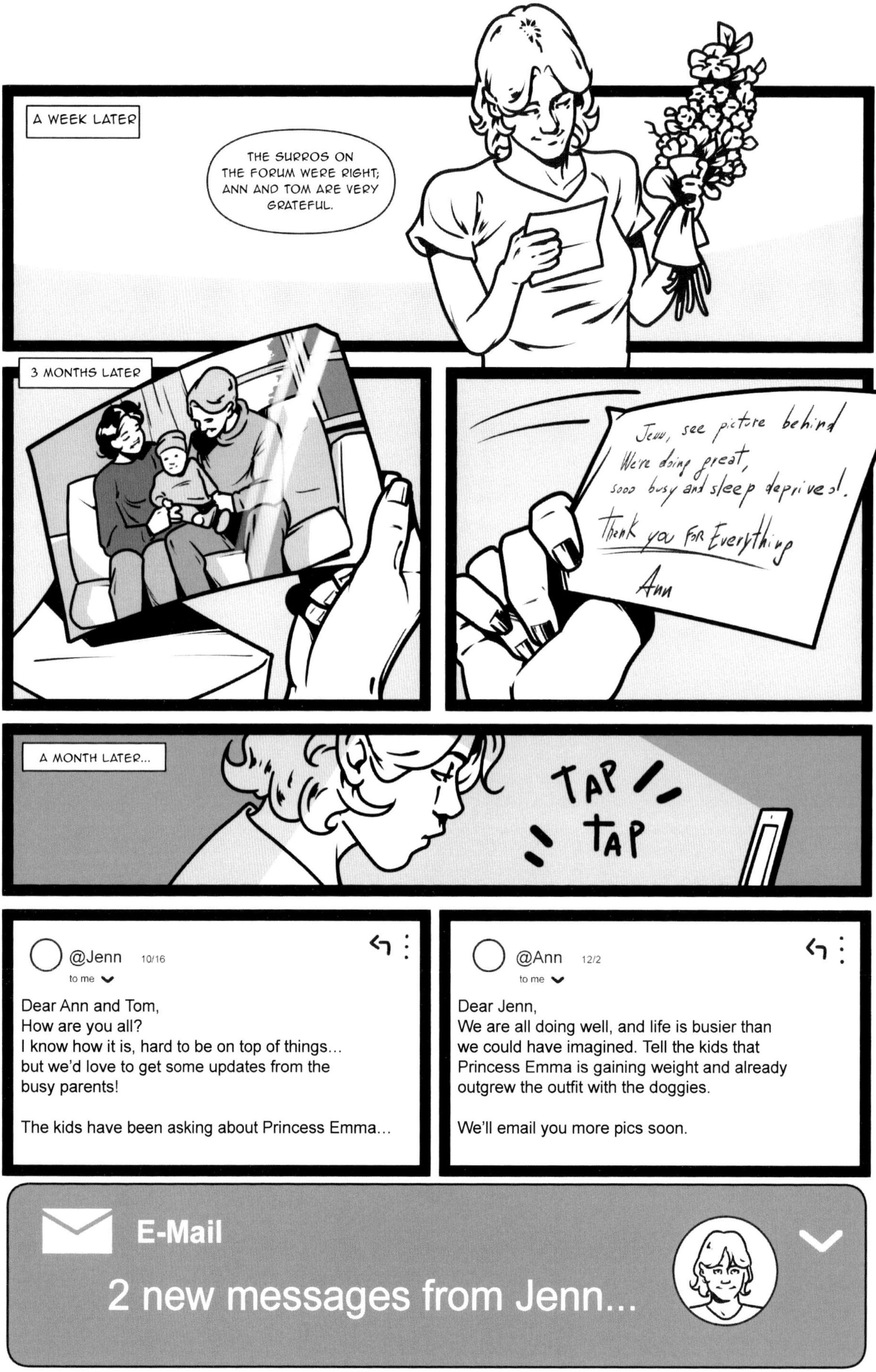
A WEEK LATER
THE SURROS ON THE FORUM WERE RIGHT; ANN AND TOM ARE VERY GRATEFUL.
3 MONTHS LATER
Jenn, see picture behind
We're doing great,
sooo busy and sleep deprived!
Thank you for Everything
Ann
A MONTH LATER...
TAP TAP
@Jenn 10/16
to me
Dear Ann and Tom,
How are you all?
I know how it is, hard to be on top of things...
but we'd love to get some updates from the busy parents!
The kids have been asking about Princess Emma...
@Ann 12/2
to me
Dear Jenn,
We are all doing well, and life is busier than we could have imagined. Tell the kids that Princess Emma is gaining weight and already outgrew the outfit with the doggies.
We'll email you more pics soon.
E-Mail
2 new messages from Jenn...

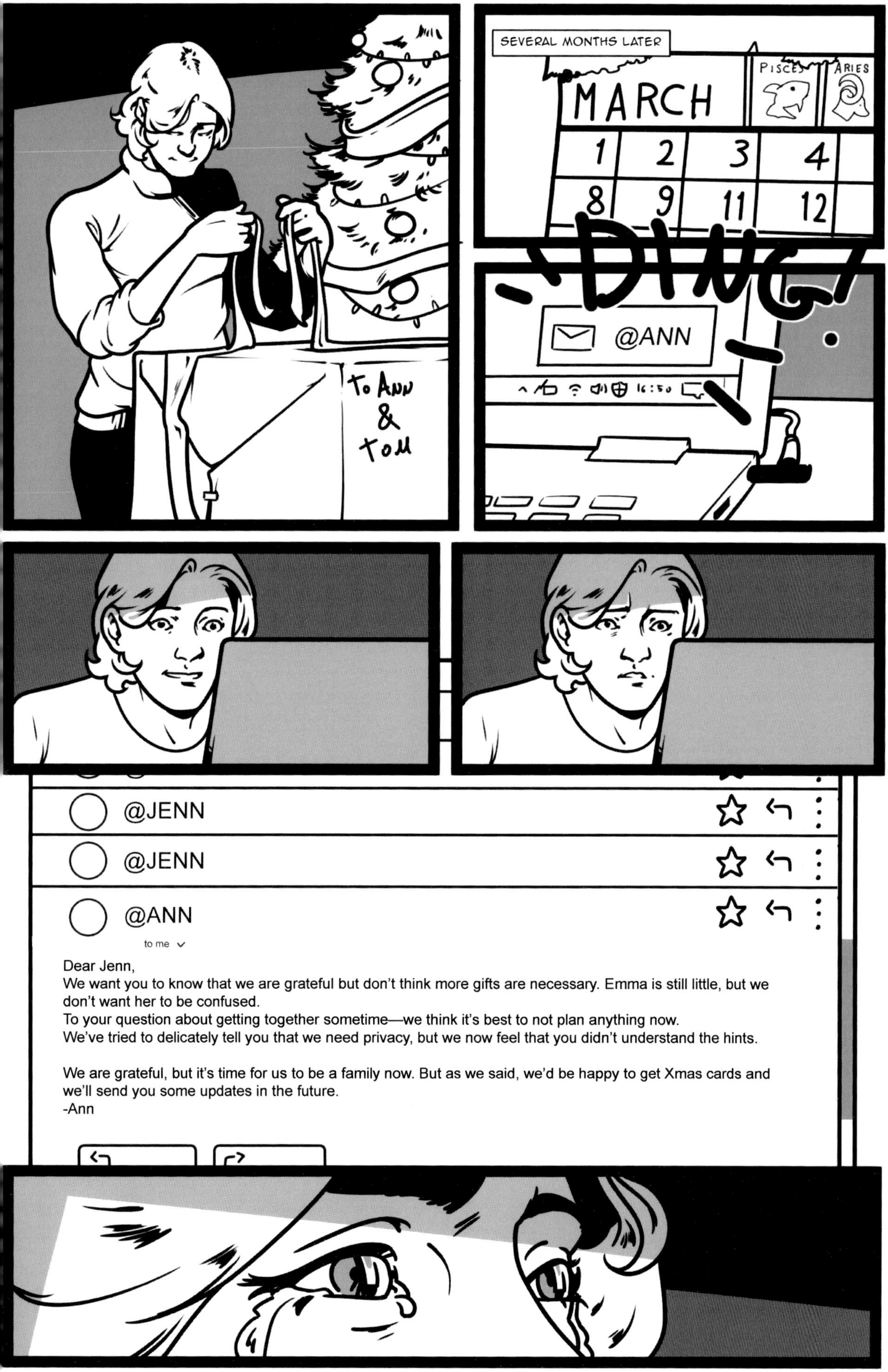
To Ann
&
Tom
SEVERAL MONTHS LATER
MARCH
PISCES
ARIES
1 2 3 4
8 9 11 12
DING!
@ANN
16:50
@JENN
@JENN
@ANN
to me
Dear Jenn,
We want you to know that we are grateful but don't think more gifts are necessary. Emma is still little, but we don't want her to be confused.
To your question about getting together sometime—we think it's best to not plan anything now.
We've tried to delicately tell you that we need privacy, but we now feel that you didn't understand the hints.

We are grateful, but it's time for us to be a family now. But as we said, we'd be happy to get Xmas cards and we'll send you some updates in the future.
-Ann

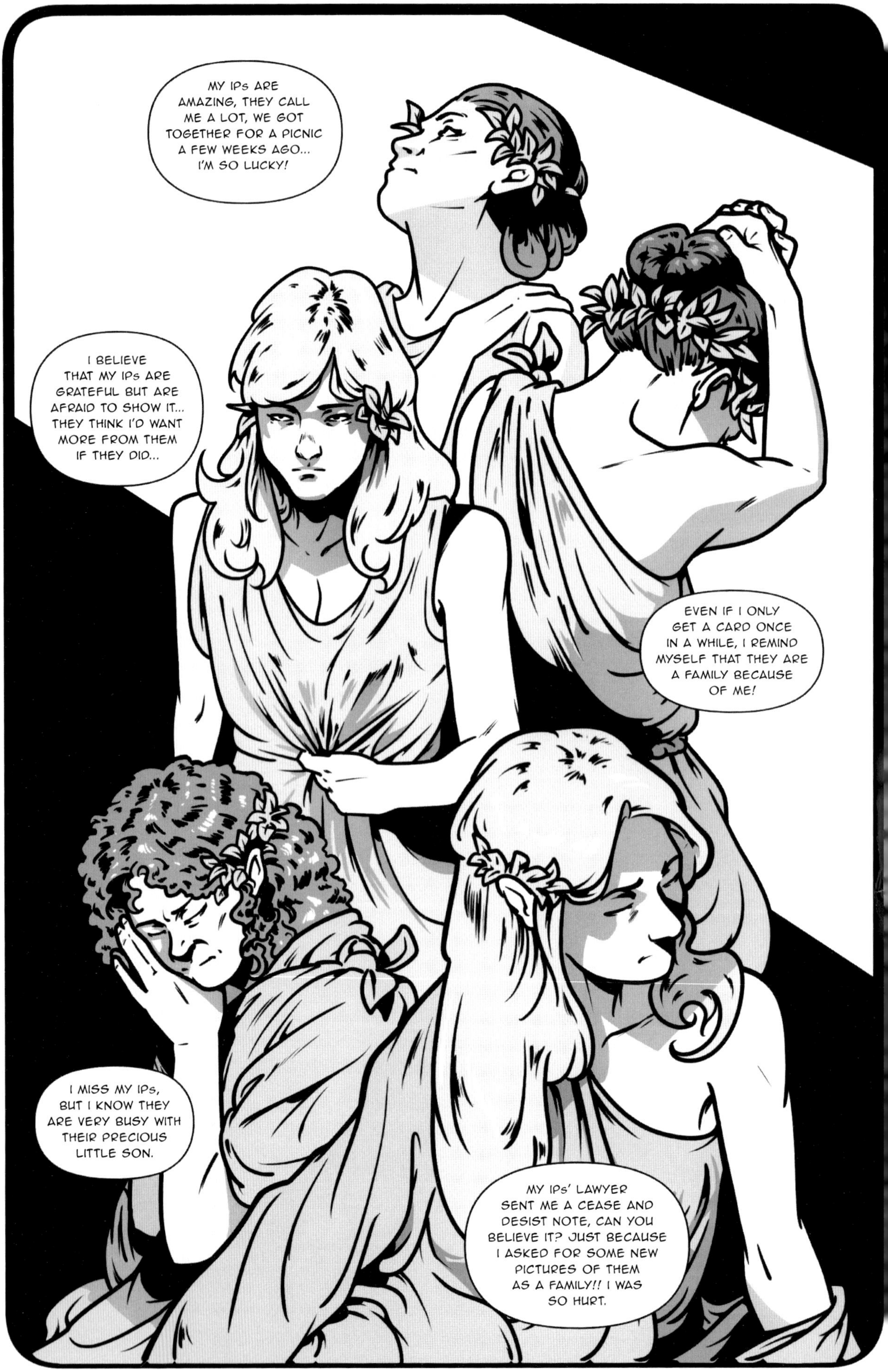
MY IPs ARE AMAZING, THEY CALL ME A LOT, WE GOT TOGETHER FOR A PICNIC A FEW WEEKS AGO... I'M SO LUCKY!
I BELIEVE THAT MY IPs ARE GRATEFUL BUT ARE AFRAID TO SHOW IT... THEY THINK I'D WANT MORE FROM THEM IF THEY DID...
EVEN IF I ONLY GET A CARD ONCE IN A WHILE, I REMIND MYSELF THAT THEY ARE A FAMILY BECAUSE OF ME!
I MISS MY IPs, BUT I KNOW THEY ARE VERY BUSY WITH THEIR PRECIOUS LITTLE SON.
MY IPs' LAWYER SENT ME A CEASE AND DESIST NOTE, CAN YOU BELIEVE IT? JUST BECAUSE I ASKED FOR SOME NEW PICTURES OF THEM AS A FAMILY!! I WAS SO HURT.

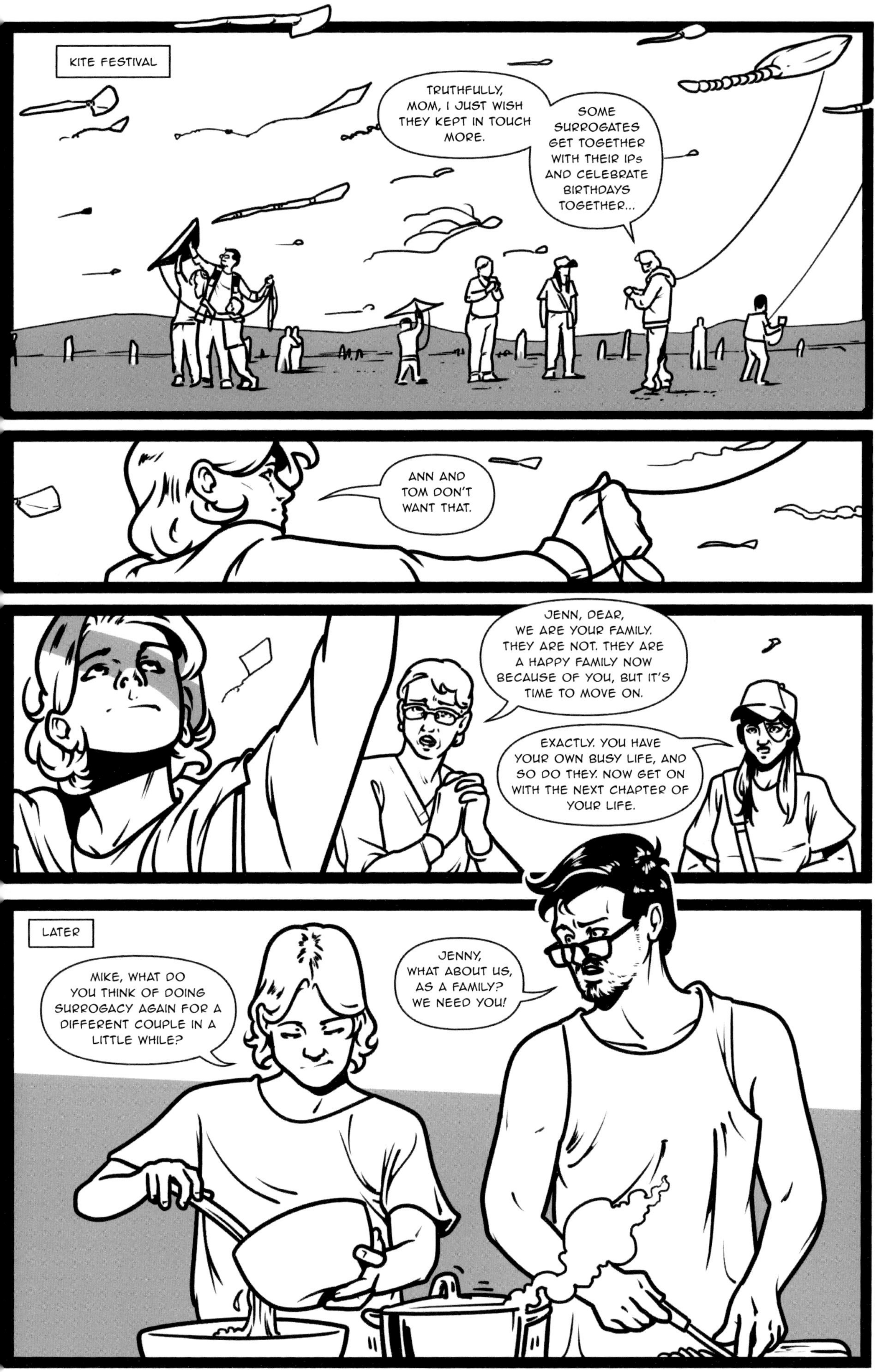

KITE FESTIVAL
TRUTHFULLY, MOM, I JUST WISH THEY KEPT IN TOUCH MORE.
SOME SURROGATES GET TOGETHER WITH THEIR IPs AND CELEBRATE BIRTHDAYS TOGETHER...
ANN AND TOM DON'T WANT THAT.
JENN, DEAR, WE ARE YOUR FAMILY. THEY ARE NOT. THEY ARE A HAPPY FAMILY NOW BECAUSE OF YOU, BUT IT'S TIME TO MOVE ON.
EXACTLY. YOU HAVE YOUR OWN BUSY LIFE, AND SO DO THEY. NOW GET ON WITH THE NEXT CHAPTER OF YOUR LIFE.
LATER
MIKE, WHAT DO YOU THINK OF DOING SURROGACY AGAIN FOR A DIFFERENT COUPLE IN A LITTLE WHILE?
JENNY, WHAT ABOUT US, AS A FAMILY? WE NEED YOU!

NTERLUDE: MARKETING MANAGER OF SURROGACY CLINIC, SOUTHERN CALIFORNIA

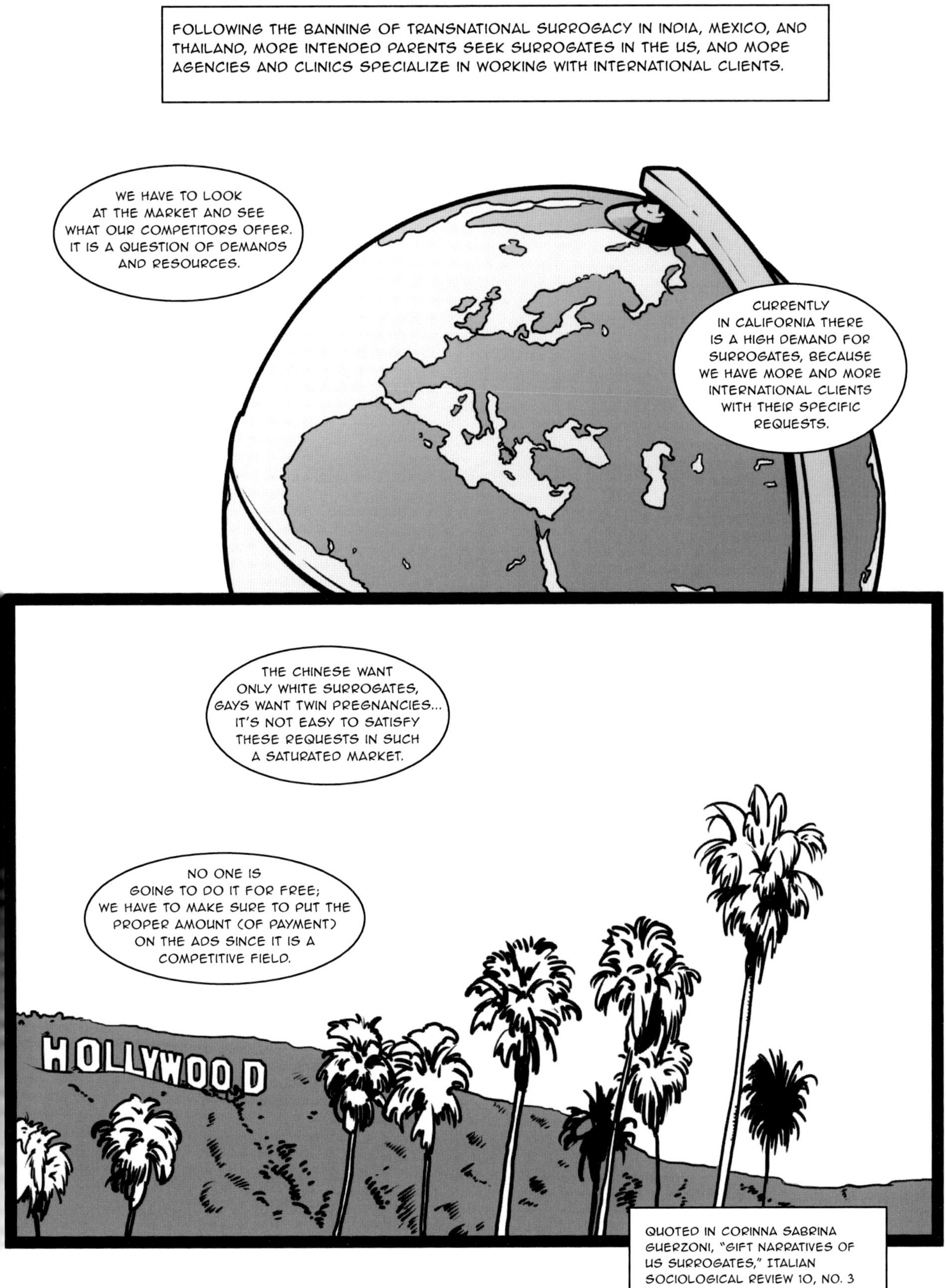
FOLLOWING THE BANNING OF TRANSNATIONAL SURROGACY IN INDIA, MEXICO, AND THAILAND, MORE INTENDED PARENTS SEEK SURROGATES IN THE US, AND MORE AGENCIES AND CLINICS SPECIALIZE IN WORKING WITH INTERNATIONAL CLIENTS.
WE HAVE TO LOOK AT THE MARKET AND SEE WHAT OUR COMPETITORS OFFER. IT IS A QUESTION OF DEMANDS AND RESOURCES.
CURRENTLY IN CALIFORNIA THERE IS A HIGH DEMAND FOR SURROGATES, BECAUSE WE HAVE MORE AND MORE INTERNATIONAL CLIENTS WITH THEIR SPECIFIC REQUESTS.
THE CHINESE WANT ONLY WHITE SURROGATES, GAYS WANT TWIN PREGNANCIES... IT'S NOT EASY TO SATISFY THESE REQUESTS IN SUCH A SATURATED MARKET.
NO ONE IS GOING TO DO IT FOR FREE; WE HAVE TO MAKE SURE TO PUT THE PROPER AMOUNT (OF PAYMENT) ON THE ADS SINCE IT IS A COMPETITIVE FIELD.
HOLLYWOOD

QUOTED IN CORINNA SABRINA GUERZONI, "GIFT NARRATIVES OF US SURROGATES," ITALIAN SOCIOLOGICAL REVIEW 10, NO. 3 (2020): 568.

-CHAPTER 21-
THE STORY

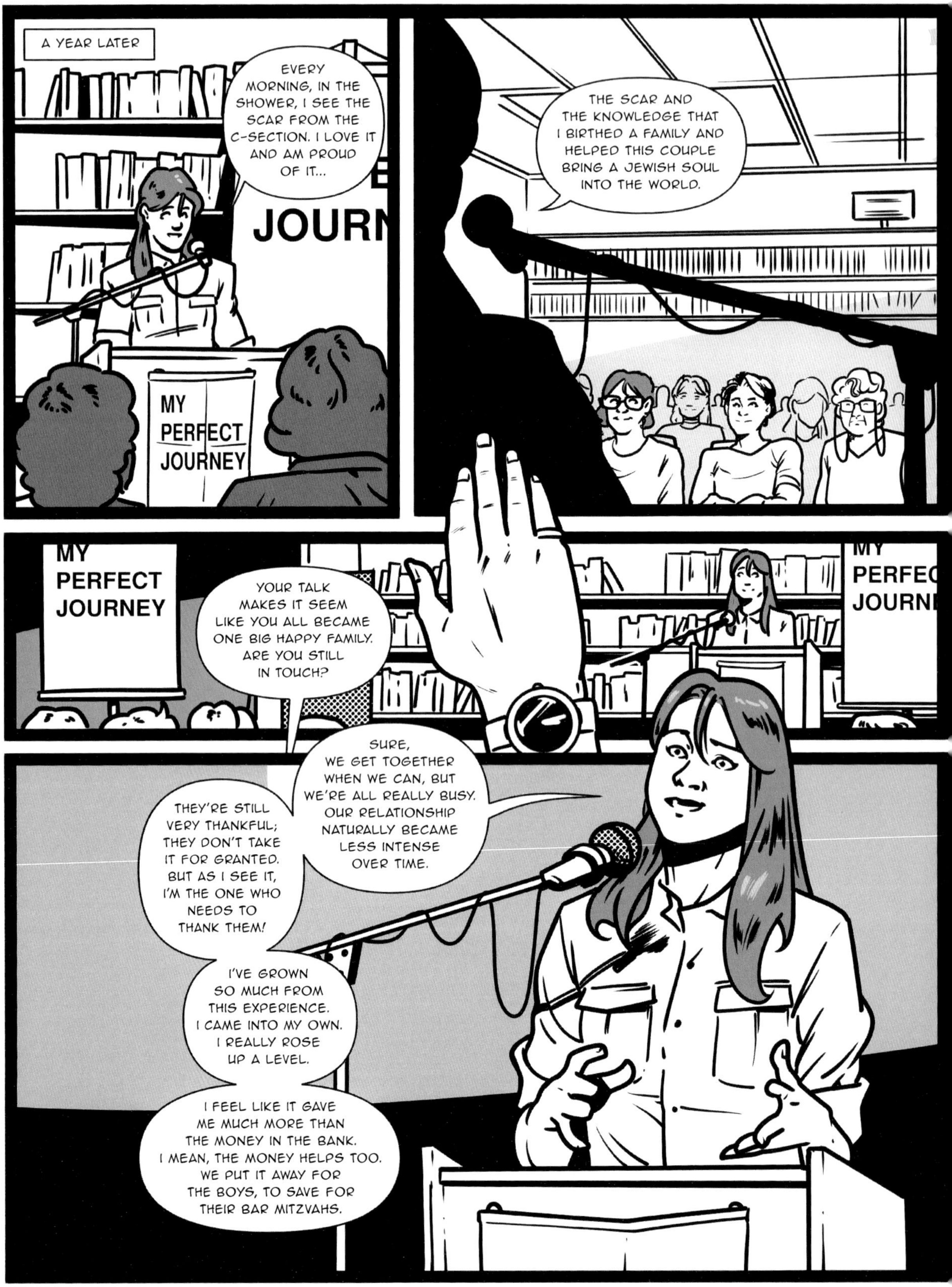
A YEAR LATER
EVERY MORNING, IN THE SHOWER, I SEE THE SCAR FROM THE C-SECTION. I LOVE IT AND AM PROUD OF IT...
JOURN
MY PERFECT JOURNEY
THE SCAR AND THE KNOWLEDGE THAT I BIRTHED A FAMILY AND HELPED THIS COUPLE BRING A JEWISH SOUL INTO THE WORLD.
MY PERFECT JOURNEY
YOUR TALK MAKES IT SEEM LIKE YOU ALL BECAME ONE BIG HAPPY FAMILY. ARE YOU STILL IN TOUCH?
MY PERFEC JOURN
SURE, WE GET TOGETHER WHEN WE CAN, BUT WE'RE ALL REALLY BUSY. OUR RELATIONSHIP NATURALLY BECAME LESS INTENSE OVER TIME.
THEY'RE STILL VERY THANKFUL; THEY DON'T TAKE IT FOR GRANTED. BUT AS I SEE IT, I'M THE ONE WHO NEEDS TO THANK THEM!
I'VE GROWN SO MUCH FROM THIS EXPERIENCE. I CAME INTO MY OWN. I REALLY ROSE UP A LEVEL.
I FEEL LIKE IT GAVE ME MUCH MORE THAN THE MONEY IN THE BANK. I MEAN, THE MONEY HELPS TOO. WE PUT IT AWAY FOR THE BOYS, TO SAVE FOR THEIR BAR MITZVAHS.

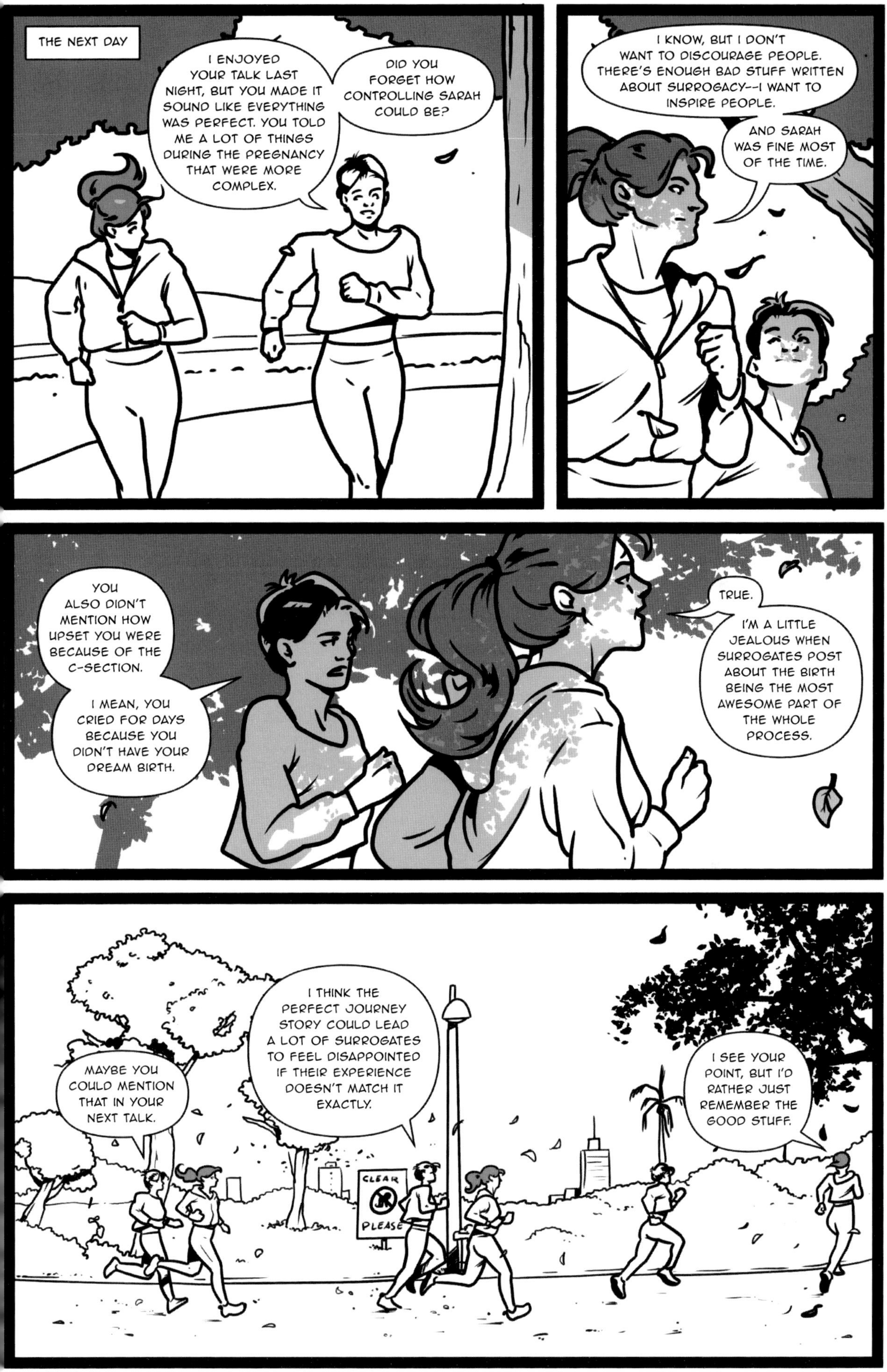
THE NEXT DAY
I ENJOYED YOUR TALK LAST NIGHT, BUT YOU MADE IT SOUND LIKE EVERYTHING WAS PERFECT. YOU TOLD ME A LOT OF THINGS DURING THE PREGNANCY THAT WERE MORE COMPLEX.
DID YOU FORGET HOW CONTROLLING SARAH COULD BE?
I KNOW, BUT I DON'T WANT TO DISCOURAGE PEOPLE. THERE'S ENOUGH BAD STUFF WRITTEN ABOUT SURROGACY--I WANT TO INSPIRE PEOPLE.
AND SARAH WAS FINE MOST OF THE TIME.
YOU ALSO DIDN'T MENTION HOW UPSET YOU WERE BECAUSE OF THE C-SECTION.
I MEAN, YOU CRIED FOR DAYS BECAUSE YOU DIDN'T HAVE YOUR DREAM BIRTH.
TRUE.
I'M A LITTLE JEALOUS WHEN SURROGATES POST ABOUT THE BIRTH BEING THE MOST AWESOME PART OF THE WHOLE PROCESS.
MAYBE YOU COULD MENTION THAT IN YOUR NEXT TALK.
I THINK THE PERFECT JOURNEY STORY COULD LEAD A LOT OF SURROGATES TO FEEL DISAPPOINTED IF THEIR EXPERIENCE DOESN'T MATCH IT EXACTLY.
CLEAR PLEASE
I SEE YOUR POINT, BUT I'D RATHER JUST REMEMBER THE GOOD STUFF.

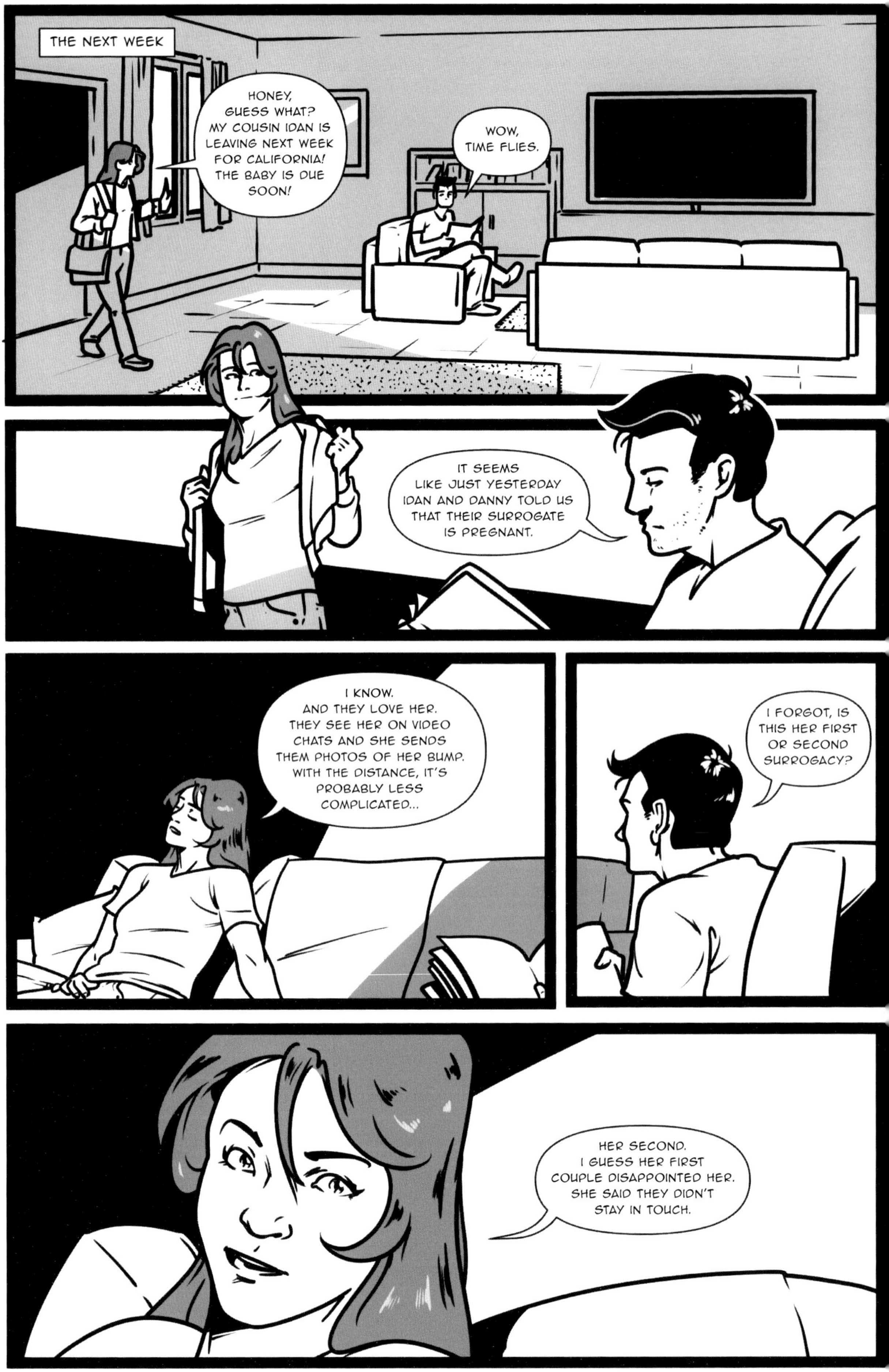
THE NEXT WEEK
HONEY, GUESS WHAT? MY COUSIN IDAN IS LEAVING NEXT WEEK FOR CALIFORNIA! THE BABY IS DUE SOON!
WOW, TIME FLIES.
IT SEEMS LIKE JUST YESTERDAY IDAN AND DANNY TOLD US THAT THEIR SURROGATE IS PREGNANT.
I KNOW. AND THEY LOVE HER. THEY SEE HER ON VIDEO CHATS AND SHE SENDS THEM PHOTOS OF HER BUMP. WITH THE DISTANCE, IT'S PROBABLY LESS COMPLICATED...
I FORGOT, IS THIS HER FIRST OR SECOND SURROGACY?
HER SECOND. I GUESS HER FIRST COUPLE DISAPPOINTED HER. SHE SAID THEY DIDN'T STAY IN TOUCH.

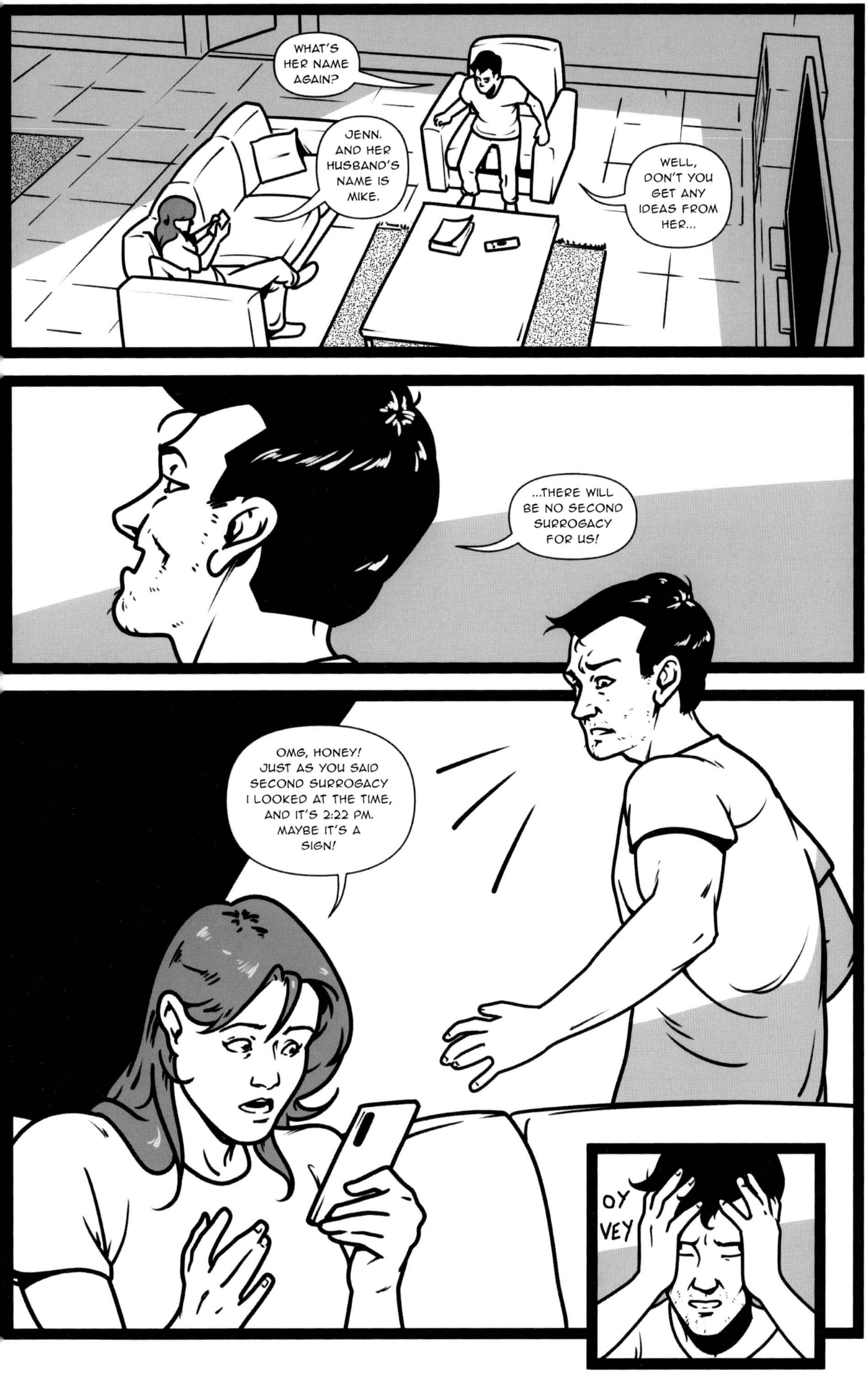
WHAT'S HER NAME AGAIN?
JENN. AND HER HUSBAND'S NAME IS MIKE.
WELL, DON'T YOU GET ANY IDEAS FROM HER...
...THERE WILL BE NO SECOND SURROGACY FOR US!
OMG, HONEY! JUST AS YOU SAID SECOND SURROGACY I LOOKED AT THE TIME, AND IT'S 2:22 PM. MAYBE IT'S A SIGN!
OY VEY

THE END

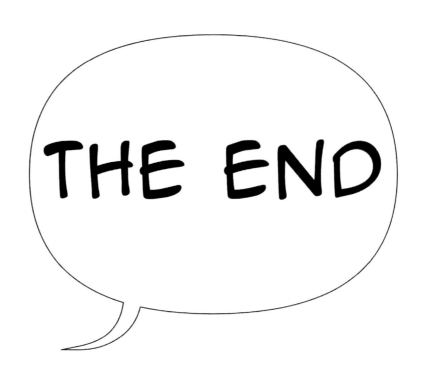

A CONCISE HISTORY OF SURROGACY AS RELEVANT TO THIS STORY

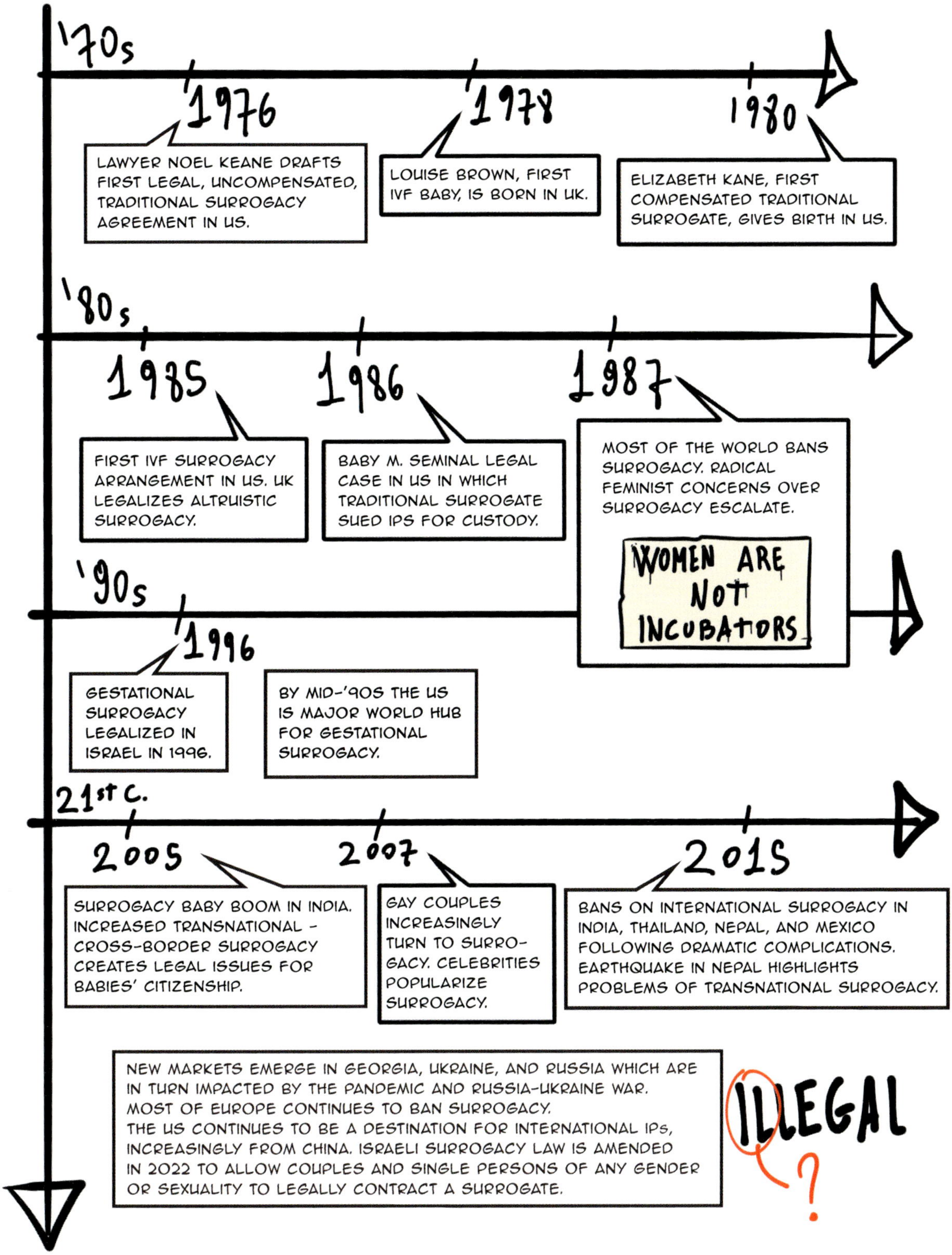
'70s
1976
LAWYER NOEL KEANE DRAFTS FIRST LEGAL, UNCOMPENSATED, TRADITIONAL SURROGACY AGREEMENT IN US.
1978
LOUISE BROWN, FIRST IVF BABY, IS BORN IN UK.
1980
ELIZABETH KANE, FIRST COMPENSATED TRADITIONAL SURROGATE, GIVES BIRTH IN US.
'80s
1985
FIRST IVF SURROGACY ARRANGEMENT IN US. UK LEGALIZES ALTRUISTIC SURROGACY.
1986
BABY M. SEMINAL LEGAL CASE IN US IN WHICH TRADITIONAL SURROGATE SUED IPS FOR CUSTODY.
1987
MOST OF THE WORLD BANS SURROGACY. RADICAL FEMINIST CONCERNS OVER SURROGACY ESCALATE.
WOMEN ARE NOT INCUBATORS
'90s
1996
GESTATIONAL SURROGACY LEGALIZED IN ISRAEL IN 1996.
BY MID-'90S THE US IS MAJOR WORLD HUB FOR GESTATIONAL SURROGACY.
21st C.
2005
SURROGACY BABY BOOM IN INDIA. INCREASED TRANSNATIONAL - CROSS-BORDER SURROGACY CREATES LEGAL ISSUES FOR BABIES' CITIZENSHIP.
2007
GAY COUPLES INCREASINGLY TURN TO SURROGACY. CELEBRITIES POPULARIZE SURROGACY.
2015
BANS ON INTERNATIONAL SURROGACY IN INDIA, THAILAND, NEPAL, AND MEXICO FOLLOWING DRAMATIC COMPLICATIONS. EARTHQUAKE IN NEPAL HIGHLIGHTS PROBLEMS OF TRANSNATIONAL SURROGACY.
NEW MARKETS EMERGE IN GEORGIA, UKRAINE, AND RUSSIA WHICH ARE IN TURN IMPACTED BY THE PANDEMIC AND RUSSIA-UKRAINE WAR. MOST OF EUROPE CONTINUES TO BAN SURROGACY. THE US CONTINUES TO BE A DESTINATION FOR INTERNATIONAL IPs, INCREASINGLY FROM CHINA. ISRAELI SURROGACY LAW IS AMENDED IN 2022 TO ALLOW COUPLES AND SINGLE PERSONS OF ANY GENDER OR SEXUALITY TO LEGALLY CONTRACT A SURROGATE.
ILLEGAL ?

Afterword

In the introduction to *A Tale of Two Surrogates*, we noted that the stories of Jenn and Dana are based on our respective research studies of surrogacy in the United States and in Israel, and we raised a number of questions to guide readers through the story. Here, we point out themes in the stories and their connections to our and others' research. This afterword is not meant to be all-encompassing, nor is it meant to cut short further thinking about the issues raised by the stories.

The narrative reflects surrogates' own responses to many of the popular critiques of surrogacy (e.g., commodification of motherhood and children, exploitation of surrogates, surrogacy as a morally wrongful pursuit). The stories also address cultural assumptions in the psychological scholarship on surrogacy. Dismissing cultural assumptions about their motivations, the characters maintain there is no deviant trait or reparative motive that explains why they want to do this "crazy" and "unnatural" thing.[1]

Both surrogates clearly refute the assumption that surrogates necessarily bond with the baby, view themselves as the baby's mother, or are traumatized by having to "give the baby up." They reflect the dominant views of surrogates in the United States and Israel that parting with the baby is a nonissue and that they are not the baby's mother.

Jenn and Dana, much like other surrogates in the two countries, conceptualize surrogacy as akin to babysitting (i.e., caring for a child before returning it to its parents). They also compare the womb to an "oven" that provides a warm place to complete the "baking" of the otherwise assembled "bun." These metaphors help portray surrogacy as a practice that provides warm, loving care but is not motherly love.

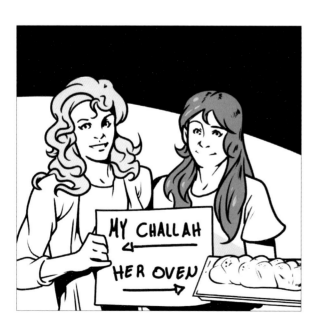

While both of these metaphors express an understanding that the baby they carry is not their own children's sibling, Jenn and Dana view the connection between genetics and relatedness differently. Dana explains familial belonging genetically: it's not her egg and she's "only carrying" the IPs' baby. Conversely, Jenn views intent, not genetics or gestation, as defining kinship and maternal identity. She does not hesitate to offer her eggs when her IPs need a donor because to her, it would still be their baby.[2]

The surrogates reject portrayals of themselves as exploited, dehumanized, and coerced, notions that are held by some feminist critics.[3] Both Dana and Jenn see surrogacy as an informed choice they willingly made. Both have a sense of personal agency and ownership of their actions and refuse to be shamed for their choices.

Both regularly communicate online with fellow surrogates. Jenn finds sisterhood and support from her online community of surrogates, depicted as the Greek chorus. Intensely involved in her journey, the surrogates in Jenn's online community encourage her, give her a sense of belonging, and teach her their ethos: "It is creating life and the journey that matter." Dana imagines her surrogacy group members as competitors in a test of endurance, reflecting her view of surrogacy as a mission that only an elite group of mentally, physically, and emotionally strong women can complete.

Money and Class

Jenn's and Dana's stories both address the popular assumption that surrogates are poor and even destitute women and that there are enormous class-based disparities between surrogates and IPs. However, class differences between surrogates and IPs can vary. The majority of surrogates in our data are middle-class mothers, as are Jenn and Dana.

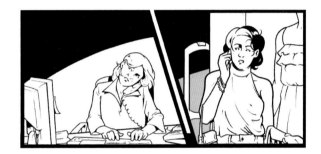

Surrogacy is not affordable for many people in the United States, but not all IPs are as well off as Ann and Tom. The illustrations subtly depict the class differences between Jenn and her IPs.

Class differences are less pronounced between Dana and her couple. Most Israeli surrogates over the past ten years have been married, middle-class working moms with an undergraduate education or even a graduate degree. In Elly's earlier research, there was a larger gap in socioeconomic status between surrogates and IPs in Israel because regulations permitted only unmarried mothers to be surrogates.[4]

Jenn's story also addresses the long-held fear among critics of surrogacy in the United States that poor minority women might be coerced into being surrogates for white women. However, by all empirical accounts, surrogates in the United States today are overwhelmingly white women. In the United States, while IPs are predominately white as well, it is more likely for a cross-racial arrangement to occur between a white surrogate and nonwhite

IPs than the opposite.[5] As the United States continues to be a major hub for international surrogacy, new demographics of surrogates and IPs are being drawn into surrogacy.[6]

Dana's story addresses the cultural assumption that Jewish-Israeli surrogates are mostly from Middle Eastern (Mizrahi) ethnic backgrounds and that IPs are largely Ashkenazi. We chose to make Dana of Ashkenazi descent and her IM from a Yemenite immigrant family to reflect the multidirectional ethnic surrogacy pairings that are actually more common.

The strong governmental and societal support for surrogacy in Israel reflects an exceptionally intense pronatalist ideology. Jewish-Israeli women have more children than women in any other developed country. Medical expenses associated with assisted reproduction are heavily subsidized by Israeli national health insurance, which covers unlimited IVF attempts for all Israeli women (regardless of religion and marital status) up to the birth of two children and all medical costs of pregnancy and hospital delivery. There is little public criticism in Israeli society for the huge national expense associated with the country's fertility policy, and Israeli women have long been the world's heaviest users of IVF technology.[7]

Dana's story also contrasts Israel's national, socialized medicine system with US privatized healthcare. Dana and her IPs have medical coverage that pays for embryo transfers, multiple doctor's visits, ultrasounds, and prenatal tests with no surrogacy exclusions. Conversely, in the United States, having health insurance is not a given, and most policies do not include coverage for IVF and contain surrogacy exclusions. Like a growing number of contemporary Israeli surrogates, Dana advocates for the embryo transfer to be done on her "natural" cycle without artificial hormones. This is possible because she knows that the nearly daily ultrasounds and blood tests it requires are covered by health insurance. Jenn, like most US surrogates, doesn't challenge the medical protocol.[8]

Regulation and Responsibility

The story contrasts the differing legal contexts in which Jenn and Dana pursue surrogacy as well as their approach to regulation.[9] There is no federal law on surrogacy in the United States, and states regulate it differently. Surrogacy agencies are unregulated and fertility clinics self-regulate.

Jenn follows the advice of fellow surrogates to "do her homework" about contracts, agencies, clinics, and procedures. She views surrogacy as a private "journey" with Ann and Tom. Jenn's story emphasizes her taking personal responsibility for making the right decisions about contractual provisions and embryo transfer.

Dana's story portrays her as feeling both "protected" and "invaded" by the paternalistic Israeli state regulation of surrogacy. Israel's surrogacy law restrictively regulates surrogacy agreements between Israeli citizens, far more comprehensively than anywhere else in the world. She undergoes extensive state-mandated medical and psychological screening before the surrogacy committee approves her contract.

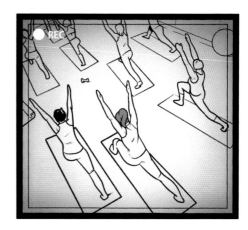

Dana exemplifies the perception among Israeli surrogates that it is the state's role to chaperone the agreement and to protect her rights in the contract. She is relieved when her attorney informs her that her contract includes standard protections that Jenn, in California, must individually advocate for. The state's differential involvement shapes how Jenn and Dana understand privacy as well as how they perceive their contribution: for Jenn, it is about helping individual families, while for Dana it also carries the national significance of creating a "continuing generation" for another family.

Comparative Contexts

The interludes show that Jenn's and Dana's experiences are not universal. While they both frame surrogacy as a choice and advocate for themselves during contract negotiations, surrogates in other countries often have few contractual protections. Sometimes the contract is only signed after conception, or written in a language they cannot understand.[10] Surrogates in Mexico, India, Thailand, and Russia may be coerced or manipulated by doctors to accept multiple embryo transfers or undergo C-section as a routine practice that helps the clinic streamline its business. They may feel shame about becoming a surrogate and keep their role secret. Often they never meet the IPs or only meet briefly following delivery.[11]

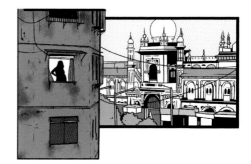

By contrasting Jenn's and Dana's stories with the interludes, we do not mean to portray surrogates in other countries as the opposites of our protagonists or suggest that they are victims and lack personal agency. We aim to illuminate how, despite the regulatory differences, there are many similarities in US and Israeli surrogacy. These similarities are more easily recognizable when the two cases are contrasted with other countries.

Negotiating Boundaries

The storyline deals with several manifestations of boundary negotiations and women's agency. Jenn's story deals with tests to her moral boundaries as she faces moral issues including selective reduction and pregnancy termination

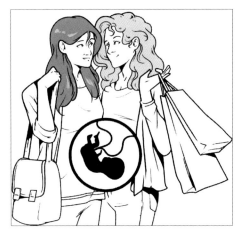

for fetal anomaly. Jenn's deliberations reflect the moral consensus among surrogates in Zsuzsa's research that "every life is precious" and surrogacy means creating life.[12]

Next, Dana's story highlights the theme of bodily boundaries in surrogacy. Dana, a workout enthusiast, embarks on this process "knowing" her body's capabilities and limits. We see her progressively reflect on losing control of her body and negotiate the boundaries of her body with Sarah. Surrogacy becomes a "dyadic body project" in which Dana actively encourages Sarah to "share" in as many aspects of the pregnancy as she can and to claim it as her own. Yet as Sarah begins to identify with the pregnancy, Dana increasingly feels that Sarah is trying to control her.[13]

The negotiation of distance and intimacy between surrogates and IPs is depicted throughout, especially in scenes that feature the use of photography. Dana records her journey with her IPs to construct surrogacy as a joint project of connectedness with her IPs, who gradually begin to believe that their baby is real. Jenn sends selfies, ultrasound pictures, and playful images in order to bridge her physical and emotional distance from her couple and to encourage them to bond with their baby.

Medicalization and Magic

The story also grapples with the problems of medicalization. Many comics in the genre of graphic medicine critique medicalization, including stories that directly challenge medicine's authority over pregnancy and birth.[14] Our story highlights the way surrogates articulate personal agency through their negotiations with the medical system.

Jenn and Dana exhibit changing stances toward medicalization, from resistance to pragmatic compliance. Their stories highlight surrogates' attitudes toward "artificial" and "natural" medical protocols, birth interventions, as well as surrogates' common critiques of doctor–patient interactions.[15] Jenn takes pride in making informed decisions about medical practices such as multiple embryo transfers but is less critical of medical interventions than Dana.

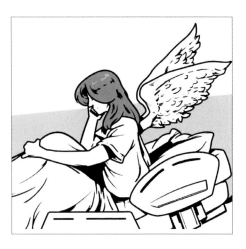

In addition, Jenn and Dana represent surrogates' collective notions and practices in both countries, which include fertility-related rituals or beliefs in good omens that coexist with highly medicalized practices. These include good luck charms, lucky numbers, and precautions against "jinxing" the process. In this highly arbitrated and medicalized endeavor, surrogates, and often IPs, too, hold onto some elements of mystery and wonder and also mystical agency. Dana "earns her angel wings" and views surrogacy as "a divine privilege" of "assisting G-d in a miracle."

Feminist scholars have widely noted that the medicalization of childbirth transformed a female domain in which women helped other women give birth at home into a mechanical process in a male, medical establishment. Women rarely put themselves in the center of the creative act, often crediting their doctor with producing the baby. In surrogacy, despite the heightened medicalization, surrogates may, paradoxically, reclaim their status in the act of creation.[16]

Gifts and Obligations

Gifts and the expectations that gifts raise for reciprocation are important themes that play out in our story. Jenn is not fully comfortable with the monetary side of surrogacy, although she sees the payment as a reward for her family, protection against risks, and also as a sign of the valuation of her contribution. She and Dana both see surrogacy as a gift relationship in which parties give and receive tangible and intangible gifts. We highlight the theme of material gifts in Jenn's story and develop the connected theme of the intangible gift (of time, trust, bodily sacrifices, etc.) in Dana's story.

In Jenn's story, we show the ritualistic practice of gift exchange that has come to be commonplace in Jenn's online community, where she learns when and how gifting is deemed appropriate in surrogacy. Jenn's multiple personalized gifts to Ann are revealed as attempts to establish a relationship and bridge the geographical and emotional distance between them. Jenn interprets Ann's standard gifts as a personal sign of care. We also learn that IPs may not know or understand that the gifts are intended to establish and maintain a relationship of ongoing reciprocity beyond the contractual obligations. Gifts create and sustain relationships, as Marcel Maus (1967) famously argued, and the refusal to accept a gift is tantamount to rejecting the giver and denying the enormity of what has been given.

One of the greatest gifts both surrogates see themselves as giving their IPs is their time, effort, and camaraderie. In contrast to Ann's lack of acknowledgment of the enormity of Jenn's gifts, Sarah acknowledges Dana's time, sacrifices, and friendship by visiting her, bringing her children gifts, and publicly thanking her. While not all Israeli IPs recognize their surrogate like Sarah does, shared cultural understandings and more similar class status often facilitates an ongoing friendship between surrogates and couples. The US geographical, class, and cultural context is more heterogeneous, and surrogacy is understood as creating private nuclear families; continued friendship, while it happens, is more difficult to achieve.

Romanticizing the Single Story

In both the United States and Israel, surrogates tend to imagine surrogacy as a "perfect" journey, of shared purpose and love with their IPs and a happy family for the IPs at the end.[17] The journey is supposed to proceed along a smooth, linear, clear path. However, in reality it is never smooth. The story illuminates disruptions on the journey through symbols such as traffic standing still and a roller coaster running off its tracks. Surrogates' romanticization of the journey is often inspired by a "single story" of a perfect journey that circulates through social media and is often perpetuated by other surrogates.[18] Our story addresses the events many of the women in our research encountered that did not align with the story they envisioned. These led to disappointment: failed embryo transfers, miscarriages, and emergency C-sections.

We also address the romanticization of surrogate–IP relationships. Dana and Jenn both hope for a "perfect match" and immediate "chemistry" with their IPs. Each relationship involved challenges: Jenn's attempts to draw Ann and Tom closer ends in disappointment, while Dana's growing intimacy with Sarah leaves her feeling stifled.

The last chapter illuminates how the "single story" is reproduced. Dana's lecture leaves out parts of her experience that do not fit with what she believes to be an inspirational account. By illuminating the discrepancies between the stories surrogates publicly tell and their lived realities, we add to the efforts of others in the graphic medicine genre to critique the romanticization of reproduction by visually representing the messiness of fertility treatments, miscarriage, and journeys that tend to be emotionally complicated.[19]

Time

The story emphasizes the role of time in the surrogacy process in order to highlight this otherwise invisible aspect of surrogacy. Comics offer many advantages in the depiction of time, such as to show synchronic time, condensed time, circular time, the lengthening of time, and time standing still.[20] Cultural time shapes the surrogacy calendar in both journeys. Israeli surrogates tend to link their stories to Jewish holidays, thus Dana's story plays out along the timeline of the Jewish calendar, including Rosh Hashanah, Hanukkah, and Passover. Jenn's story cycles twice through the Fourth of July, Halloween, Thanksgiving, two Christmases, and Valentine's Day.

This passing of seasons highlights the longtime commitment surrogates and their families make to this process, which usually takes longer than it does in our story because of delays in gathering initial paperwork, screening, matching, contract negotiations, failed embryo transfers, searching for egg donors, and so on. We highlight these long waiting periods during surrogacy in symbolic scenes such as one depicting Jenn and Mike waiting in a slow checkout line.

Sequential panels also enable us to evoke the perception of time lengthening and slowing through the surrogacy process.[21] Using condensed imagery, we can therefore show the lengthy processes of hormonal preparation for embryo transfer and of Jenn's frustration with not making progress in the Ferris wheel imagery. Likewise, half- and full-page spreads are used to depict emotional moments when time stands still, such as when Jenn is under pressure to agree to a multiple embryo transfer or Dana regroups for the journey that lies ahead.

This story has portrayed Jenn and Dana throughout their surrogacy "journeys" as they overcame various obstacles. There is no tragic turn of events in our story; rather, we represented the more common scenarios we found during our years of research. Like most of the surrogates in our wider studies, Jenn and Dana were supported and encouraged to persevere by their husbands and other surrogates in their online or social media support groups. Throughout their journeys they learned to attach meaning to the practice and shape their own emotional approach and response to whatever they encountered, including miscommunications and challenges in their relationships with their IPs. Jenn and Dana, however, both give birth at the end of the story, unlike many surrogates in both countries who share the goal of "making IPs' dream come true" but never reach the "finish line." We purposely left the future of their relationships with their IPs ambiguous, indicating that Jenn expected more of a friendship, while Dana romanticizes her story and "forgets" the more complex emotional and physical parts.

The interludes, however, make it clear that our ethnographic research is grounded in the local sociocultural, political, and economic contexts of the United States and Israel and that our findings are not broadly generalizable to the continuously evolving international surrogacy "market," especially in very different economic contexts. Banning assisted practices in some countries simply redirects those practices elsewhere as long as there is demand for surrogacy. Thus, as countries such as those depicted in the interludes close their doors to foreign or commercial surrogacy, new markets emerge, such as Ukraine and Georgia in recent years. The US surrogacy market also continues to evolve as it continues to be a central magnet for international surrogacy travel.

We end this discussion with the so-true but also somewhat clichéd notion that surrogacy is not *one* thing. It cannot be understood by using concepts such as exploitation or self-realization, false consciousness or informed choice, and so forth, across different contexts. Even within one context or one country, institutional, cultural, and political histories matter. Yet most people approach surrogacy in this one-size-fits-all, and often overly moralized and normative, framework.

We hope our contribution to graphic medicine will take conversations about surrogacy beyond the common dichotomies and inspire readers to think further about the single stories, the wider stories, the contexts of their telling, and their consequences.

Discussion Guide

What are some of the stereotypes and misconceptions about surrogacy that the surrogates encounter?

What were the differences in each surrogate's screening process?

Describe the differences in the way surrogacy is regulated in Israel and in the United States.

Discuss the contract negotiations. Which issues were the surrogates not in agreement about with the IPs?

Which issues about embryo transfer emerged from the stories?

What kind of issues arose surrounding termination or selective reduction?

What degree of privacy does each surrogate have to give up?

What criteria did each surrogate consider during the "matching" process?

Discuss the surrogate–IP relationship in each journey.

What is the surrogate's husband's role in the journey?

Both surrogates encouraged their IPs to attend the transfer and appointments. Why was this important to them?

Discuss doctor–patient interactions in the two stories. What issues arose, and how could they have been resolved?

Discuss how each of the surrogates responds to medicalization.

Jenn undergoes a miscarriage. How does she handle this?

Describe each surrogate's support system for her "journey."

What do the surrogates' families consider to be "sacrifices"?

How do the surrogates and IPs negotiate boundaries with one another?

What are the surrogates' expectations regarding the birth? What issues can come up during the birth?

Discuss what happens after the birth in the two stories.

In what ways does surrogacy differ in the countries portrayed in the interludes? What issues do the interludes illuminate?

Notes

Introduction

1. For more on each of our research methods, see Teman, *Birthing*; Teman, "Power of the Single Story"; Berend, *Online World*; Teman and Berend, "Surrogate Non-Motherhood"; Teman and Berend, "Surrogacy as a Family Project"; and Teman and Berend, "Individual Responsibility."
2. For more on the international surrogacy industry, see Whittaker, *International Surrogacy*.
3. New York's new surrogacy legislation is an exception, but overall the United States does not have much regulation on surrogacy in comparison with Israel.
4. For a fuller description of the Israeli law, its history, and how it was influenced by Jewish law, see Kahn, *Reproducing Jews*; Teman and Berend, "Individual Responsibility"; Teman, "Case for Restrictive Regulation"; and Teman, "Last Outpost."
5. For statistical information about US surrogacy, see Birenbaum-Carmeli and Montebruno, "Incidence of Surrogacy"; Dongarwar et al., "Racial/Ethnic Disparities"; Jacobson, *Labor of Love*; Jacobson and Rozeé, "Inequalities"; Smietana, "Affective De-Commodifying"; and Ziff, "'Honey.'"
6. See note 5.
7. The interludes are based on published ethnographies of surrogacy, including Deomampo, *Transnational Reproduction*; Hovav, "Cutting Out the Surrogate"; Nilsson, "Merit Making"; Khvorostyanov and Yeshua-Katz, "Bad, Pathetic and Greedy"; Pande, *Wombs in Labor*; Rudrappa, *Discounted Life*; Weis, *Surrogacy in Russia*; Whittaker, *International Surrogacy*; and Guerzoni, "Gift Narratives."
8. For more about graphic medicine, see Czerwiec et al., *Graphic Medicine Manifesto*. For volumes in this series that deal with reproductive issues, see Czerwiec, *Menopause*; Johnson, introduction to *Graphic Reproduction*; and Knight, *Facts of Life*. Some other comic memoirs dealing with reproduction are Potts, *Good Eggs*, and Steinberg, "Broken Eggs."
9. See Ginsburg and Rapp, "Politics of Reproduction," a pivotal text that helped birth the anthropology of reproduction as a subfield of anthropology. For a review of developments in this field, see Han and Tomori, *Handbook of Anthropology and Reproduction*. For some recent works that use comics to communicate ethnographic research, see Boum and Berber, *Undesirables*; Hamdy and Nye, *Lissa*; Sopranzetti et al., *King of Bangkok*; Sousanis, *Unflattening*; and White, *Turkish Kaleidoscope*.

Afterword

1. For a critique of cultural assumptions about surrogates' motivations, see Teman, "Social Construction of Surrogacy Research."
2. For a discussion of the differing kinship understandings of US and Israeli surrogates, see Teman and Berend, "Surrogate Non-Motherhood."
3. For a summary of feminist critiques of reproductive technologies and of surrogacy, see Thompson, "Fertile Ground."
4. Teman, *Birthing*, and Teman, "Power of the Single Story."
5. See Berend, *Online World*, and Jacobson and Rozeé, "Inequalities."
6. See Guerzoni, "Gift Narratives."
7. Birenbaum-Carmeli and Montebruno, "Incidence of Surrogacy."
8. For more on how surrogates in the United States and Israel respond to medicalization, see Teman, *Birthing*; Teman, "Power of the Single Story"; Berend,

Online World; and Ziff, "Surrogacy and Medicalization."

9. For more on how surrogates in the United States and Israel think about regulation, see Teman and Berend, "Individual Responsibility." For more on the Israeli surrogacy law, see Teman, "Last Outpost."

10. Deomampo, *Transnational Reproduction*; Pande, *Wombs in Labor*; Rudrappa, *Discounted Life*.

11. Hovav, "Cutting out the Surrogate"; Weis, *Surrogacy in Russia*; Whittaker, *International Surrogacy*; Lustenberger, *Judaism in Motion*; Khvorostyanov and Yeshua-Katz, "Bad, Pathetic, and Greedy."

12. Berend, *Online World*.

13. Teman, "Embodying Surrogate Motherhood."

14. See, for example, the stories included in Johnson, *Graphic Reproduction*.

15. Berend, *Online World*; Teman, "Medicalization of 'Nature'"; Teman, *Birthing*; Teman, "Power of the Single Story"; Ziff, "Surrogacy and Medicalization."

16. Teman, *Birthing*.

17. Berend, *Online World*; Teman, *Birthing*; Teman, "Power of the Single Story."

18. See Adichie, "Danger of a Single Story," and Teman, "Power of the Single Story."

19. Potts, *Good Eggs*; Knight, *Facts of Life*; Johnson, *Graphic Reproduction*; Steinberg, "Broken Eggs"; Czerwiec, *Menopause*.

20. Czerwiec et al., *Graphic Manifesto*, 46.

21. For more on how panels can be used to communicate time passing, see McCloud, *Understanding Comics*.

Bibliography

Adichie, Chimamanda Ngozi. "The Danger of a Single Story." TEDGlobal, July 2009. https://www.ted.com/talks/chimamanda_adichie_the_danger_of_a_single_story.

Berend, Zsuzsa. "The Emotion Work of a 'Labor of Love.'" In *Handbook of Gestational Surrogacy: International Clinical Practice and Policy Issues,* edited by E. Scott Sills, 62–69. Cambridge: Cambridge University Press, 2016.

———. *The Online World of Surrogacy.* London: Berghan Books, 2016.

———. "The Romance of Surrogacy." *Sociological Forum* 27, no. 4 (2012): 913–36.

Birenbaum-Carmeli, Daphna, Marcia C. Inhorn, Mira D. Vale, and Pasquale Patrizio. "Cryopreserving Jewish Motherhood: Egg Freezing in Israel and the United States." *Medical Anthropology Quarterly* 35, no. 3 (2021): 346–63.

Birenbaum-Carmeli, Daphna, and Piero Montebruno. "Incidence of Surrogacy in the USA and Israel and Implications on Women's Health: A Quantitative Comparison." *Journal of Assisted Reproduction and Genetics* 36, no. 12 (2019): 2459–69.

Boum, Aomar, and Nadjib Berber. *Undesirables: A Holocaust Journey to North Africa.* Stanford, CA: Stanford University Press, 2023.

Czerwiec, MaryKay, ed. *Menopause: A Comic Treatment.* University Park: Penn State University Press, 2021.

Czerwiec, MaryKay, Ian Williams, Susan Merrill Squier, Michael J. Green, Kimberly R. Myers, and Scott T. Smith. *Graphic Medicine Manifesto.* University Park: Penn State University Press, 2020.

Deomampo, Daisy. *Transnational Reproduction: Race, Kinship and Commercial Surrogacy in India.* New York: NYU Press, 2016.

Dongarwar, Deepa, Vicki Mercado-Evans, Sylvia Adu-Gyamfi, Mei-Li Laracuente, and Hamisu M. Salihu. "Racial/Ethnic Disparities in Infertility Treatment Utilization in the US, 2011–2019." *Systems Biology in Reproductive Medicine* 68 (2022): 1–10.

Ginsburg, Faye, and Rayna Rapp. "The Politics of Reproduction." *Annual Review of Anthropology* 20 (1991): 311–43.

Guerzoni, Corinna Sabrina. 2020. "Gift Narratives of US Surrogates." *Italian Sociological Review* 10, no. 3 (2020): 561–77.

Hamdy, Sherine, and Coleman Nye. *Lissa: A Story About Medical Promise, Friendship, and Revolution.* Toronto: University of Toronto Press, 2017.

Han, Sallie, and Cecília Tomori, eds. *The Routledge Handbook of Anthropology and Reproduction.* London: Routledge, 2021.

Hovav, April. "Cutting Out the Surrogate: Caesarean Sections in the Mexican Surrogacy Industry." *Social Science and Medicine* 256 (2020): 113063.

Jacobson, Heather. *Labor of Love: Gestational Surrogacy and the Work of Making Babies.* New Brunswick, NJ: Rutgers University Press, 2016.

Jacobson, Heather, and Virginie Rozée. "Inequalities in (Trans)national Surrogacy: A Call for Examining Complex Lived Realities with an Empirical Lens." *International Journal of Comparative Sociology* 63, nos. 5–6 (2022): 285–303.

Johnson, Jenell. Introduction to *Graphic Reproduction: A Comics Anthology,* edited by Jenell Johnson. University Park: Penn State University Press, 2018.

Kahn, Susan M. *Reproducing Jews: A Cultural Account of Assisted Conception in Israel.* Durham, NC: Duke University Press, 2000.

Khvorostyanov, Natalia, and Daphna Yeshua-Katz. "Bad, Pathetic and Greedy Women: Expressions of Surrogate Motherhood Stigma in a Russian Online Forum." *Sex Roles* 83, no. 7 (2020): 474–84.

Knight, Paula. *The Facts of Life.* University Park: Penn State University Press, 2017.

Lustenberger, Sibylle. *Judaism in Motion: The Making of Same-Sex Parenthood in Israel.* London: Palgrave Macmillan, 2020.

Mauss, Marcel. *The Gift: Forms and Functions of Exchange in Archaic Societies.* New York: Norton, 1967.

McCloud, Scott. *Understanding Comics: The Invisible Art.* New York: HarperCollins, 1993.

Nilsson, Elina. "Merit Making, Money and Motherhood: Women's Experiences of Commercial Surrogacy in Thailand." MA thesis, Uppsala University, 2015.

Pande, Amrita. *Wombs in Labor: Transnational Commercial Surrogacy in India*. New York: Columbia University Press, 2014.

Potts, Phoebe. *Good Eggs*. New York: Harper Collins, 2010.

Rudrappa, Sharmila. *Discounted Life: The Price of Global Surrogacy in India*. New York: NYU Press, 2015.

Smietana, Marcin. "Affective De-Commodifying, Economic De-Kinning: Surrogates' and Gay Fathers' Narratives in US Surrogacy." *Sociological Research Online* 22, no. 2 (2017): 1–13.

Sopranzetti, Claudio, Sara Fabbri, and Chiara Natalucci. *The King of Bangkok*. Toronto: University of Toronto Press, 2021.

Sousanis, Nick. *Unflattening*. Cambridge, MA: Harvard University Press, 2015.

Steinberg, Emily. "Broken Eggs: A Visual Narrative." *Cleaver: Philadelphia's International Literary Magazine* 7 (2014). https://www.cleavermagazine.com /broken-eggs-by-emily-steinberg/.

Teman, Elly. *Birthing a Mother: The Surrogate Body and the Pregnant Self*. Berkeley: University of California Press, 2010.

———. "A Case for Restrictive Regulation of Surrogacy? An Indo-Israeli Comparison of Ethnographic Studies." In *Cross-Cultural Comparisons on Surrogacy and Egg Donation: Interdisciplinary Perspectives from India, Germany and Israel*, edited by Sayani Mitra, Silke Schicktanz, and Tulsi Patel, 57–81. London: Palgrave Macmillan, 2018.

———. "Embodying Surrogate Motherhood: Pregnancy as a Dyadic Body Project." *Body and Society* 15, no. 3 (2009): 47–69.

———. "The Last Outpost of the Nuclear Family: A Cultural Critique of Israeli Surrogacy Policy." In *Kin, Gene, Community: Reproductive Technologies Among Jewish Israelis*, edited by Daphna Birenbaum-Carmeli and Yoram Carmeli, 107–26. New York: Berghahn Books, 2009.

———. "The Medicalization of 'Nature' in the 'Artificial Body': Surrogate Motherhood in Israel." *Medical Anthropology Quarterly* 17, no. 1 (2003): 78–98.

———. "The Power of the Single Story: Surrogacy and Social Media in Israel." *Medical Anthropology* 38, no. 3 (2019): 282–94.

———. "The Social Construction of Surrogacy Research: An Anthropological Critique of the Psychosocial Scholarship on Surrogate Motherhood." *Social Science and Medicine* 67, no. 7 (2008): 1104–12.

Teman, Elly, and Zsuzsa Berend. "Individual Responsibility or Trust in the State: A Comparison of Surrogates' Legal Consciousness." *International Journal of Comparative Sociology* 42, no. 6 (2022): 265–84.

———. "Surrogacy as a Family Project: How Surrogates Articulate Familial Identity and Belonging." *Journal of Family Issues* 42, no. 6 (2021): 1143–65.

———. "Surrogate Non-Motherhood: Israeli and US Surrogates Speak About Kinship and Parenthood." *Anthropology and Medicine* 25, no. 3 (2018): 296–310.

———. "Unsustainable Surrogacy Practices: What We Can Learn from a Comparative Assessment." In *Sustainable Birth in Disruptive Times*, edited by Kim Guttshow and Robbie Davis-Floyd, 115–27. London: Springer, 2021.

Thompson, Charis. "Fertile Ground: Feminists Theorize Infertility." In *Infertility Around the Globe: New Thinking on Childlessness, Gender, and Reproductive Technologies*, edited by Marcia Inhorn and Frank van Balen, 52–78. Berkeley: University of California Press, 2002.

Weis, Christina. *Surrogacy in Russia: An Ethnography of Reproductive Labour, Stratification and Migration*. Bingley, UK: Emerald, 2021.

White, Jenny. *Turkish Kaleidoscope: Fractured Lives in a Time of Violence*. Princeton, NJ: Princeton University Press, 2021.

Whittaker, Andrea. *International Surrogacy as Disruptive Industry in Southeast Asia*. New Brunswick, NJ: Rutgers University Press, 2018.

Ziff, Elizabeth. "'Honey, I Want to Be a Surrogate': How Military Spouses Negotiate and Navigate Surrogacy with Their Service Member Husbands." *Journal of Family Issues* 40, no. 18 (2019): 2774–800.

———. "Surrogacy and Medicalization: Navigating Power, Control, and Autonomy in Embodied Labor." *Sociological Quarterly* 62, no. 3 (2021): 510–27.

Creator Bios

PROF. ELLY TEMAN is Associate Professor of Social Anthropology in the Department of Behavioral Sciences at Ruppin Academic Center in Israel. She is the author of the ethnography of surrogacy *Birthing a Mother: The Surrogate Body and the Pregnant Self* and of academic articles on the surrogate–intended mother relationship, the surrogate's embodiment of the pregnancy, and the stories surrogates tell about their "journey."

PROF. ZSUZSA BEREND teaches sociology at the University of California, Los Angeles. She is the author of the ethnography *The Online World of Surrogacy* and of academic articles on surrogates' online interactions and collective meaning-making, as well as their understandings of kinship, pregnancy loss, and emotion work.

ANDREA SCEBBA is a comic artist and illustrator. He is a graduate of the three-year comic graphics and illustration program Graffinated Cartoon in Palermo, Italy, and is skilled in drawing, inking, coloring, and lettering. He recently graduated with a BA from the University of Palermo.